Drug Metabolism/Transport and Pharmacokinetics

Drug Metabolism/Transport and Pharmacokinetics

Editor

Im-Sook Song

MDPI • Basel • Beijing • Wuhan • Barcelona • Belgrade • Manchester • Tokyo • Cluj • Tianjin

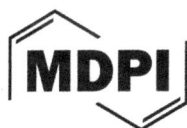

Editor
Im-Sook Song
Department of Pharmaceutics
Kyungpook National University
Daegu
Korea

Editorial Office
MDPI
St. Alban-Anlage 66
4052 Basel, Switzerland

This is a reprint of articles from the Special Issue published online in the open access journal *Pharmaceutics* (ISSN 1999-4923) (available at: www.mdpi.com/journal/pharmaceutics/special-issues/dmp).

For citation purposes, cite each article independently as indicated on the article page online and as indicated below:

LastName, A.A.; LastName, B.B.; LastName, C.C. Article Title. *Journal Name* **Year**, *Volume Number*, Page Range.

ISBN 978-3-0365-2459-7 (Hbk)
ISBN 978-3-0365-2458-0 (PDF)

© 2021 by the authors. Articles in this book are Open Access and distributed under the Creative Commons Attribution (CC BY) license, which allows users to download, copy and build upon published articles, as long as the author and publisher are properly credited, which ensures maximum dissemination and a wider impact of our publications.

The book as a whole is distributed by MDPI under the terms and conditions of the Creative Commons license CC BY-NC-ND.

Contents

About the Editor vii

Preface to "Drug Metabolism/Transport and Pharmacokinetics" ix

Ji Sang Lee and So Hee Kim
Dose-Dependent Pharmacokinetics of Tofacitinib in Rats: Influence of Hepatic and Intestinal First-Pass Metabolism
Reprinted from: *Pharmaceutics* 2019, 11, 318, doi:10.3390/pharmaceutics11070318 1

Ji-Hyeon Jeon, Bitna Kang, Sowon Lee, Sojeong Jin, Min-Koo Choi and Im-Sook Song
Pharmacokinetics and Intestinal Metabolism of Compound K in Rats and Mice
Reprinted from: *Pharmaceutics* 2020, 12, 129, doi:10.3390/pharmaceutics12020129 15

In Yong Bae, Min Sun Choi, Young Seok Ji, Sang-Ku Yoo, Kyungil Kim and Hye Hyun Yoo
Species Differences in Stereoselective Pharmacokinetics of HSG4112, A New Anti-Obesity Agent
Reprinted from: *Pharmaceutics* 2020, 12, 127, doi:10.3390/pharmaceutics12020127 31

Sung Hun Bae, Sun-Young Chang and So Hee Kim
Slower Elimination of Tofacitinib in Acute Renal Failure Rat Models: Contribution of Hepatic Metabolism and Renal Excretion
Reprinted from: *Pharmaceutics* 2020, 12, 714, doi:10.3390/pharmaceutics12080714 45

Min-Koo Choi, So Jeong Nam, Hye-Young Ji, Mi Jie Park, Ji-Soo Choi and Im-Sook Song
Comparative Pharmacokinetics and Pharmacodynamics of a Novel Sodium-Glucose Cotransporter 2 Inhibitor, DWP16001, with Dapagliflozin and Ipragliflozin
Reprinted from: *Pharmaceutics* 2020, 12, 268, doi:10.3390/pharmaceutics12030268 61

Deok-Kyu Hwang, Ju-Hyun Kim, Yongho Shin, Won-Gu Choi, Sunjoo Kim, Yong-Yeon Cho, Joo Young Lee, Han Chang Kang and Hye Suk Lee
Identification of Catalposide Metabolites in Human Liver and Intestinal Preparations and Characterization of the Relevant Sulfotransferase, UDP-glucuronosyltransferase, and Carboxylesterase Enzymes
Reprinted from: *Pharmaceutics* 2019, 11, 355, doi:10.3390/pharmaceutics11070355 77

Won-Gu Choi, Ria Park, Dong Kyun Kim, Yongho Shin, Yong-Yeon Cho and Hye Suk Lee
Mertansine Inhibits mRNA Expression and Enzyme Activities of Cytochrome P450s and Uridine 5-Diphospho-Glucuronosyltransferases in Human Hepatocytes and Liver Microsomes
Reprinted from: *Pharmaceutics* 2020, 12, 220, doi:10.3390/pharmaceutics12030220 91

Seung Yon Han and Young Hee Choi
Pharmacokinetic Interaction between Metformin and Verapamil in Rats: Inhibition of the OCT2-Mediated Renal Excretion of Metformin by Verapamil
Reprinted from: *Pharmaceutics* 2020, 12, 468, doi:10.3390/pharmaceutics12050468 107

Yoo-Kyung Song, Jin-Ha Yoon, Jong Kyu Woo, Ju-Hee Kang, Kyeong-Ryoon Lee, Seung Hyun Oh, Suk-Jae Chung and Han-Joo Maeng
Quercetin Is a Flavonoid Breast Cancer Resistance Protein Inhibitor with an Impact on the Oral Pharmacokinetics of Sulfasalazine in Rats
Reprinted from: *Pharmaceutics* 2020, 12, 397, doi:10.3390/pharmaceutics12050397 123

Dong-Gyun Han, Jinsook Kwak, Seong-Wook Seo, Ji-Min Kim, Jin-Wook Yoo, Yunjin Jung, Yun-Hee Lee, Min-Soo Kim, Young-Suk Jung, Hwayoung Yun and In-Soo Yoon
Pharmacokinetic Evaluation of Metabolic Drug Interactions between Repaglinide and Celecoxib by a Bioanalytical HPLC Method for Their Simultaneous Determination with Fluorescence Detection
Reprinted from: *Pharmaceutics* **2019**, *11*, 382, doi:10.3390/pharmaceutics11080382 137

Yiting Yang and Xiaodong Liu
Imbalance of Drug Transporter-CYP450s Interplay by Diabetes and Its Clinical Significance
Reprinted from: *Pharmaceutics* **2020**, *12*, 348, doi:10.3390/pharmaceutics12040348 151

Jinfeng Chen, Xiaoyu Guo, Yingyuan Lu, Mengling Shi, Haidong Mu, Yi Qian, Jinlong Wang, Mengqiu Lu, Mingbo Zhao, Pengfei Tu, Yuelin Song and Yong Jiang
Large Volume Direct Injection Ultra-High Performance Liquid Chromatography–Tandem Mass Spectrometry-Based Comparative Pharmacokinetic Study between Single and Combinatory Uses of *Carthamus tinctorius* Extract and Notoginseng Total Saponins
Reprinted from: *Pharmaceutics* **2020**, *12*, 180, doi:10.3390/pharmaceutics12020180 179

Yunhai Cui, Stephanie Claus, David Schnell, Frank Runge and Caroline MacLean
In-Depth Characterization of EpiIntestinal Microtissue as a Model for Intestinal Drug Absorption and Metabolism in Human
Reprinted from: *Pharmaceutics* **2020**, *12*, 405, doi:10.3390/pharmaceutics12050405 191

Jan F. Joseph, Leonie Gronbach, Jill García-Miller, Leticia M. Cruz, Bernhard Wuest, Ulrich Keilholz, Christian Zoschke and Maria K. Parr
Automated Real-Time Tumor Pharmacokinetic Profiling in 3D Models: A Novel Approach for Personalized Medicine
Reprinted from: *Pharmaceutics* **2020**, *12*, 413, doi:10.3390/pharmaceutics12050413 207

Seung-Hyun Jeong, Ji-Hun Jang, Hea-Young Cho and Yong-Bok Lee
Population Pharmacokinetic Analysis of Tiropramide in Healthy Korean Subjects
Reprinted from: *Pharmaceutics* **2020**, *12*, 374, doi:10.3390/pharmaceutics12040374 221

About the Editor

Im-Sook Song

Im-Sook Song received her undergraduate degree in Manufacturing Pharmacy, College of Pharmacy, from Seoul National University in 1996 and her master's degree in Pharmaceutics, College of Pharmacy, from Seoul National University in 1998. In 2001, she completed her PhD degree in Biopharmaceutics, College of Pharmacy, Seoul National University. Then, she trained in the Department of Molecular Pathology, University of Texas MD Anderson Cancer Center, Houston, Texas, as a postdoctoral fellow. She then joined the Pharmacogenomics Research center, Inje University School of Medicine, Korea, in 2006 as an assistant professor. In 2012, she joined the College of Pharmacy, Kyungpook National University, Korea, as a Professor.

She has published more than 50 papers over the past five years in the area of pharmacokinetics, including on drug transport, drug metabolism, and drug interaction and also in the area of pharmaceutical formulations to increase the bioavailability of drugs.

Preface to "Drug Metabolism/Transport and Pharmacokinetics"

Clinically important phase I and II metabolizing enzymes, such as the cytochrome P450s (CYP) and UDP-glucuronosyltransferase (UGT) families, and drug transporters from two major superfamilies, ATP binding cassette (ABC) and Solute carrier (SLC) transporters, play pivotal roles in the pharmacokinetics, pharmacogenomics, and the drug–drug interactions of therapeutic drugs, as well as herbal medicines. Therefore, researchers and regulatory agencies have made great efforts to understand the underlying mechanisms for the pharmacokinetic determinants, pharmacogenomic features, and drug–drug interactions of drugs, with a focus on the metabolism and transport characteristics of drugs and drug candidates. With a trend of polypills with different mode of action mechanisms and the increased use of medicinal food, the concurrent administration of therapeutic drugs and herbal drugs can cause serious adverse reactions with substrate drugs for drug-metabolizing enzymes and transporters by the inhibition or induction of their activities. Therefore, the prediction and evaluation of the contribution of drug-metabolizing enzymes and transporters to the pharmacokinetics and drug–drug interaction potential of drugs or drug candidates are important in clinics and in the drug development process.

This book serves to highlight pharmacokinetics/drug–drug interactions and mechanistic understanding in relation to drug-metabolizing enzymes and drug transporters.

This book presents a series of drug metabolism and transport mechanisms that govern the pharmacokinetic features of therapeutic drugs, as well as natural herbal medicines. It also deals the pharmacokinetic interaction caused by inhibiting or inducing the metabolic or transport activities under disease states or the coadministration of potential inhibitors. It also deals with microenvironmental pharmacokinetic profiles as well as population pharmacokinetics, which gives new insights regarding the pharmacokinetic features with regard to the drug metabolism and transporters.

Im-Sook Song
Editor

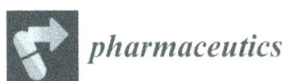

Article

Dose-Dependent Pharmacokinetics of Tofacitinib in Rats: Influence of Hepatic and Intestinal First-Pass Metabolism

Ji Sang Lee and So Hee Kim *

College of Pharmacy and Research Institute of Pharmaceutical Science and Technology, Ajou University, 206 Worldcup-ro, Yeongtong-gu, Suwon 16499, Korea
* Correspondence: shkim67@ajou.ac.kr; Tel.: +82-31-219-3451; Fax: +82-31-219-3435

Received: 3 June 2019; Accepted: 4 July 2019; Published: 5 July 2019

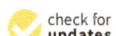

Abstract: This study investigated the pharmacokinetics of tofacitinib in rats and the effects of first-pass metabolism on tofacitinib pharmacokinetics. Intravenous administration of 5, 10, 20, and 50 mg/kg tofacitinib showed that the dose-normalized area under the plasma concentration-time curve from time zero to infinity (AUC) was significantly higher at 50 mg/kg than at lower doses, a difference possibly due to saturation of the hepatic metabolism of tofacitinib. Oral administration of 10, 20, 50, and 100 mg/kg tofacitinib showed that the dose-normalized AUC was significantly higher at 100 mg/kg than at lower doses, a difference possibly due to saturation of the intestinal metabolism of tofacitinib. Following oral administration of 10 mg/kg tofacitinib, the unabsorbed fraction from the rat intestine was 3.16% and the bioavailability (F) was 29.1%. The AUC was significantly lower (49.3%) after intraduodenal, compared to intraportal, administration, but did not differ between intragastric and intraduodenal administration, suggesting that approximately 46.1% of orally administered tofacitinib was metabolized through an intestinal first-pass effect. The AUC was also significantly lower (42%) after intraportal, compared to intravenous, administration, suggesting that the hepatic first-pass effect on tofacitinib after entering the portal vein was approximately 21.3% of the oral dose. Taken together, these findings suggest that the low F of tofacitinib is due primarily to intestinal first-pass metabolism.

Keywords: tofacitinib; dose-dependent pharmacokinetics; hepatic and intestinal first-pass effect; rats

1. Introduction

Tofacitinib (3-[(3R,4R)-4-methyl-3-[methyl-(7H-pyrrolo[2,3-day]pyrimidin-4-l)amino]piperidin-1-yl]-3-oxopropanenitril, Figure 1) potently and selectively inhibits Janus kinases (JAK) 1 and 3 through blocking the signal transducer and activator of transcription 1 (STAT1) signaling pathway, thereby suppressing the production of inflammatory mediators, including interleukins-2, -4, -7, -9, -15 and -21 [1–3]. These findings led to the use of tofacitinib in the treatment of diseases involving the immune system and to its approval for the treatment of rheumatoid arthritis, particularly in patients intolerant to methotrexate therapy [4]. Tofacitinib was also approved by the US Food and Drug Administration in 2018 for the treatment of moderate to severe ulcerative colitis [5], making it the first oral JAK inhibitor for chronic use in patients with ulcerative colitis [6].

Oral administration of 10 mg tofacitinib to healthy volunteers resulted in an absolute oral bioavailability (F) of approximately 74% [7]. Pharmacokinetic analysis showed that its volume of distribution was 87 L, and its terminal half-life was 3.2 h [3,7,8]. Studies found that 40% of oral tofacitinib bound to plasma proteins [3,8], and that approximately 70% of eliminated tofacitinib was excreted in urine after being metabolized, with the remaining 30% eliminated unmetabolized through the kidneys [3,7,8]. Tofacitinib is metabolized through hepatic oxidation and N-demethylation, primarily by cytochrome P450 (CYP) 3A4, but also by CYP2C19 and glucuronide conjugation [3]. Although the dose-dependent pharmacokinetics of tofacitinib have been described in humans [7,8], the mechanisms underlying its incomplete absorption have not yet been characterized. However, it is difficult to get the information from clinical settings for evaluating the mechanisms of its incomplete absorption. Instead, using a rat model has been considered, but the basic pharmacokinetic characteristics of tofacitinib in rats has not been thoroughly investigated yet.

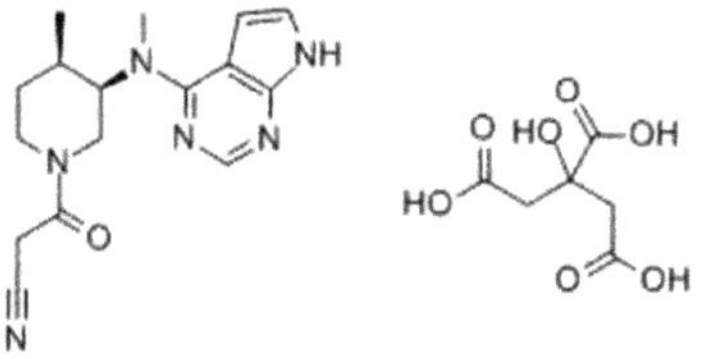

Figure 1. Structure of tofacitinib citrate.

The present study assessed the dose-dependent pharmacokinetics of tofacitinib administered both intravenously and orally in rats by evaluating the total area under the plasma concentration–time curve from time zero to infinity (AUC). This study also investigated the effects of first-pass hepatic, gastric, and intestinal metabolism on tofacitinib administered to rats intravenously, intraportally, intragastrically, and intraduodenally. Furthermore, biliary excretion and tissue distribution of intravenously administered tofacitinib were evaluated in rats.

2. Materials and Methods

2.1. Chemicals

Tofacitinib citrate and hydrocortisone, the internal standard for high-performance liquid chromatography (HPLC) analysis, were obtained from Sigma-Aldrich (St. Louis, MO, USA), and ethyl acetate was from J.T. Baker (Phillipsburg, NJ, USA). Heparin and 0.9% NaCl-injectable solution were purchased from JW Pharmaceutical Corporation (Seoul, Korea), and β-cyclodextrin was from Wako (Osaka, Japan). All other chemicals were HPLC grade and were used without further purification.

2.2. Animals

Male Sprague-Dawley rats, aged 7–8 weeks and weighing 240–260 g, were purchased from OrientBio Korea (Seongnam, Korea), housed individually in a clean room, and maintained at a temperature of 22 ± 1 °C, with 12-h light (07:00–19:00) and 12-h dark (19:00–07:00) cycles at a relative humidity of 50 ± 5% with air filtration (Laboratory Animal Research Center of Ajou University Medical Center, Suwon, Korea). The rats had access to food (Purina Korea, Pyeongtaek, Korea) and water *ad libitum*. All experimental procedures and protocols were reviewed and approved by the Institutional Animal Care and Use Committee (IACUC No. 2017-0074, 2018) of the Laboratory Animal Research Center of Ajou University Medical Center.

2.3. Estimation of the Appropriate Number of Animals

The appropriate number of animals in each group (n) and total number of animals in each experimental setting (N) were calculated based on the statistics [9]. For statistical analysis, the degree of freedom should range from 10 to 20. The minimum and maximum number of animals in each group were calculated as:

$$\text{Minimum } n = 10/k + 1 \tag{1}$$

$$\text{Maximum } n = 20/k + 1 \tag{2}$$

where k is the number of groups in each setting. The minimum and maximum n were rounded up and down, respectively. The total minimum and maximum N required were minimum n multiplied by k and maximum n multiplied by k, respectively.

2.4. Intravenus and Oral Administration of Tofacitinib

The pretreatment and surgical procedures for oral and intravenous administration were similar to those described previously [10,11]. For oral administration, the rats were fasted overnight with free access to water. The rats were anesthetized with ketamine (200 mg/kg), and their carotid arteries were cannulated using polyethylene tubing (Clay Adams, Parsippany, NJ, USA) for blood sampling. For intravenous administration, the rats were anesthetized with ketamine (200 mg/kg), and their jugular veins and carotid arteries were cannulated for drug administration and blood sampling, respectively. Rats were allowed to recover for 4–5 h after surgical procedures. The rats were not restrained during the experimental period and had free access to water and food.

For intravenous administration, tofacitinib, dissolved in 0.9% NaCl-injectable solution containing 0.5% β-cyclodextrin, was injected via the jugular vein for 1 min at doses of 5 ($n = 9$), 10 ($n = 8$), 20 ($n = 7$), and 50 ($n = 7$) mg/kg. Blood samples (110–220 µL) were collected via the carotid artery at times 0 (prior to drug administration), 1 (at the end of drug infusion), 5, 15, 30, 45, 60, 90, 120, 180, 240, 360, 480, and 600 min. The total amount of blood collected from each rat did not exceed 10% of the total blood volume during the entire experimental period so as not to alter the pharmacokinetics and physiological functions. These blood samples were immediately centrifuged at 8000× g for 10 min, and plasma was collected and stored at −80 °C until HPLC analysis of tofacitinib [12]. To prevent blood clotting, 0.3 mL of heparinized 0.9% NaCl-injectable solution (20 IU/mL) was immediately injected into the carotid artery after each blood sampling. Urine samples were collected over 24 h; in addition, each metabolic cage was rinsed with 20 mL of distilled water 24 h after drug administration, and the rinses were combined with their corresponding 24-h urine samples. The volumes of the combined urine samples were measured, and two 100 µL aliquots of each were stored at −80 °C until HPLC analysis of tofacitinib [12]. At 24-h, each rat was exsanguinated, followed by cervical dislocation. The abdomen of each rat was opened and the entire gastrointestinal tract, including its contents and feces, was removed, transferred to a beaker containing 50 mL methanol, and cut into small pieces using scissors. The contents of each beaker were stirred manually with a glass rod for 1 min, and two 100 µL aliquots of each supernatant were collected and stored at −80 °C until HPLC analysis of tofacitinib [12].

For oral administration, approximately 1.0 mL tofacitinib was administered to rats at doses of 10 ($n = 7$), 20 ($n = 8$), 50 ($n = 9$), and 100 ($n = 7$) mg/kg. Blood samples (110–220 µL) were collected via the carotid artery at times 0 (prior to drug administration), 5, 15, 30, 45, 60, 90, 120, 180, 240, 360, 480, 600, and 720 min. Urine and gastrointestinal tract samples were also obtained over 24 h were processed as described above for the corresponding samples collected after intravenous administration.

2.5. Hepatic First-Pass Effects of Tofacitinib

The carotid artery and jugular vein were handled as described previously [10,11]. In addition, the vein from the cecum was cannulated and the cannula was pushed forward about 4 cm toward the liver through the portal vein to minimize the damage from blood flowing into the portal vein [13,14]. Using a peristaltic pump (BT-300CA, JIH Pump, Chongqing, China), 10 mg/kg tofacitinib was infused over 30 min into the jugular vein ($n = 7$) and an equal volume of 0.9% NaCl-injectable solution containing 0.5% β-cyclodextrin was infused simultaneously over 30-min into the portal vein. In another group of rats, 10 mg/kg tofacitinib was infused over 30 min into the portal vein ($n = 7$) and an equal volume of 0.9% NaCl-injectable solution containing 0.5% β-cyclodextrin was infused simultaneously over 30 min into the jugular vein. Blood samples were collected from the carotid artery at times 0, 15, 30 (at the end of the infusion), 31, 35, 45, 60, 90, 150, 210, 270, 390, 510, and 630 min, with all sample collection and processing procedures identical to those described above.

2.6. Gastric and Intestinal First-Pass Effect of Tofacitinib

Rats were fasted overnight with free access to water. Cannulae were inserted into the carotid artery and the cecal vein [13,14]. Using the peristaltic pump, 10 mg/kg tofacitinib was infused over 30 min into the portal vein ($n = 6$), and equal volumes of 0.9% NaCl-injectable solution containing 0.5% β-cyclodextrin were instilled into both the stomach and duodenum using a 23-gauge needle. In addition, 10 mg/kg tofacitinib was instilled into the duodenum ($n = 5$), and equal volumes of 0.9% NaCl-injectable solution containing 0.5% β-cyclodextrin were instilled into the stomach and infused via the portal vein over 30 min. Furthermore, 10 mg/kg tofacitinib was instilled into the stomach ($n = 5$), and equal volumes of 0.9% NaCl-injectable solution containing 0.5% β-cyclodextrin were instilled into the duodenum and infused via the portal vein over 30 min. Blood samples were collected from the carotid artery at times 0, 15, 30, 31, 35, 45, 90, 150, 270, 390, 510, 630, and 750 min after the start of intraportal infusion of tofacitinib, and at times 0, 5, 15, 30, 60, 120, 180, 240, 360, 480, 600, and 720 min after intragastric and intraduodenal instillations of the drug. All sample collection and processing procedures were identical to those described above.

2.7. Tissue Distribution of Tofacitinib

Rats were handled and processed as described previously [10]. Tofacitinib (10 mg/kg) was administered intravenously to rats for 1 min. After 30 min and 2 h ($n = 4$ each), as much blood as possible was collected from the carotid artery. Blood samples were immediately centrifuged, and plasma was collected. The rats were sacrificed by cervical dislocation, approximately 1 g of each brain, fat, heart, kidney, large intestine, liver, lung, mesentery, muscle, small intestine, spleen, and stomach was removed, rinsed with phosphate-buffered solution (pH 7.4), and blotted dry with paper towels to remove any remaining blood. Each tissue sample was added to four volumes of homogenizing buffer, homogenized using a tissue homogenizer (T25 Ultra-Turrax, IKA Labortechnik, Staufen, Germany) and centrifuged at $8000 \times g$ for 10 min. A 100 μL aliquot of each supernatant was collected and stored at −80 °C until HPLC analysis of tofacitinib [12].

2.8. Biliary Excretion of Tofacitinib

The jugular vein of each rat was cannulated. The abdomen was opened and the bile duct was cannulated with polyethylene tubing [14]. The incision was closed with surgical sutures and each rat was kept warm under an electric light. Each rat was maintained in the supine position during the entire experiment. Tofacitinib (10 mg/kg) was infused for 1 min via the jugular vein ($n = 3$). Bile samples were collected over various time periods, from 0–1, 1–2, 2–4, 4–6, and 6–24 h. The volume of each bile sample was measured, and an aliquot of each was stored at −80 °C until HPLC analysis of tofacitinib [12].

2.9. HPLC Analysis of Tofacitinib

Two microliters of hydrocortisone (5 mg/mL) and 40 μL of 20% ammonia solution were added to 100 μL aliquots of biological samples and vortex-mixed for 30 s using a vortex mixer. Each solution was extracted with 1.5 mL of ethyl acetate by centrifugation at 12,000 rpm for 5 min. The organic layer was collected and dried (Dry Thermobath, Eyela, Tokyo, Japan) under a gentle stream of nitrogen gas at 40 °C. The samples were reconstituted in 130 μL of 20% acetonitrile, and 50 μL of resuspended samples were analyzed by HPLC [12].

The concentrations of tofacitinib in the prepared biological samples were determined using a Shimadzu Prominence LC-20A HPLC system (Kyoto, Japan), consisting of a pump (LC-20A), an auto-sampler (SIL-20A), a column oven, and a detector (SPD-20A/20AD), controlled by the CBM-20A system controller. The samples were filtered through 0.45-μm filters (Millipore, Billerica, MA, USA), followed by separation of tofacitinib on a reversed-phase column (AegisPak C_{18}; 25 cm × 4.6 mm, 5 μm; Young Jin Biochrom, Seongnam, Korea). The mobile phase consisted of a 69.5:30.5 (v/v) mixture of 10 mM ammonium acetate buffer (pH 5.0) and acetonitrile, respectively, with a flow rate of 1.0 mL/min.

Column effluent was monitored by a UV detector at 287 nm. The retention times of tofacitinib and the internal standard (hydrocortisone) were approximately 7.2 and 11.3 min, respectively. The lower limits of quantitation of tofacitinib in rat plasma, urine, and tissue homogenates were 0.01, 0.1, and 0.1 µg/mL, respectively, with intraday assay precision (coefficients of variation) in these samples being 3.69–5.88%, 4.21–6.18%, and 0.0205–8.74%, respectively. The interday assay precision was 5.06% for rat plasma and 5.46% for rat urine.

2.10. Pharmacokinetics Analysis

Pharmacokinetic parameters, including AUC, apparent volume of distribution at steady state (V_{ss}), mean residence time (MRT), and time-averaged total body (CL), renal (CL_R), and nonrenal (CL_{NR}) clearances, were calculated by noncompartmental analysis (WinNonlin, Pharsight Corporation, Mountain View, CA, USA) using standard methods [15]. AUC values were calculated using the trapezoidal rule–extrapolation method [16]. The peak plasma concentration (C_{max}) and time to reach C_{max} (T_{max}) were obtained directly from the experimental data. The mean values of clearance [17], terminal half-life [18], and V_{ss} [19] were calculated using the harmonic mean method.

2.11. Statistical Analysis

All results are expressed as mean ± standard deviation (SD), except that T_{max} is expressed as median (range). Comparisons between two means were evaluated using Student's *t*-tests and comparisons among three or more means by analysis of variance (ANOVA) with Tukey's post-test. A *p* value <0.05 was considered statistically significant.

3. Results

3.1. Pharmacokinetics of Tofacitinib after Intravenous and Oral Administration to Rats

Figure 2A shows the mean arterial plasma concentration-time profiles after intravenous infusion of 5, 10, 20, and 50 mg/kg tofacitinib over 1 min, and Table 1 shows the associated pharmacokinetic parameters. At all four doses, the mean arterial plasma concentrations of tofacitinib showed a polyexponential decrease. The dose-normalized AUCs following intravenous infusion of 5, 10, 20, and 50 mg/kg tofacitinib were 282, 342, 404, and 705 µg·min/mL, respectively (Table 1 and Supplementary Figure S1A). The dose-normalized AUC at 50 mg/kg was 2.50-, 2.06-, and 1.75-fold greater than the dose-normalized AUCs at 5, 10, and 20 mg/kg, respectively ($p < 0.001$ each). CL and CL_{NR} at 50 mg/kg were significantly slower than at 5, 10, and 20 mg/kg ($p < 0.01$ each). Thus, the terminal half-life and MRT were significantly longer following infusion of 50 mg/kg tofacitinib than the other doses ($p < 0.001$ each), whereas V_{ss} and the percentage of intravenous tofacitinib excreted unchanged in 24-h urine ($Ae_{0-24\,h}$) did not differ significantly among the four intravenous doses (Table 1). The CL_R was 69%, 71%, and 71% slower at 50 mg/kg than at 5, 10, and 20 mg/kg, respectively, because the $Ae_{0-24\,h}$ was smaller and AUC was greater at 50 mg/kg than at the other doses. However, the percentages of tofacitinib recovered unchanged from the entire gastrointestinal tract (including its contents and feces) at 24 h ($GI_{24\,h}$) were negligible for all four intravenous doses (data not shown). Taken together, these findings indicate that the pharmacokinetic parameters of intravenous tofacitinib in rats were dependent on dose.

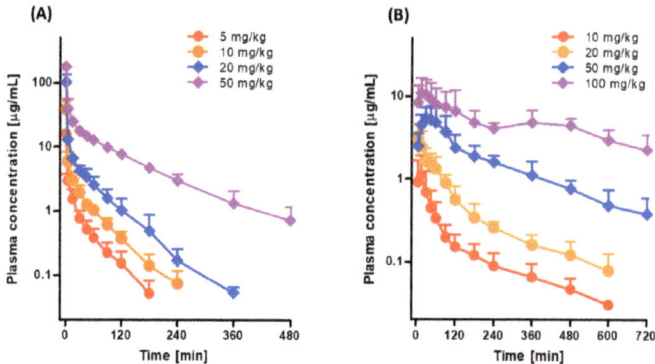

Figure 2. Mean arterial plasma concentration-time profiles of tofacitinib in Sprague-Dawley rats after (**A**) 1-min intravenous infusion of 5 ($n = 9$), 10 ($n = 8$), 20 ($n = 7$), and 50 ($n = 7$) mg/kg tofacitinib and (**B**) oral administration of 10 ($n = 7$), 20 ($n = 8$), 50 ($n = 9$), and 100 ($n = 7$) mg/kg tofacitinib. Bars represent standard deviations (SD).

Table 1. Pharmacokinetic parameters of tofacitinib after 1-min intravenous infusion of the drug at various doses to male Sprague-Dawley rats. Data are expressed as mean ± standard deviation (SD).

Parameters.	5 mg/kg ($n = 9$)	10 mg/kg ($n = 8$)	20 mg/kg ($n = 7$)	50 mg/kg ($n = 7$)
Body weight (g)	337 ± 39.2	347 ± 11.0	317 ± 15.9	356 ± 22.0
AUC (μg·min/mL) [a]	141 ± 23.0	342 ± 33.1	807 ± 146	3526 ± 572
Dose-normalized AUC (μg·min/mL) [a]	282 ± 46.0	342 ± 33.1	404 ± 73.0	705 ± 114
Terminal half-life (min) [b]	38.2 ± 11.7	41.6 ± 7.86	48.1 ± 5.56	97.8 ± 19.2
MRT (min) [b]	35.2 ± 11.4	41.1 ± 20.2	35.5 ± 7.50	105 ± 21.4
CL (mL/min/kg) [c]	36.3 ± 6.02	29.5 ± 2.99	25.4 ± 4.26	14.5 ± 2.33
CL_R (mL/min/kg)	2.69 ± 1.70	2.80 ± 1.69	2.80 ± 1.17	0.824 ± 0.651
CL_{NR} (mL/min/kg) [d]	32.9 ± 7.72	26.3 ± 2.16	22.6 ± 3.90	13.7 ± 2.12
V_{ss} (mL/kg)	1258 ± 460	1208 ± 579	900 ± 218	1489 ± 134
$Ae_{0-24\,h}$ (% of dose)	7.62 ± 5.08	9.40 ± 5.06	11.0 ± 3.72	5.55 ± 3.91

AUC values were normalized to tofacitinib dose of 10 mg/kg for statistical analysis. [a] 20 mg/kg was significantly different ($p < 0.05$) from 5 mg/kg. 50 mg/kg was significantly different ($p < 0.001$) from 5, 10 and 20 mg/kg. [b] 50 mg/kg was significantly different ($p < 0.001$) from 5, 10 and 20 mg/kg. [c] 5 mg/kg was significantly different from 10 ($p < 0.05$) and 20 ($p < 0.001$) mg/kg, respectively. 50 mg/kg was significantly different ($p < 0.001$) from 5, 10 and 20 mg/kg. [d] 5 mg/kg was significantly different from 10 ($p < 0.05$), 20 ($p < 0.01$) and 50 ($p < 0.001$) mg/kg, respectively. 50 mg/kg was significantly different from 10 ($p < 0.001$) and 20 ($p < 0.01$) mg/kg, respectively.

Figure 2B shows the mean arterial plasma concentration-time profiles following oral administration of 10, 20, 50, and 100 mg/kg tofacitinib, and Table 2 shows the associated pharmacokinetic parameters. Orally administered tofacitinib, at all four doses, was rapidly absorbed by the rat gastrointestinal tract, with tofacitinib detected in plasma within 5 min. After reaching T_{max}, the plasma concentrations of tofacitinib showed a polyexponential decrease for all four doses. The dose-normalized AUCs following oral administration of 10, 20, 50, and 100 mg/kg tofacitinib were dose dependent, being 99.4, 135, 238, and 407 μg·min/mL, respectively (Table 2 and Supplementary Figure S1B). The dose-normalized AUC at 100 mg/kg was 4.09-, 3.01-, and 1.71-fold greater than those at 10, 20, and 50 mg/kg, respectively ($p < 0.01$ each). The CL_R was much slower at 100 mg/kg than at the other doses because AUC was significantly greater at 100 mg/kg. T_{max} was significantly longer at 100 mg/kg than at 10, 20 and 50 mg/kg ($p < 0.05$ each). The dose-normalized C_{max} (based on 10 mg/kg dose), $GI_{24\,h}$, and $Ae_{0-24\,h}$ did not differ significantly among the four oral doses studied (Table 2). Based on the AUC of 10 mg/kg intravenous tofacitinib, the F values for oral doses of 10, 20, 50, and 100 mg/kg were 29.1%, 39.3%, 69.7%, and 119%, respectively. These findings indicated that the pharmacokinetic parameters of orally administered tofacitinib in rats were dependent on dose.

Table 2. Pharmacokinetic parameters of tofacitinib after oral administration of the drug at various doses to male Sprague-Dawley rats.

Parameters	10 mg/kg (n = 7)	20 mg/kg (n = 8)	50 mg/kg (n = 9)	100 mg/kg (n = 7)
Body weight (g)	312 ± 19.8	308 ± 24.5	284 ± 22.3	286 ± 17.7
AUC (µg·min/mL) [a]	99.4 ± 35.5	269 ± 53.7	1192 ± 280	4073 ± 1787
Dose-normalized AUC (µg·min/mL) [a]	99.4 ± 35.5	135 ± 26.9	238 ± 56.0	407 ± 179
C_{max} (µg/mL)	1.13 ± 0.774	3.13 ± 1.27	5.62 ± 2.18	13.1 ± 5.48
T_{max} (min) [b]	15.7 ± 7.32	15.7 ± 15.9	34.4 ± 26.7	170 ± 192
CL_R (mL/min/kg) [c]	11.6 ± 2.87	6.97 ± 3.95	7.61 ± 2.82	3.37 ± 2.52
$Ae_{0-24\,h}$ (% of dose)	11.3 ± 4.60	10.0 ± 6.51	17.2 ± 3.98	13.0± 9.47
$GI_{24\,h}$ (% of dose)	3.16 ± 5.12	3.13 ± 3.27	2.77 ± 3.96	0.772± 0.905
F (%)	29.1	39.3	69.7	119

Data are expressed as mean ± standard deviation (SD). AUC and C_{max} values were normalized to tofacitinib dose of 10 mg/kg for statistical analysis. F was calculated by dose-normalized AUC (based on 10 mg/kg) after oral administration of tofacitinib divided by AUC after intravenous administration of the drug at dose of 10 mg/kg. [a] 10 mg/kg was significantly different ($p < 0.05$) from 50 mg/kg. 100 mg/kg was significantly different from 10 ($p < 0.001$), 20 ($p < 0.001$) and 50 ($p < 0.01$) mg/kg, respectively. [b] 100 mg/kg was significantly different ($p < 0.05$) from 10, 20 and 50 mg/kg. [c] 10 mg/kg was significantly different from 20 ($p < 0.05$) and 100 ($p < 0.001$) mg/kg, respectively.

3.2. Hepatic First-Pass Effect of Tofacitinib in Rats

Figure 3A shows the mean arterial plasma concentration-time profiles following intravenous and intraportal administration of 10 mg/kg tofacitinib, and Table 3 shows the associated pharmacokinetic parameters. The mean arterial plasma concentrations of tofacitinib administered intravenously and intraportally showed polyexponential reductions. The AUCs were 417 and 242 µg·min/mL, respectively, demonstrating considerable hepatic first-pass metabolism of tofacitinib after absorption into the portal vein, with 42.0% of the intravenous dose metabolized in the liver before entering the systemic circulation. As a result, the CL and CL_{NR} of tofacitinib were 67% and 60% faster, respectively, after intraportal administration. Furthermore, V_{ss} was 50% higher after intraportal than after intravenous administration of tofacitinib ($p < 0.05$).

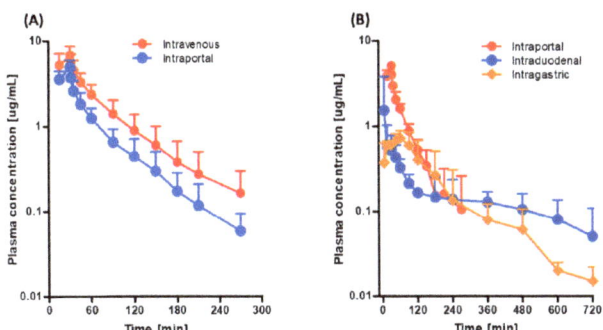

Figure 3. Mean arterial plasma concentration-time profiles of tofacitinib in Sprague-Dawley rats after (**A**) 30-min intravenous (n = 7) and intraportal (n = 7) infusions of 10 mg/kg tofacitinib and (**B**) 30-min intraportal (n = 6) infusion, and intraduodenal (n = 5) and intragastric (n = 5) instillations of 10 mg/kg tofacitinib. Bars represent standard deviations (SD).

Table 3. Pharmacokinetic parameters of tofacitinib after 30-min intravenous and intraportal infusion of the drug at dose of 10 mg/kg to male Sprague-Dawley rats.

Parameter	Intravenous (n = 7)	Intraportal (n = 7)
Body weight (g)	292 ± 18.0	299 ± 28.6
AUC (μg·min/mL)	417 ± 136	242 ± 66.0 **
Terminal half-life (min)	46.2 ± 12.5	42.4 ± 10.4
MRT (min)	67.5 ± 26.8	59.6 ± 13.9
CL (mL/min/kg)	26.3 ± 8.85	43.8 ± 11.0 **
CL_R (mL/min/kg)	2.34 ± 2.90	5.00 ± 4.69
CL_{NR} (mL/min/kg)	24.0 ± 6.46	38.5 ± 10.4 **
V_{ss} (mL/kg)	1695 ± 737	2549 ± 720 *
$Ae_{0-24\,h}$ (% of dose)	12.5 ± 5.20	10.7 ± 9.42

Data are expressed as mean ± standard deviation (SD). * $p < 0.05$; ** $p < 0.01$.

3.3. Gastric and Intestinal First-Pass Effects of Tofacitinib in Rats

Figure 3B shows the mean arterial plasma concentration-time profiles following intragastric, intraduodenal, and intraportal administration of 10 mg/kg tofacitinib, and Table 4 shows the associated pharmacokinetic parameters. The AUCs of intragastrically and intraduodenally administered tofacitinib did not differ significantly (134 and 138 μg·min/mL), suggesting that the gastric first-pass effect of tofacitinib was negligible. In contrast, AUC was significantly lower after intraduodenal (138 μg·min/mL) than after intraportal (272 μg·min/mL) administration, indicating that the intestinal first-pass effect of tofacitinib was significant, with approximately 49.3% of the orally administered drug removed prior to entry into the portal vein.

Table 4. Pharmacokinetic parameters of tofacitinib after 30-min intraportal infusion, intraduodenal and intragastric instillation of the drug at dose of 10 mg/kg to male Sprague-Dawley rats.

Parameter	Intraportal (n = 6)	Intraduodenal (n = 5)	Intragastric (n = 5)
Body weight (g)	287 ± 10.6	282 ± 6.30	285 ± 4.97
AUC (μg·min/mL) [a]	272 ± 62.7	138 ± 33.2	134 ± 44.6
Terminal half-life (min)	44.8 ± 14.2		
C_{max} (μg/mL) [b]	5.18 ± 0.586	1.55 ± 1.93	0.716 ± 0.255
T_{max} (min)	27.5 ± 6.12	38.8 ± 38.2	63.8 ± 18.9
MRT (min)	53.0 ± 22.3		
CL (mL/min/kg)	38.4 ± 8.47		
CL_R (mL/min/kg)	2.44 ± 1.23	5.72 ± 2.62	7.08 ± 2.91
CL_{NR} (mL/min/kg)	38.3 ± 6.16		
V_{ss} (mL/kg)	1900 ± 369		
$Ae_{0-24\,h}$ (% of dose)	5.82 ± 2.32	8.30 ± 5.10	8.90 ± 3.00

Data are expressed as mean ± standard deviation (SD). [a] Intraportal infusion was significantly different ($p < 0.05$) from intraduodenal and intragastric instillation. [b] Intraportal infusion was significantly different ($p < 0.001$) from intraduodenal and intragastric instillation.

3.4. Tissue Distribution of Tofacitinib in Rats

Figure 4 shows the concentrations of tofacitinib in plasma (μg/mL) and in tissue samples (μg/g) and its tissue-to-plasma (T/P) ratios 30 min (distribution phase) and 2 h (elimination phase) after intravenous administration of 10 mg/kg tofacitinib. Tofacitinib was widely distributed in all rat tissues, with T/P ratios greater than 1.0 in every tissue except the brain, mesentery, and fat, both 30 min and 2 h after intravenous administration. At 30 min, tofacitinib was exclusively distributed in the kidneys, small intestine, and large intestine, with its concentrations remaining stable until 2 h after intravenous administration.

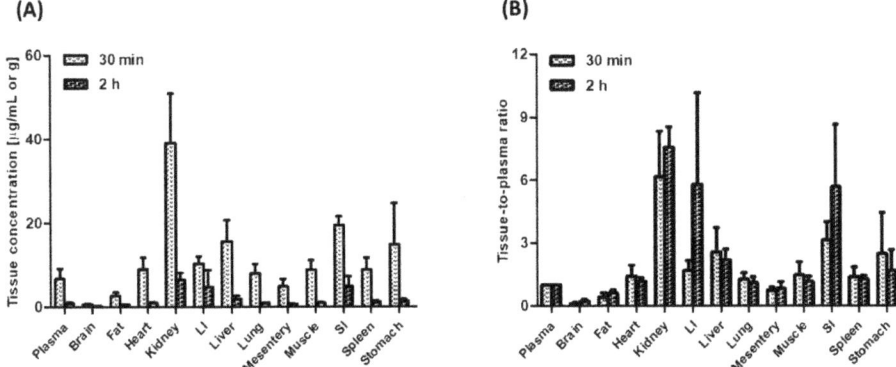

Figure 4. (**A**) Mean plasma and tissue/organ concentrations of tofacitinib and (**B**) tissue-to-plasma (T/P) ratios of tofacitinib 30 min ($n = 4$) and 2 h ($n = 4$) in Sprague-Dawley rats after 1-min intravenous infusion of 10 mg/kg tofacitinib. Data are expressed means ± standard deviations (SD). LI; large intestine, SI; small intestine.

3.5. Biliary Excretion of Tofacitinib in Rats

Following a 1-min intravenous infusion of 10 mg/kg tofacitinib, less than 1% of the intravenous dose (0.703 ± 0.303%) was excreted in bile of each of the three rats studied, suggesting that biliary excretion of tofacitinib is a minor elimination pathway.

4. Discussion

The present study found that the dose-normalized AUC of tofacitinib was dependent on the administered dose. Plots of AUC versus dose for intravenous and oral tofacitinib yielded slopes of 2.74 and 4.65, respectively (Supplementary Figure S2). Several factors may account for the observed dose-dependent characteristics of tofacitinib. First, V_{ss} values did not differ significantly among the four intravenous doses, suggesting that the tofacitinib distribution process did not affect its dose-dependency. Thus, the contribution of V_{ss} to the dose-dependency of tofacitinib was negligible. Second, the contribution of CL_R to CL was not significant. $Ae_{0-24\,h}$ was less than 11.0% for all intravenous doses and less than 17.2% for all oral doses, with no significant differences among doses, suggesting that the contribution of renal excretion to the dose-dependent characteristics of tofacitinib is also low.

The renal extraction ratios (CL_R/renal plasma flow rate) for urinary excretion of unchanged tofacitinib were estimated in rats based on its CL_R, a reported renal blood flow rate of 36.8 mL/min/kg [20], and a hematocrit of approximately 45% [21]. The estimated renal extraction ratios following intravenous administration of 5, 10, 20, and 50 mg/kg tofacitinib were 13.3%, 13.8%, 13.8%, and 4.07%, respectively. These findings indicate that, in rats, tofacitinib has a low renal extraction ratio and that little tofacitinib is excreted via the kidneys. Therefore, most of the administered tofacitinib was eliminated via nonrenal pathways (CL_{NR}).

The CL_{NR} of tofacitinib was affected by gastrointestinal (including biliary) excretion of unchanged drug and metabolic clearance. The contribution of gastrointestinal excretion to CL_{NR} was negligible, with no tofacitinib detected in the gastrointestinal tract 24 h after intravenous administration. The observed CL_{NR} of tofacitinib may therefore represent metabolic clearance of the drug, suggesting that changes in its CL_{NR} in rats may be due to changes in its metabolism. The increases in the dose-normalized AUC after intravenous and oral administration of tofacitinib may have been due to saturation of its metabolism, in agreement with the inverse relationship between slower CL_{NR} and higher intravenous dose. Oral tofacitinib also showed a dose-dependent AUC in humans, as evidenced by dose-dependent increases in dose-normalized AUCs [8,22].

Although the F values of tofacitinib differed in humans (74%) [7] and rats (29.1–33.8%), based on calculations using the same intravenous and oral doses, F values were not 100% in either species. Because it is difficult to measure first-pass metabolism in humans, first-pass metabolism in the liver and gastrointestinal tract was measured in rats. The F and $GI_{24\,h}$ of 10 mg/kg tofacitinib administered orally were 29.1% and 3.16%, respectively. The level of unchanged drug in the gastrointestinal tract (3.16%) may be due in part to the gastrointestinal (including biliary) excretion of absorbed drug. For comparison, the mean "true" fraction of unabsorbed dose (F_{unabs}) following oral administration could be estimated using the equation [23];

$$GI_{24\,h,\,oral} = F_{unabs} + (F \times GI_{24\,h,\,intravenous}) \tag{3}$$

where $GI_{24\,h,\,oral}$ and $GI_{24\,h,\,intravenous}$ are the percentages of oral and intravenous doses, respectively, remaining in the gastrointestinal tract after 24 h. Because $GI_{24\,h,\,intravenous}$ in the present study was negligible, F_{unabs} was almost equal to $GI_{24\,h,\,oral}$, indicating that gastrointestinal (including biliary) excretion of absorbed tofacitinib contributed little to the total drug recovered from the gastrointestinal tract after oral administration. Thus, approximately 96.8% of orally administered tofacitinib (10 mg/kg) was absorbed from the gastrointestinal tract in rats. Because only 3.16% of oral tofacitinib was not absorbed from the gastrointestinal tract at 24 h and the F value was 29.1%, approximately 67.7%·[100% − (3.16% + 29.1%)] of orally administered tofacitinib may have been eliminated by first-pass metabolism.

After intravenous administration of tofacitinib, the CL values of 14.5–36.3 mL/min/kg based on plasma data were considerably lower than the reported cardiac output of 296 mL/min/kg based on blood data [20] and a hematocrit of approximately 45% [21] in rats. These findings suggested that the first-pass effects of tofacitinib in the lungs and heart were negligible.

The AUCs were similar after intragastric and intraduodenal instillation of 10 mg/kg tofacitinib, suggesting that gastric first-pass effects on tofacitinib were negligible. However, the AUC after intraduodenal instillation of 10 mg/kg tofacitinib was 50.7% of that after intraportal administration, suggesting that approximately 49.3% of orally administered drug was not absorbed into the portal vein and that approximately 46.1%·[100% − (50.7% + 3.16%)] of orally administered tofacitinib was metabolized in the intestine before entering the portal vein. The AUC after intraportal administration of 10 mg/kg tofacitinib was 58.0% of that after intravenous administration, suggesting that the hepatic first-pass metabolism of tofacitinib after absorption into the portal vein was approximately 42.0%. Moreover, approximately 21.3% of the oral dose (42% of 50.7% of orally administered tofacitinib) was metabolized in the rat liver and 29.4% (50.7−21.3%) of the oral dose was absorbed into the systemic circulation. The latter percentage (29.4%) was close to the F value of 29.1%. Even though there is a species difference of bioavailability between human and rats, we could presume that 26%·(100−74%) of oral tofacitinib in humans was first-pass metabolized in the intestine and the liver with a similar ratio as rats. If a drug was not first-pass metabolized in the liver of the rat model, no hepatic first-pass metabolism was expected in humans. Considerable hepatic and intestinal first-pass metabolism has also been reported for other drugs, including ipriflavone [24], oltipraz [25], and sildenafil [26] in rats, and midazolam [27] in humans.

The AUCs were similar after intragastric and intraduodenal instillation of 10 mg/kg tofacitinib, suggesting that gastric first-pass effects on tofacitinib were negligible. However, the AUC after intraduodenal instillation of 10 mg/kg tofacitinib was 50.7% of that after intraportal administration, suggesting that approximately 49.3% of orally administered drug was not absorbed into the portal vein and that approximately 46.1%·[100% − (50.7% + 3.16%)] of orally administered tofacitinib was metabolized in the intestine before entering the portal vein. The AUC after intraportal administration of 10 mg/kg tofacitinib was 58.0% of that after intravenous administration, suggesting that the hepatic first-pass metabolism of tofacitinib after absorption into the portal vein was approximately 42.0%. Moreover, approximately 21.3% of the oral dose (42% of 50.7% of orally administered tofacitinib) was metabolized in the rat liver and 29.4% (50.7−21.3%) of the oral dose was absorbed into the systemic circulation. The latter percentage (29.4%) was close to the F value of 29.1%. Even though there is a species difference of bioavailability between human and rats, we could presume that 26% (100−74%) of oral tofacitinib in humans was first-pass metabolized in the intestine and the liver with a similar ratio as rats. If a drug was not first-pass metabolized in the liver of the rat model, no hepatic first-pass metabolism was expected in humans. Considerable hepatic and intestinal first-pass metabolism has also been reported for other drugs, including ipriflavone [24], oltipraz [25], and sildenafil [26] in rats, and midazolam [27] in humans.

In humans, hepatic microsomal CYP3A4 and to a lesser extent CYP2C19 are involved in the metabolism of tofacitinib, oxidizing the pyrrolopyrimidine moiety and producing a carbonyl moiety, the major metabolite of tofacitinib [3]. CYP3A1(23)/2 and CYP2C11 are the main enzymes involved in drug metabolism in rats and are highly expressed in the rat liver and small intestine [28,29]. Human liver and intestinal CYP2C19 and rat CYP2C11 are highly homologous and human liver and gastrointestinal CYP3A4 and rat CYP3A1(23) share 73% homology [28,30]. We recently observed [31] that CYP3A1(23)/2 and CYP2C11 are the main CYPs responsible for the metabolism of tofacitinib in rats, as evidenced by a 46% greater AUC in rats pretreated with ketoconazole, an inhibitor of CYP3A1/2 [32], and a 39% greater AUC in rats pretreated with fluconazole, an inhibitor of CYP2C11 [33]. In contrast, the AUC of tofacitinib reduced by 56% in rats pretreated with dexamethasone, an inducer of CYP3A1/2 [34], and 26% in rats pretreated with rifampin, an inducer of CYP2C11 [35]. The AUCs of tofacitinib in rats pretreated with specific inhibitors or inducers of different CYP isoforms did not differ significantly [31]. Therefore, the dose dependent increases in AUCs of tofacitinib after intravenous and oral administration to rats suggested that hepatic first-pass metabolism of tofacitinib (42%) was saturated after intravenous administration, whereas its intestinal (46.1%) and/or hepatic (23.1%) first-pass metabolism was saturated after oral administration. This saturation may have been due to the saturable metabolism of tofacitinib by CYP3A1/2 and/or CYP2C11 in rat liver and intestine.

The distribution process of tofacitinib did not contribute to its dose-dependent profiles, as V_{ss} values did not differ significantly among the four intravenous doses. However, tofacitinib was widely distributed in rat tissues, especially in the small and large intestines, with the T/P ratios being higher for the intestines than for other tissues at both 30 min and 2 h. These findings suggest a mechanism for the effectiveness of tofacitinib in the treatment of ulcerative colitis, resulting in its approval in 2018 as the first oral drug for the treatment of chronic ulcerative colitis [6]. Tofacitinib is undergoing evaluation in clinical trials for the treatment of various diseases, including psoriasis [36,37], alopecia [38], atopic dermatitis [39], and ankylosing spondylitis [40].

Recently, several studies on tofacitinib pharmacokinetics were reported in patients with various diseases, including hepatic injury [41], renal failure [42], psoriasis [43], as well as inflammatory bowel disease [44], and most of them focused on the relationship between the drug concentration and the therapeutic efficacy. It was not well explained that the changes of plasma concentration according to diseases was related to the pharmacokinetic basis. In addition, pharmacokinetic drug interaction of tofacitinib is also expected since tofacitinib is mainly metabolized by CYP3A and is a substrate of P-glycoprotein [45]. Some pharmacokinetic drug interactions with tofacitinib were reported [46–48]. However, it is difficult to get the information from the clinical settings in order to evaluate the pharmacokinetic mechanism of the drug–disease or drug-drug interaction. Therefore, we need to further investigate the pharmacokinetic mechanism of the drug-disease or drug-drug interaction of tofacitinib in the rat model based on our pharmacokinetic characteristics of the drug in rats.

5. Conclusions

In conclusion, the low F of 10 mg/kg tofacitinib (29.1%) after oral administration to rats was mainly due to significant intestinal (46.1%) and hepatic (23.1%) first-pass metabolism. Our observation that the dose-normalized AUCs of tofacitinib in rats increased with increasing intravenous and oral doses, suggests that the hepatic and intestinal first-pass metabolism of tofacitinib was saturated by increasing its intravenous and oral doses.

Supplementary Materials: The following are available online at http://www.mdpi.com/1999-4923/11/7/318/s1, **Figure S1:** Mean dose (mg/kg) versus dose-normalized AUC (µg·min/mL) of tofacitinib in Sprague-Dawley rats after (**A**) 1-min intravenous infusion of 5 ($n = 9$), 10 ($n = 8$), 20 ($n = 7$), and 50 ($n = 7$) mg/kg tofacitinib and (**B**) oral administration of 10 ($n = 7$), 20 ($n = 8$), 50 ($n = 9$), and 100 ($n = 7$) mg/kg tofacitinib. Bars represent standard deviations (SD). (**A**) 20 mg/kg was significantly different ($p < 0.05$) from 5 mg/kg. 50 mg/kg was significantly different ($p < 0.001$) from 5, 10 and 20 mg/kg. (**B**) 10 mg/kg was significantly different ($p < 0.05$) from 50mg/kg. 100 mg/kg was significantly different from 10 ($p < 0.001$), 20 ($p < 0.001$) and 50 ($p < 0.01$) mg/kg, respectively, **Figure S2:** Plots of dose versus AUC of tofacitinib in Sprague-Dawley rats after (**A**) 1-min intravenous infusion of 5, 10, 20, and 50 mg/kg tofacitinib and (**B**) oral administration of 10, 20, 50, and 100 mg/kg tofacitinib. Dose and AUC ratios were calculated based on 5 and 10 mg/kg dose and respective AUC for intravenous and oral administration, respectively.

Author Contributions: J.S.L. performed all of the animal experiments and the HPLC analysis of tofacitinib in the biological samples and estimated the pharmacokinetic parameters. S.H.K. designed the experiments, performed the statistical analysis and graphic works, and drafted the manuscript. All authors have read and approved the final manuscript.

Funding: This work was supported by the Korea Health Technology R&D Project (HI16C0992) through the Korea Health Industry Development Institute (KHIDI) funded by the Ministry of Health and Welfare, Korea.

Conflicts of Interest: The authors declare no competing financial interests.

References

1. Fleischmann, R.; Kremer, J.; Cush, J.; Schulze-Koops, H.; Connell, C.A.; Bradley, J.D.; Kanik, K.S. Placebo-controlled trial of tofacitinib monotherapy in rheumatoid arthritis. *N. Engl. J. Med.* **2012**, *367*, 495–507. [CrossRef] [PubMed]
2. Strand, V.; van Vollenhoven, R.F.; Lee, E.B.; Fleischmann, R.; Zwillich, S.H.; Gruben, D.; Wallenstein, G. Tofacitinib or adalimumab versus placebo: Patient-reported outcomes from a phase 3 study of active rheumatoid arthritis. *Rheumatology* **2016**, *55*, 1031–1041. [CrossRef] [PubMed]
3. Dowty, M.E.; Lin, J.; Ryder, T.F.; Wang, W.; Walker, G.S.; Vaz, A.; Prakash, C. The pharmacokinetics, metabolism, and clearance mechanisms of tofacitinib, a janus kinase inhibitor, in humans. *Drug Metab. Dispos.* **2014**, *42*, 759–773. [CrossRef] [PubMed]
4. Claxton, L.; Taylor, M.; Soonasra, A.; Bourret, J.A.; Gerber, R.A. An economic evaluation of tofacitinib treatment in rheumatoid arthritis after methotrexate or after 1 or 2 TNF inhibitors from a U.S. payer perspective. *J. Manag. Care Spec. Pharm.* **2018**, *24*, 1010–1017. [CrossRef] [PubMed]
5. Fukuda, T.; Naganuma, M.; Kanai, T. Current new challenges in the management of ulcerative colitis. *Intest. Res.* **2019**, *17*, 36–44. [CrossRef] [PubMed]
6. Antonelli, E.; Villanacci, V.; Bassotti, G. Novel oral-targeted therapies for mucosal healing in ulcerative colitis. *World. J. Gastroenterol.* **2018**, *24*, 5322–5330. [CrossRef] [PubMed]
7. Scott, L.J. Tofacitinib: A review of its use in adult patients with rheumatoid arthritis. *Drugs* **2013**, *73*, 857–874. [CrossRef]
8. Cada, D.J.; Demaris, K.; Levien, T.L.; Baker, D.E. Tofacitinib. *Hosp. Pharm.* **2013**, *48*, 413–424. [CrossRef]
9. Arifin, W.N.; Zahiruddin, W.M. Sample size calculation in animal studies using resource equation approach. *Malays. J. Med. Sci.* **2017**, *24*, 101–105.
10. Du, E.S.; Moon, H.S.; Lim, S.J.; Kim, S.H. Pharmacokinetics of YJC-10592, a novel chemokine receptor 2 (CCR-2) antagonist, in rats. *Arch. Pharm. Res.* **2016**, *39*, 833–842. [CrossRef]
11. Kim, S.H.; Choi, Y.M.; Lee, M.G. Pharmacokinetics and pharmacodynamics of furosemide in protein-calorie malnutrition. *J. Pharmacokinet. Biopharm.* **1993**, *21*, 1–17. [CrossRef] [PubMed]
12. Kim, J.E. Simple Determination of Tofacitinib, A Jak Inhibitor, in Plasma, Urine and Tissue Homogenates by Hplc and Its Application to A Pharmacokinetic Study. Master's Thesis, Ajou University, Suwon, Korea, February 2018.
13. Murakami, T.; Nakanishi, M.; Yoshimori, T.; Okamura, N.; Norikura, R.; Mizojiri, K. Separate assessment of intestinal and hepatic first-pass effects using a rat model with double cannulation of the portal and jugular veins. *Drug Metab. Pharmacokinet.* **2003**, *18*, 252–260. [CrossRef] [PubMed]
14. Choi, Y.H.; Lee, Y.K.; Lee, M.G. Effects of 17α-ethynylestradiol-induced cholestasis on the pharmacokinetics of doxorubicin in rats: Reduced biliary excretion and hepatic metabolism of doxorubicin. *Xenobiotica* **2013**, *43*, 901–907. [CrossRef] [PubMed]
15. Gibaldi, M.; Perrier, D. *Pharmacokinetics*, 2nd ed.; Marcel-Dekker: New York, NY, USA, 1982.

16. Chiou, W.L. Critical evaluation of the potential error in pharmacokinetic studies of using the linear trapezoidal rule method for the calculation of the area under the plasma level-time curve. *J. Pharmacokinet. Biopharm.* **1978**, *6*, 539–546. [CrossRef] [PubMed]
17. Chiou, W.L. New calculation method of mean total body clearance of drugs and its application to dosage regimens. *J. Pharm. Sci.* **1980**, *69*, 90–91. [CrossRef] [PubMed]
18. Eatman, F.B.; Colburn, W.A.; Boxenbaum, H.G.; Posmanter, H.N.; Weinfeld, R.E.; Ronfeld, R.; Kaplan, S.A. Pharmacokinetics of diazepam following multiple-dose oral administration to healthy human subjects. *J. Pharmacokinet. Biopharm.* **1977**, *5*, 481–494. [CrossRef]
19. Chiou, W.L. New calculation method for mean apparent drug volume of distribution and application to rational dosage regimens. *J. Pharm. Sci.* **1979**, *68*, 1067–1069. [CrossRef]
20. Davies, B.; Morris, T. Physiological parameters in laboratory animals and humans. *Pharm. Res.* **1993**, *10*, 1093–1095. [CrossRef]
21. Mitruka, B.M.; Rawnsley, H.M. *Clinical Biomedical and Hematological Reference Values in Normal Experimental Animals and Normal Humans*, 2nd ed.; Masson Publishing USA Inc.: New York, NY, USA, 1981.
22. Caporali, R.; Zavaglia, D. Real-World Experience with Tofacitinib for Treatment of Rheumatoid Arthritis. Available online: https://www.ncbi.nlm.nih.gov/pubmed/30183607 (accessed on 29 August 2018).
23. Lee, M.G.; Chiou, W.L. Evaluation of potential causes for the incomplete bioavailability of furosemide: Gastric first-pass metabolism. *J. Pharmacokinet. Biopharm.* **1983**, *11*, 623–640. [CrossRef]
24. Kim, S.H.; Lee, M.G. Pharmacokinetics of ipriflavone, an isoflavone derivative, after intravenous and oral administration to rats hepatic and intestinal first-pass effects. *Life Sci.* **2002**, *70*, 1299–1315. [CrossRef]
25. Bae, S.K.; Kim, J.W.; Kim, Y.H.; Kim, Y.G.; Kim, S.G.; Lee, M.G. Hepatic and intestinal first-pass effects of oltipraz in rats. *Biopharm. Drug Dispos.* **2005**, *26*, 129–134. [CrossRef] [PubMed]
26. Shin, H.S.; Bae, S.K.; Lee, M.G. Pharmacokinetics of sildenafil after intravenous and oral administration in rats: Hepatic and intestinal first-pass effects. *Int. J. Pharm.* **2006**, *320*, 64–70. [CrossRef] [PubMed]
27. Thummel, K.E.; O'shea, D.; Paine, M.F.; Shen, D.D.; Kunze, K.L.; Perkins, J.D.; Wilkinson, G.R. Oral first-pass elimination of midazolam involves both gastrointestinal and hepatic CYP3A-mediated metabolism. *Clin. Pharmacol. Ther.* **1996**, *59*, 491–502. [CrossRef]
28. Hurst, S.; Loi, C.M.; Brodfuehrer, J.; El-Kattan, A. Impact of physiological, physicochemical and biopharmaceutical factors in absorption and metabolism mechanisms on the drug oral bioavailability of rats and humans. *Expert Opin. Drug Metab. Toxicol.* **2007**, *3*, 469–489. [CrossRef] [PubMed]
29. Lindell, M.; Lang, M.; Lennernas, H. Expression of genes encoding for drug metabolizing cytochrome P450 enzymes and P-glycoprotein the rat small intestine: Comparison to the liver. *Eur. J. Drug Metab. Pharmacokinet.* **2003**, *28*, 41–48. [CrossRef]
30. Lewis, D.F.V. P450 Substrate Specificity and Metabolism. Cytochromes 450. In *Structure, Function and Mechanism*; Taylor & Francis Inc.: Philadelphia, PA, USA, 1996; pp. 102–116.
31. Park, M.Y. Effects of Cytochrome P450 (CYP) Inducers and Inhibitors on Tofacitinib Pharmacokinetics in Rats. Master's Thesis, Ajou University, Suwon, Korea, February 2018.
32. Correia, M.A.; Appendix, B. Rat and human liver cytochromes P450. In *Substrate and Inhibitor Specificities and Functional Markers*, 2nd ed.; Ortiz de Montellano, P.R., Ed.; Plenum Press: New York, NY, USA; London, UK, 1995; pp. 607–630.
33. Ogiso, T.; Iwaki, M.; Tanaka, H.; Kobayashi, E.; Tanino, T.; Sawada, A.; Uno, S. Pharmacokinetic drug interactions between ampiroxicam and sulfaphenazole in rats. *Biol. Pharm. Bull.* **1999**, *22*, 191–196. [CrossRef]
34. De Martin, S.; Gabbia, D.; Albertin, G.; Sfriso, M.M.; Mescoli, C.; Albertoni, L.; Palatini, P. Differential effect of liver cirrhosis on the pregnane X receptor-mediated induction of CYP3A1 and 3A2 in the rat. *Drug Metab. Dispos.* **2014**, *42*, 1617–1626. [CrossRef]
35. Dixit, V.; Moore, A.; Tsao, H.; Hariparsad, N. Application of micropatterned cocultured hepatocytes to evaluate the inductive potential and degradation rate of major xenobiotic metabolizing enzymes. *Drug Metab. Dispos.* **2016**, *44*, 250–261. [CrossRef]
36. Papp, K.A.; Menter, M.A.; Abe, M.; Elewski, B.; Feldman, S.R.; Gottlieb, A.B.; Gupta, P. Tofacitinib, an oral Janus kinase inhibitor, for the treatment of chronic plaque psoriasis: Results from two, randomized, placebo-controlled, Phase 3 trials. *Br. J. Dermatol.* **2015**, *173*, 949–961. [CrossRef]

37. Bachelez, H.; Van de Kerkhof, P.C.; Strohal, R.; Kubanov, A.; Valenzuela, F.; Lee, J.H.; Gupta, P. Tofacitinib versus etanercept or placebo in moderate-to-severe chronic plaque psoriasis: A phase 3 randomized non-inferiority trial. *Lancet* **2015**, *386*, 552–561. [CrossRef]
38. Crispin, M.K.; Ko, J.M.; Craiglow, B.G.; Li, S.; Shankar, G.; Urban, J.R.; Marinkovich, M.P. Safety and efficacy of the JAK inhibitor tofacitinib citrate in patients with alopecia areata. *JCI Insight* **2016**, *1*, e89776.
39. Levy, L.L.; Urban, J.; King, B.A. Treatment of recalcitrant atopic dermatitis with the oral Janus kinase inhibitor tofacitinib citrate. *J. Am. Acad. Dermatol.* **2015**, *73*, 395–399. [CrossRef]
40. Tahir, H. Therapies in ankylosing spondylitis-from clinical trials to clinical practice. *Rheumatology* **2018**, *57* (Suppl. 6), vi23–vi28. [CrossRef]
41. Lawendy, N.; Lamba, M.; Chan, G.; Wang, R.; Alvey, C.W.; Krishnaswami, S. The effect of mild and moderate hepatic impairment on the pharmacokinetics of tofacitinib, an orally active Janus kinase inhibitor. *Clin. Pharmacol. Drug Dev.* **2014**, *3*, 421–427. [CrossRef] [PubMed]
42. Krishnaswami, S.; Chow, V.; Boy, M.; Wang, C.; Chan, G. Pharmacokinetics of tofacitinib, a janus kinase inhibitor, in patients with impaired renal function and end-stage renal disease. *J. Clin. Pharmacol.* **2014**, *54*, 46–52. [CrossRef] [PubMed]
43. Ma, G.; Xie, R.; Strober, B.; Langley, R.; Ito, K.; Krishnaswami, S.; Wolk, R.; Valdez, H.; Rottinghaus, S.; Tallman, A.; et al. Pharmacokinetic characteristics of tofacitinib in adult patients with moderate to severe chronic plaque psoriasis. *Clin. Pharmacol. Drug Dev.* **2018**, *7*, 587–596. [CrossRef] [PubMed]
44. Ma, C.; Battat, R.; Jairath, V.; Vande Casteele, N. Advances in therapeutic drug monitoring for small-molecule and biologic therapies in inflammatory bowel disease. *Curr. Treat. Options Gastroenterol.* **2019**, *17*, 127–145. [CrossRef]
45. Hussa, D.A. 2013 new drug update: What do new approvals hold for the elderly? *Consult. Pharm.* **2014**, *29*, 224–238. [CrossRef]
46. Gupta, P.; Chow, V.; Wang, R.; Kaplan, I.; Chan, G.; Alvey, C.; Ni, G.; Ndongo, M.N.; LaBadie, R.R.; Krishnaswami, S. Evaluation of the effect of fluconazole and ketoconazole on the pharmacokinetics of tofacitinib in healthy adult subjects. *Clin. Pharmacol. Drug Dev.* **2014**, *3*, 72–77. [CrossRef] [PubMed]
47. Cohen, S.; Zwillich, S.H.; Chow, V.; Labadie, R.R.; Wilkinson, B. Co-administration of the JAK inhibitor CP-690,550 and methotrexate is well tolerated in patients with rheumatoid arthritis without need for dose adjustment. *Br. J. Clin. Pharmacol.* **2010**, *69*, 143–151. [CrossRef] [PubMed]
48. Menon, S.; Riese, R.; Wang, R.; Alvey, C.; Shi, H.; Petit, W.; Krishnaswami, S. Evaluation of the effect of tofacitinib on the pharmacokinetics of oral contraceptive steroids in healthy female volunteers. *Clin. Pharmacol. Drug Dev.* **2016**, *5*, 336–342. [CrossRef] [PubMed]

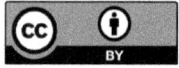

© 2019 by the authors. Licensee MDPI, Basel, Switzerland. This article is an open access article distributed under the terms and conditions of the Creative Commons Attribution (CC BY) license (http://creativecommons.org/licenses/by/4.0/).

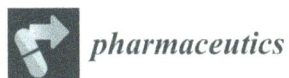

Article

Pharmacokinetics and Intestinal Metabolism of Compound K in Rats and Mice

Ji-Hyeon Jeon [1], Bitna Kang [2], Sowon Lee [1], Sojeong Jin [2], Min-Koo Choi [2,*] and Im-Sook Song [1,*]

1. College of Pharmacy and Research Institute of Pharmaceutical Sciences, Kyungpook National University, Daegu 41566, Korea; kei7016@naver.com (J.-H.J.); okjin917@hanmail.net (S.L.)
2. College of Pharmacy, Dankook University, Cheon-an 31116, Korea; qlcska8520@naver.com (B.K.); astraea327@naver.com (S.J.)
* Correspondence: minkoochoi@dankook.ac.kr (M.-K.C.); isssong@knu.ac.kr (I.-S.S.); Tel.: +82-41-550-1432 (M.-K.C.); +82-53-950-8575 (I.-S.S.)

Received: 10 December 2019; Accepted: 31 January 2020; Published: 3 February 2020

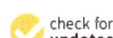

Abstract: We aimed to investigate the plasma concentration, tissue distribution, and elimination of compound K following the intravenous administration of compound K (2 mg/kg) in rats and mice. The plasma concentrations of compound K in mice were much higher (about five-fold) than those in rats. In both rats and mice, compound K was mainly distributed in the liver and underwent biliary excretion. There was 28.4% fecal recovery of compound K in mice and 13.8% in rats, whereas its renal recovery was less than 0.1% in both rats and mice. Relative quantification of compound K and its metabolite protopanaxadiol (PPD) in rat bile and intestinal feces indicated that the metabolism from compound K into PPD occurred in the intestine but not in the plasma. Therefore, PPD detected in the plasma samples could have been absorbed from the intestine after metabolism in control rats, while PPD could not be detected in the plasma samples from bile duct cannulated rats. In conclusion, mice and rats shared common features such as exclusive liver distribution, major excretion pathway via biliary route, and intestinal metabolism to PPD. However, there were significant differences between rats and mice in the plasma concentrations of compound K and the fecal recovery of compound K and PPD.

Keywords: compound K; protopanaxadiol (PPD); pharmacokinetics; biliary excretion; intestinal metabolism

1. Introduction

Compound K, which belongs to the protopanaxadiol (PPD)-type ginsenoside group, was first discovered in 1972 from a hydrolase mixture of ginsenosides (Rb1, Rb2, and Rc) and soil bacteria [1]. Since then, compound K has attracted special attention among the various ginsenosides because it is reported as a major pharmacologically active component that has hepatoprotective, chemo-preventive, anti-diabetic, anti-inflammatory, anti-arthritic, neuroprotective, and immune stimulating effects [1,2]. The therapeutic benefit of compound K has been demonstrated in both in vitro studies and in vivo disease models [1]. Paek et al. [3] investigated the dose-dependent bioavailability of compound K by comparing its oral and intravenous administration in rats. The area under plasma concentration (AUC) of compound K increased linearly following intravenous injection at a dose range of 1–10 mg/kg (dose increase 10-fold; AUC increase 11.6-fold), but the AUC of compound K following oral administration did not increase linearly at a dose range of 5–20 mg/kg (dose increase four-fold; AUC increase 75.8-fold) [3]. The AUC of compound K was significantly increased (23.5-fold) in P-glycoprotein (P-gp) knock-out mice compared to wild-type mice after a single oral dose (10 mg/kg) [4]. Therefore,

P-gp-mediated efflux during intestinal absorption could be a possible explanation for non-linear oral bioavailability of compound K.

The safety, pharmacokinetics, and preliminary efficacy of compound K in tablet form as an anti-rheumatoid arthritis drug are under clinical investigation in China (Study No. NCT03755258) [5]. In this study, Chen et al. [5] investigated the pharmacokinetics of compound K and PPD, a metabolite of compound K, following a single oral administration of a 200 mg compound K tablet. This was the first pharmacokinetic study in humans using pure compound K. The maximum plasma concentration (C_{max}) of compound K was 796.8 ng/mL with a time to reach C_{max} (T_{max}) of 3.6 h. On the other hand, the C_{max} of PPD was 5.7 ng/mL with a T_{max} of 24.5 h. The results suggested that the formation of PPD from compound K occurred slowly. The AUC ratio of PPD to compound K was calculated as 0.04 [5]. They also investigated the effect of high-fat meal on the pharmacokinetics of compound K. The high-fat meal consumption increased C_{max} (2.0-fold) and AUC (2.2-fold) of compound K but decreased T_{max} (3.6 h in fasting group vs. 2.5 h in high-fat meal group, $p < 0.05$) compared with fasting group, suggesting that the high-fat meal accelerated the absorption of compound K [5].

Other pharmacokinetic studies of compound K have been reported in human subjects following oral administration of ginseng product [2,6–9]. The C_{max} of compound K was 41.5 ng/mL in 12 Japanese subjects following a single oral administration of fermented ginseng tablet (274.4 mg total; 2.2 mg as compound K) [6]. The mean C_{max} (254.5 ng/mL) was substantially higher and less variable in subjects who were orally administered fermented Korean red ginseng (3 g total; 10.9 mg as compound K) than the C_{max} (3.2–24.8 ng/mL) in subjects who received non-fermented Korean red ginseng extract (3 g total; 0 mg as compound K) [2,7,9]. The results suggested that the consumption of ginseng product with higher compound K content resulted in higher plasma concentrations of compound K. The compound K in the plasma was absorbed after the metabolism from Rb1, Rb2, Rc, and Rd (major components of red ginseng product) to compound K following oral administration of non-fermented red ginseng product [7,10]. Therefore, the variability in the gut metabolism and intestinal absorption of compound K could be attributed to the variable plasma concentrations of compound K. However, little information is available on the distribution and elimination of compound K. Therefore, the purpose of this study was to investigate the pharmacokinetics of compound K in rats and mice with a focus on tissue distribution, elimination, and metabolism to PPD.

2. Materials and Methods

2.1. Materials

Compound K and 20(S)-protopanaxadiol (PPD) was purchased from the Ambo Institute (Daejeon, Korea). To be used as internal standards (IS), 13C-caffeine was purchased from Sigma-Aldrich Chemical Co. (St. Louis, MO, USA). All other chemicals and solvents were of reagent or analytical grade.

2.2. Animals and Ethical Approval

Male Institute of Cancer Research (ICR) mice (7 or 8-weeks-old, weighing 34–37 g) and male Sprague-Dawley (SD) rats (7 or 8-weeks-old, 230–270 g) were purchased from Samtako Co. (Osan, Korea). The animals were acclimatized for 1 week at an animal facility at Kyungpook National University. Food and water were available ad libitum. All animal procedures were approved by the Animal Care and Use Committee of Kyungpook National University (Approval No. KNU 2018-192, 19 December 2018) and carried out in accordance with the National Institutes of Health guidance for the care and use of laboratory animals. An overview of the study design and methods is provided in Table 1.

Table 1. Overview of the study design and methods.

Study Name	SD Rats	ICR Mice	Remarks
Pharmacokinetics of compound K ($n = 4$)	• Compound K IV 2 mg/kg • Blood sampling: 0.17–48 h • Feces collection for 48 h • Urine collection for 48 h	• Compound K IV 2 mg/kg • Blood sampling: 0.17–48 h • Feces collection for 48 h • Urine collection for 48 h	• Comparison between rats and mice • PK parameters of compound K • Fecal and urine recovery of compound K and PPD
Tissue distribution of compound K ($n = 4$)	• Compound K IV 2 mg/kg • Blood and tissue collection: 0.17–24 h • Liver, kidney, brain, heart, lung, spleen, testis	• Compound K IV 2 mg/kg • Blood and tissue collection: 0.17–24 h • Liver, kidney, brain, heart, lung, spleen, testis	• Comparison between rats and mice • Tissue to plasma AUC ratios of compound K
Inhibition of hepatic uptake of compound K ($n = 3$)	• Compound K IV 2 mg/kg • Rifampin pretreatment PO 20 mg/kg • Blood and liver collection at 0.5 and 2 h	• Compound K IV 2 mg/kg • Rifampin pretreatment PO 20 mg/kg • Blood and liver collection at 0.5 and 2 h	• Comparison between groups with/without rifampin pretreatment • Tissue to plasma concentration ratios of compound K
Biliary excretion of compound K ($n = 4$)	• Compound K IV 2 mg/kg • Blood sampling: 0.25–8 h • Bile collection: for 12 h		• PK parameters of compound K • Biliary excretion of compound K
Metabolism of compound K ($n = 4$)	• Compound K IV 2 mg/kg • Bile collection for 0-2 h and 2–12 h • Intestinal feces collection at 2 and 12 h		• PPD quantification in plasma, bile, and intestinal feces samples

IV, intravenous injection; PO, per oral administration, PPD, 20(S)-protopanaxadiol; PK parameters, pharmacokinetic parameters; AUC, area under plasma concentration.

2.3. Pharmacokinetic Study

ICR mice and SD rats received compound K intravenously at a single dose of 2 mg/kg via the tail vein and were returned to the metabolic cage with water and chow ad libitum. Before administration, the compound K was dissolved in a vehicle containing DMSO: saline (2:8, v/v) (vehicle volume, 1 mL/kg for mice and 0.4 mL/kg for rats). Blood samples (approximately 100 µL) were collected at 0, 0.17, 0.5, 1, 2, 4, 8, 24, and 48 h following intravenous injection of compound K with no sign of hemoglobinemia and hemoglobinuria. Blood sampling was performed using a sparse sampling method (time schedule is given in Table 2). The blood samples were centrifuged at $16,000 \times g$ for 10 min to separate the plasma. An aliquot (50 µL) of each plasma sample was stored at −80 °C until the analysis. Urine and feces samples were collected from 0–24 h and 24–48 h following the compound K administration. Aliquots (50 µL) of urine and 10% feces homogenates were stored at −80 °C until the analysis.

SD rats were randomly divided into two groups: the non-bile cannulated control group and the bile cannulated group. For the bile cannulated rats, the femoral artery, femoral vein, and bile duct were cannulated with polyethylene tubes (PE-50 and PE-10; Jungdo, Seoul, Korea) under light anesthesia with isoflurane. For the control group, the femoral artery and femoral vein were cannulated with PE-50. Compound K was injected intravenously via the femoral vein at 2 mg/kg. Blood samples (approximately 200 µL) were collected from the femoral artery at 0, 0.25, 0.5, 1, 2, 4, and 8 h after the compound K injection. After each blood sampling, normal saline was injected into the femoral vein to compensate for blood loss. Bile samples were collected every 2 h for a total of 12 h. The blood samples were centrifuged at $16,000 \times g$ for 10 min, and 50 µL aliquots of plasma and 50 µL aliquots of bile were stored at −80 °C until the compound K analysis. In the non-bile cannulated rats, the complete contents of the entire gastrointestinal tract were collected using a 10 mL syringe filled with 30 mL pre-warmed saline. The contents were homogenized with tissue homogenizer, and 50 µL aliquots of intestinal fecal homogenates were stored at −80 °C until the analysis.

The 50 µL samples of plasma, urine, 10% fecal homogenates, bile, and intestinal fecal homogenates were each mixed with 60 µL of IS (20 ng/mL 13C-caffeine in water) and 600 µL of methyl *tert*-butyl ether (MTBE). The mixtures were vortexed vigorously for 10 min and centrifuged at 16,000× *g* for 5 min. After centrifugation, the samples were frozen at −80 °C for 2 h. For each sample, the upper layer was transferred to a clean tube and evaporated to dryness under a nitrogen stream. The residue was reconfigured with 200 µL of 80% methanol consisting of 0.1% formic acid, and a 10 µL aliquot was injected into the liquid chromatography–tandem mass spectrometry (LC–MS/MS) system.

Table 2. Blood sampling schedule for the pharmacokinetic study of compound K in mice and rats following intravenous injection of compound K.

Sampling Time (h)	Group 1 (n = 4)	Group 2 (n = 4)	Group 3 (n = 4)	Sampling Method	Anesthesia
0	O			RO-right [1]	O
0.17		O		RO-right	O
0.5			O	RO-right	O
1	O			RO-left [2]	O
2		O		RO-left	O
4			O	RO-left	O
8	O			AA [3]	O
24		O		AA	O
48			O	AA	O

[1] RO-right: retro-orbital blood sampling—right eye under anesthesia with isoflurane; [2] RO-left: retro-orbital blood sampling—left eye under anesthesia with isoflurane; [3] AA: abdominal artery blood sampling.

2.4. Tissue Distribution Study

ICR mice and SD rats received compound K intravenously at a single dose of 2 mg/kg via tail vein and were returned to the metabolic cage with water and chow ad libitum. The animals were euthanized and blood samples (approximately 200 µL) were collected from the abdominal artery at 0.17, 0.5, 2, 4, 8, and 24 h after intravenous injection. The liver, kidney, brain, heart, lung, spleen, and testis were immediately excised, gently washed with ice-cold saline, and weighed. The tissue samples were homogenized with 4 volumes of saline. Aliquots (50 µL) of plasma and 20% tissue homogenates were stored at −80 °C until the analysis of compound K.

To investigate the effect of rifampin (a representative inhibitor of the organic anion-transporting polypeptide (Oatp) transporters [11]) on the hepatic distribution of compound K, ICR mice and SD rats were randomly divided into either control or rifampin groups. The rifampin group was orally administered with rifampin solution (20 mg/kg, dissolved in DMSO: saline = 2:8, *v/v*) and the control group received only the vehicle via oral gavage. One hour after rifampin treatment, mice and rats received compound K intravenously at a single dose of 2 mg/kg via tail vein. The animals were euthanized and blood samples (approximately 200 µL) were collected from the abdominal artery at 0.5 and 2 h after intravenous injection. The liver tissues were immediately excised, gently washed with ice-cold saline, and homogenized with 4 volumes of saline. Aliquots (50 µL) of plasma and 20% liver homogenates were stored at −80 °C until the analysis of compound K.

The plasma samples and 20% tissue homogenates samples were each mixed with 60 µL of IS (20 ng/mL 13C-caffeine in water) and 600 µL of MTBE. The mixtures were vortexed vigorously for 10 min and centrifuged at 16,000× *g* for 5 min. After centrifugation, the samples were frozen at −80 °C for 2 h. The upper layer was transferred to a clean tube and evaporated to dryness under a nitrogen stream. The residue was reconfigured with 200 µL of 80% methanol consisting of 0.1% formic acid, and a 10 µL aliquot was injected into the LC-MS/MS system.

2.5. LC-MS/MS Analysis of Compound K

Compound K and PPD concentrations were analyzed using a modified LC-MS/MS method of Jin et al. [8] with an Agilent 6430 triple quadrupole LC-MS/MS system (Agilent, Wilmington, DE, USA). Compound K and PPD were separated using an Eclipse Plus C18 RRHD (1.8 μm particle size, 3.0 × 5.0 mm, Agilent, Wilmington, DE, USA). The mobile phase consisted of 0.1% formic acid in water (8%) and 0.1% formic acid in methanol (92%) at a flow rate of 0.15 mL/min.

Quantification of a separated analyte peak was performed at m/z 645.5 → 203.1 for compound K (T_R (retention time) 6.9 min), m/z 425.3 → 109.1 for PPD (T_R 13.9 min), and m/z 198.2 → 140.1 for 13C-caffeine (IS) (T_R 2.9 min) in the positive ionization mode with collision energy (CE) of 35, 25 and 20 eV, respectively. The analytical data were quantified using Mass Hunter (version B.06.00, Agilent, Wilmington, DE, USA).

The calibration standards and quality control (QC) samples were prepared by spiking a 5 μL aliquot of the working solution with 45 μL aliquot of blank matrix (plasma, liver, kidney, heart, lung, pancreas, brain, testis, and urine). The final concentrations of the compound K and PPD calibration standards for plasma and urine samples were 5, 10, 20, 50, 200, 500, 2000 ng/mL, and the concentrations of QC samples of compound K and PPD were 15, 100, and 1500 ng/mL. The concentrations of calibration standards and QC samples of compound K and PPD for bile and fecal homogenates were 25, 50, 100, 250, 1000, 2500, and 10,000 ng/mL and 75, 500, and 7500 ng/mL, respectively. The concentrations of calibration standards and QC samples of compound K for liver, kidney, heart, lung, pancreas, brain, and testis homogenates were 5, 10, 20, 50, 200, 500, and 2000 ng/mL and 15, 100, and 1500 ng/mL, respectively. The standard calibration curves for compound K and PPD was linear in the concentration range of 5–2000 ng/mL in the plasma, urine, and tissue homogenates samples and in the concentration range of 25–10,000 ng/mL in the bile and feces homogenates samples, respectively. The inter-day and intra-day precision and accuracy (%CV) for compound K and PPD in all biological samples was less than 15%.

2.6. Data Analysis

Pharmacokinetic parameters were estimated using non-compartmental methods (WinNonlin version 2.0, Pharsight Co., Certara, NJ, USA).

All pharmacokinetic parameters are given as the mean ± standard deviation. All statistical analyses were performed using SAS (ver. 9.4; SAS Institute Inc., Cary, NC, USA). A *p*-value < 0.05 was considered statistically significant.

3. Results

3.1. Comparative Pharmacokinetics of Compound K in Rats and Mice

The plasma concentration-time profile of compound K was compared between the mice and the rats. Since the intestinal absorption of compound K is low and variable [3,4], intravenous injection of compound K was used in this study intead of oral administration. The plasma concentrations of compound K in mice were greater than those in rats (Figure 1). The pharmacokinetic parameters of compound K such as AUC and plasma concentration were about 5–6-fold greater in mice than in rats, while there was no significant difference in the half-life ($T_{1/2}$) and mean residence time (MRT) between rats and mice (Table 3). However, the clearance (CL) and volume of distribution (Vd) values were about five-fold larger in rats than in mice (Table 3). Taken together, the results suggest that the distribution and elimination of compound K differ between rats and mice.

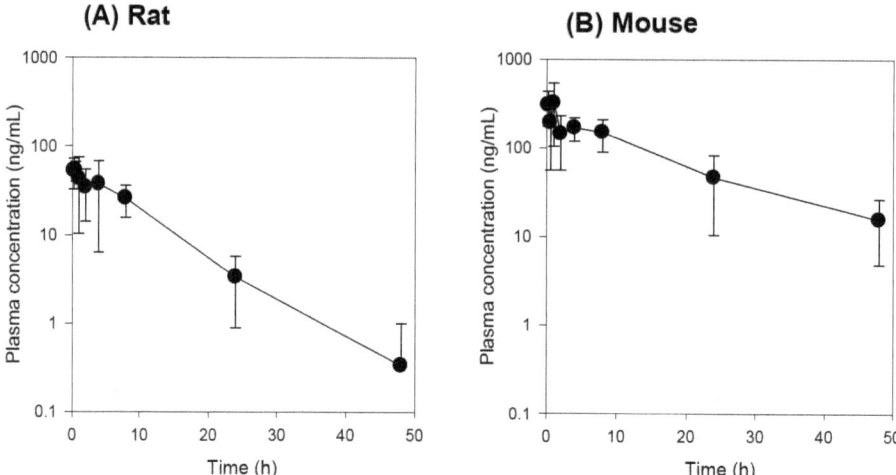

Figure 1. (**A**) Plasma concentration vs. time profile of compound K following intravenous injection of compound K at a single dose of 2 mg/kg in rats (**A**) and mice (**B**). Plasma concentration of compound K (Y-axis) was represented using a logarithmic scale. Data expressed as mean± standard deviation from four rats or four mice at different time points.

Table 3. Pharmacokinetic parameters of compound K in rat and mouse.

Characteristics	Parameters	Rat	Mouse
Plasma	C_0 (ng/mL)	75.3 ± 23.3	400 ± 137 *
	$AUC_{48\,h}$ (ng·h/mL)	638.8 ± 298.6	3756.3 ± 1636 *
	AUC_∞ (ng·h/mL)	670.1 ± 284.1	4025.1 ± 1836 *
	$T_{1/2}$ (h)	7.3 ± 0.4	11.4 ± 1.5
	MRT (h)	8.9 ± 0.4	11.8 ± 2.0
	CL (mL/min/kg)	59.0 ± 21.8	10.4 ± 4.9 *
	Vd (L/kg)	31.8 ± 3.1	7.08 ± 2.6 *
Excretion	$Feces_{48\,h}$ (% of dose)	13.8 ± 7.1	28.4 ± 5.9 *
	$Urine_{48\,h}$ (% of dose)	0.01 ± 0.01	0.02 ± 0.01

$AUC_{48\,h}$ or AUC_∞: area under the plasma concentration-time curve from 0 to 48 h or to infinity; C_0: initial plasma concentration; $T_{1/2}$: half-life; MRT: mean residence time; CL: clearance; Vd: Volume of distribution. Data expressed as mean ± standard deviation ($n = 4$). *: $p < 0.05$ compared with the rat group.

To compare the elimination pathway of compound K, we measured the renal and fecal recovery of compound K following intravenous administration of compound K in both rats and mice. The recovery of compound K from the urine was about 0.02% of the intravenous dose in both mice and rats. In contrast, the fecal recovery of compound K was about 28.4 ± 5.9% in mice and 13.8 ± 7.1% in rats (Table 1). The results suggest that fecal excretion is a major excretion route for compound K in both rats and mice but also that compound K may undergo in vivo metabolism in both rats and mice.

3.2. Tissue Distribution of Compound K

To analyze the tissue distribution of compound K, we measured the temporal profile of compound K in various tissues in rats and mice following intravenous administration of compound K. As shown in Figures 2 and 3, the tissue distribution pattern of compound K was comparable in both mice and rats. Compound K was predominantly distributed to the liver in both rats and mice, and the liver to plasma AUC ratio was 11.1 in rats and 16.7 in mice. The AUC ratios of other tissues (i.e., kidney, heart, lung, pancreas, testis, and brain) to plasma, however, were much lower than the liver/plasma AUC ratio for both species (Figures 2B and 3B). These results suggest the involvement of the uptake transport system, which is dominantly expressed in the liver. Previously, Jiang et al. [12] reported the involvement of the Oatp transporters (OATP1B3 in humans and Oatp1b2 in rats) in the hepatic uptake of ginsenosides Rg1, Re, and R1. Therefore, we investigated the effect of rifampin, a representative inhibitor of the Oatp transporter [11], on the liver distribution of compound K to further assess the involvement of the Oatp uptake transporter.

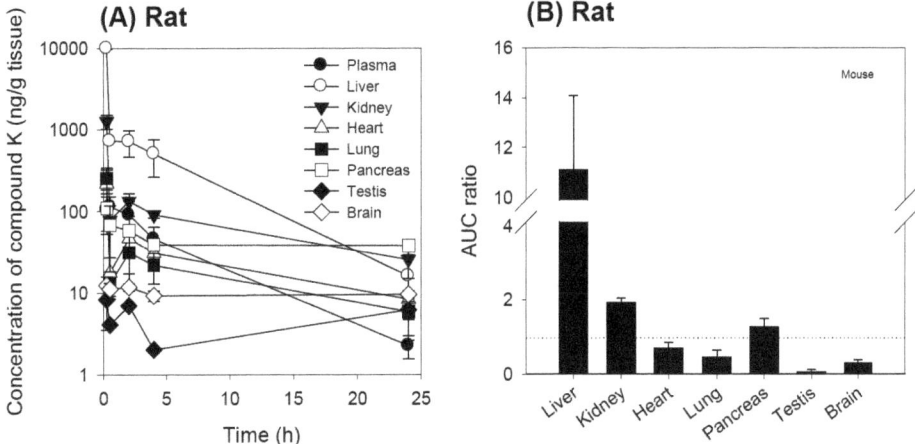

Figure 2. (**A**) Tissue concentration vs. time profile of compound K following intravenous injection of compound K at a single dose of 2 mg/kg in rats. (**B**) AUC ratios ($AUC_{tissue}/AUC_{plasma}$) of compound K in the liver, kidney, heart, lung, pancreas, testis, and brain following intravenous injection (2 mg/kg) in rats. AUC was calculated from the data shown in (**A**) and the dotted line in (**B**) represents unity. Data are expressed as mean± standard deviation from four rats at different time points.

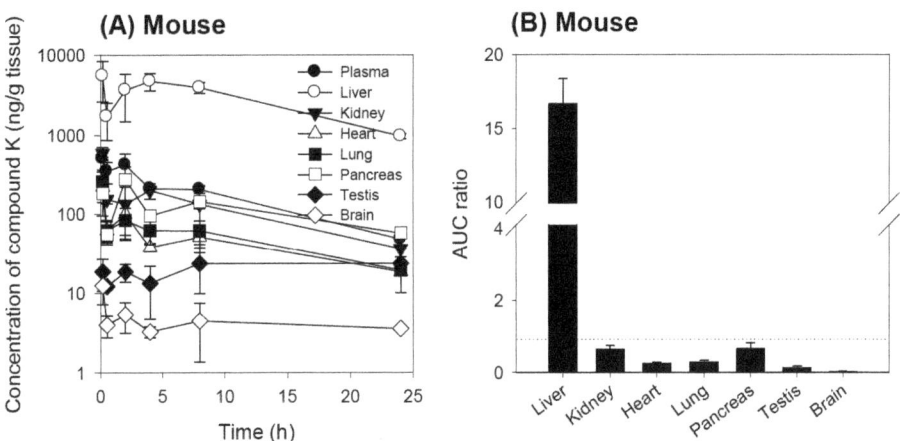

Figure 3. (**A**) Tissue concentration vs. time profile of compound K following intravenous injection of compound K at a single dose of 2 mg/kg in mice. (**B**) AUC ratios of compound K in the liver, kidney, heart, lung, pancreas, testis, and brain to plasma following intravenous injection (2 mg/kg) in mice. AUC was calculated from the data shown in (**A**) and the dotted line in (**B**) represents unity. Data are expressed as mean ± standard deviation from four rats at different time points.

When rifampin was given orally at 1 h prior to compound K injection, the plasma concentration of compound K increased and the liver to plasma concentration ratios decreased when compared to the control group (no rifampin pre-treatment) in both mice and rats (Figure 4). This can be explained by the blocking of Oatp-mediated hepatic uptake of compound K by the rifampin pre-treatment.

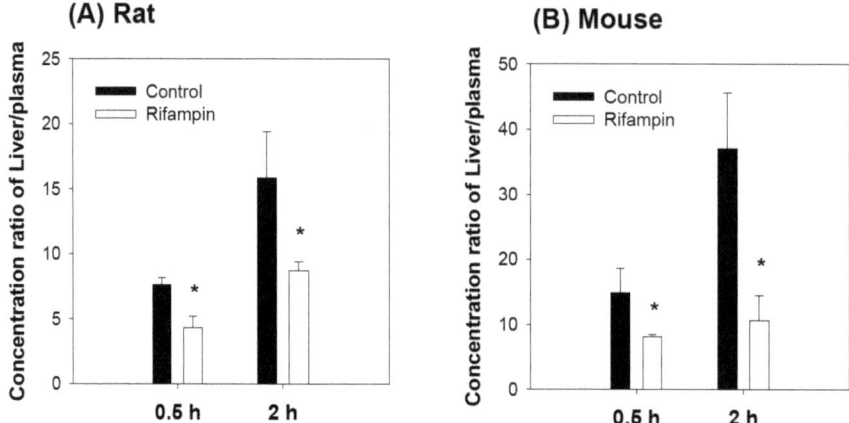

Figure 4. Effect of rifampin pre-treatment on the liver to plasma concentration ratios of compound K in (**A**) rats and (**B**) mice. Liver and plasma compound K concentration were measured following intravenous injection of compound K at a single dose of 2 mg/kg in the presence or absence of rifampin pre-treatment (20 mg/kg, per oral). Data expressed as mean ± standard deviation from four rats or four mice at different time points. *: $p < 0.05$ compared with control group.

3.3. Intestinal Metabolism of Compound K

To understand the metabolism of compound K, we measured PPD levels in the plasma, urine, and feces samples from rats and mice. Previous studies have demonstrated that compound K is metabolized to PPD via β-glucosidase in intestinal microbacterium (Figure 5) [1,13]. As shown in Figure 6, PPD was detected in the plasma and fecal samples from both mice and rats following intravenous injection of compound K (2 mg/kg). However, PPD was not detected in the rat and mouse urine samples. These results suggest that compound K was metabolized to PPD in both rats and mice.

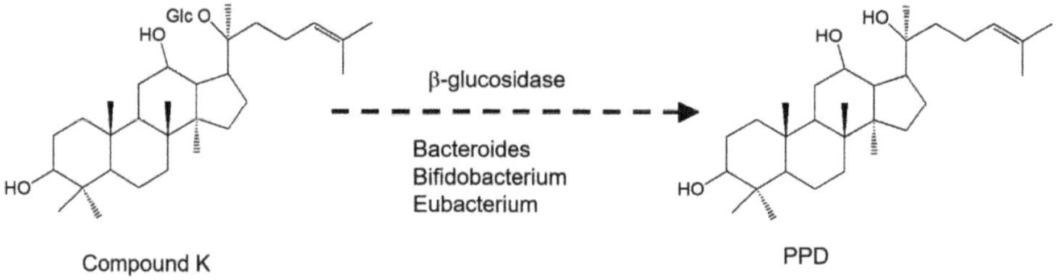

Figure 5. Structure and reported metabolic pathway of compound K to PPD. Glc: glucose; PPD: 20(S)-protopanaxadiol.

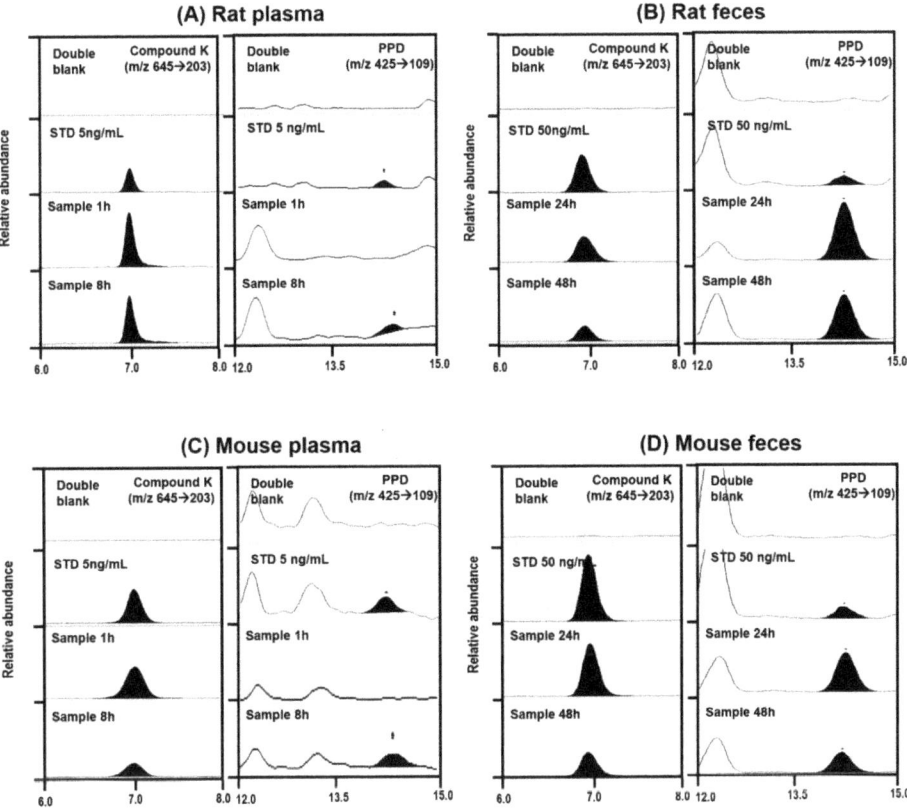

Figure 6. Representative multiple reaction monitoring chromatogram of compound K and PPD in plasma and feces samples collected from rats (**A,B**) and mice (**C,D**) following intravenous injection of compound K at a dose of 2 mg/kg.

The concentrations of compound K and PPD in plasma and feces samples are shown in Figure 7. Following intravenous injection of compound K, the PPD peak was detected in the mouse plasma samples between 4 and 24 h and in the rat plasma samples between 8 and 24 h (Figure 7A,B), suggesting that the metabolism of compound K to PPD might be a slow process. The PPD concentration in the plasma samples at 48 h was below the lower limit of quantification (LLOQ; 5 ng/mL). The metabolic ratio calculated from the PPD to compound K ratio was much greater in rat plasma than in mouse plasma (0.02–0.08 in mouse vs. 0.2–1.6 in rat; Figure 7A,B). Similarly, the ratio of PPD to compound K in the feces samples was also significantly greater in rats than in mice (Figure 7C,D). The recovery of PPD was 3.4-fold higher than that of compound K in rat feces, whereas the recovery of PPD was 1.2-fold higher than that of compound K in mouse feces. As shown in Table 4, compound K and its metabolite PPD were exclusively recovered from feces but not from urine. The higher percentage of PPD recovery in rats compared to mice suggest the higher metabolism of compound K to PPD in rats compared to mice (Figure 1 and Table 3).

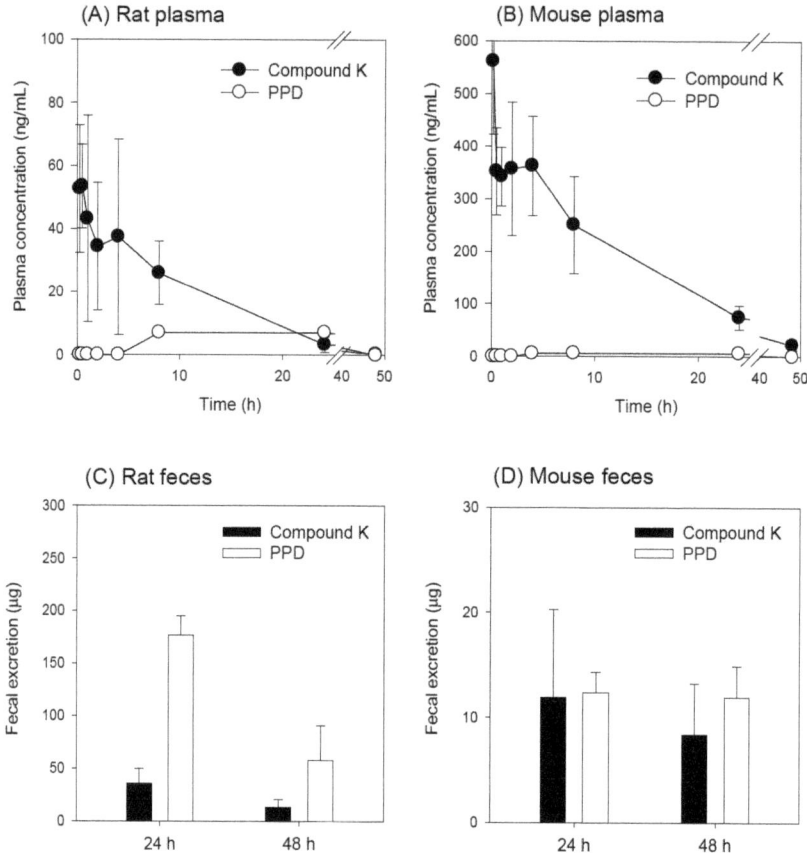

Figure 7. Plasma concentration vs. time profile of compound K and PPD (a metabolite of compound K) following intravenous injection of compound K at a single dose of 2 mg/kg in (**A**) rats and (**B**) mice. Fecal excretion of compound K and PPD following intravenous injection of compound K at a single dose of 2 mg/kg in (**C**) rats and (**D**) mice. Data expressed as mean± standard deviation of four samples for each time point.

Table 4. Recovery of compound K and PPD from urine and feces over the 48 h period following intravenous injection of compound K at a single dose of 2 mg/kg.

Species	Compounds	Recovery$_{48\,h}$ (% of Dose)	
		Feces	Urine
Rat	Compound K	13.8 ± 7.1	0.05 ± 0.03
	PPD	46.6 ± 4.9	ND
Mouse	Compound K	28.4 ± 5.9	0.02 ± 0.01
	PPD	34.4 ± 5.8	ND

ND: Not detected. Data expressed as mean ± standard deviation from four rats and mice per group.

Next, we compared the pharmacokinetic features of compound K between the bile-cannulated rats and the non-bile-cannulated rats. In the bile-cannulated rats, biliary excretion of compound K was very fast and most of the excreted compound K was collected during the 0–2 h period (Figure 8B), which could be due to high and fast distribution of compound K to the liver (Figure 2). Because of the fast distribution to the liver and biliary excretion, the plasma concentration of compound K disappeared rapidly and was best fitted to the one-compartment model. The elimination constant was estimated using 5 points and yielded 0.90 h^{-1} with an r^2 value of 0.92 (Figure 8A). The $T_{1/2}$ was calculated as 0.78 ± 0.11 h in the bile-cannulated rats. In contrast, the AUC value for compound K in the non-bile-cannulated rats was significantly greater than that of the non-bile cannulated control rats (Table 5). The plasma concentration profile of compound K in the control group showed 2-exponential decay. The elimination constant was estimated using 3 points and yielded 0.29 h^{-1} with r^2 value of 0.94 (Figure 9A). As results, $T_{1/2}$ was calculated as 2.40 ± 0.61 h in the non-bile cannulated rats, which is significantly greater than that in bile cannulated rats. The results suggest that the compound K enters into the systemic circulation from other compartments.

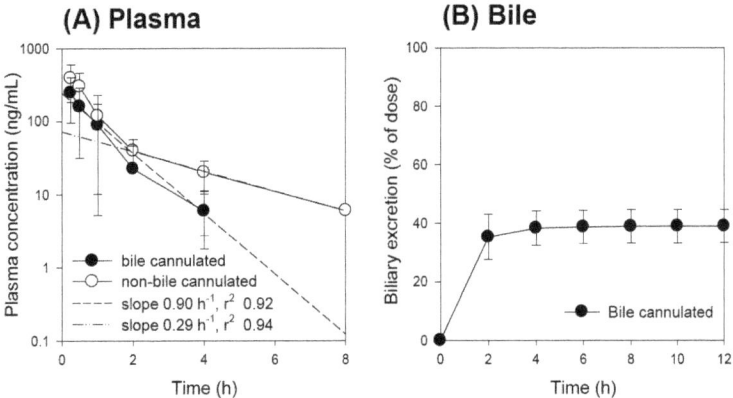

Figure 8. (**A**) Plasma concentration and (**B**) biliary excretion of compound K following intravenous injection at a single dose of 2 mg/kg in the bile-cannulated rats (●) and in the non-bile-cannulated rats (○). Dotted lines represent the regression line of the elimination constant from the plasma concentrations of compound K. Data expressed as mean ± standard deviation from four rats per group.

Table 5. Pharmacokinetic parameters of compound K in rats of bile cannulation and non-bile cannulation.

Characteristics	Parameters	Non-Bile Cannulated Rat	Bile Cannulated Rat
Plasma	C_0 (ng/mL)	451.13 ± 192.5	436.25 ± 325.8
	AUC_{12h} (ng·h/mL)	496.38 ± 253.1	211.09 ± 87.32 *
	AUC_∞ (ng·h/mL)	517.19 ± 248.6	234.78 ± 125.6 *
	$T_{1/2}$ (h)	2.40 ± 0.61	0.78 ± 0.11 *
Excretion	$Bile_{12h}$ (% of dose)	-	39.1 ± 5.7

C_0: initial plasma concentration; AUC_{12h} or AUC_∞: area under the plasma concentration-time curve from 0 to last sampling time or infinity; $T_{1/2}$: half-life. Data expressed as mean ± standard deviation from four rats. *: $p < 0.05$ compared with non-bile cannulated rat group.

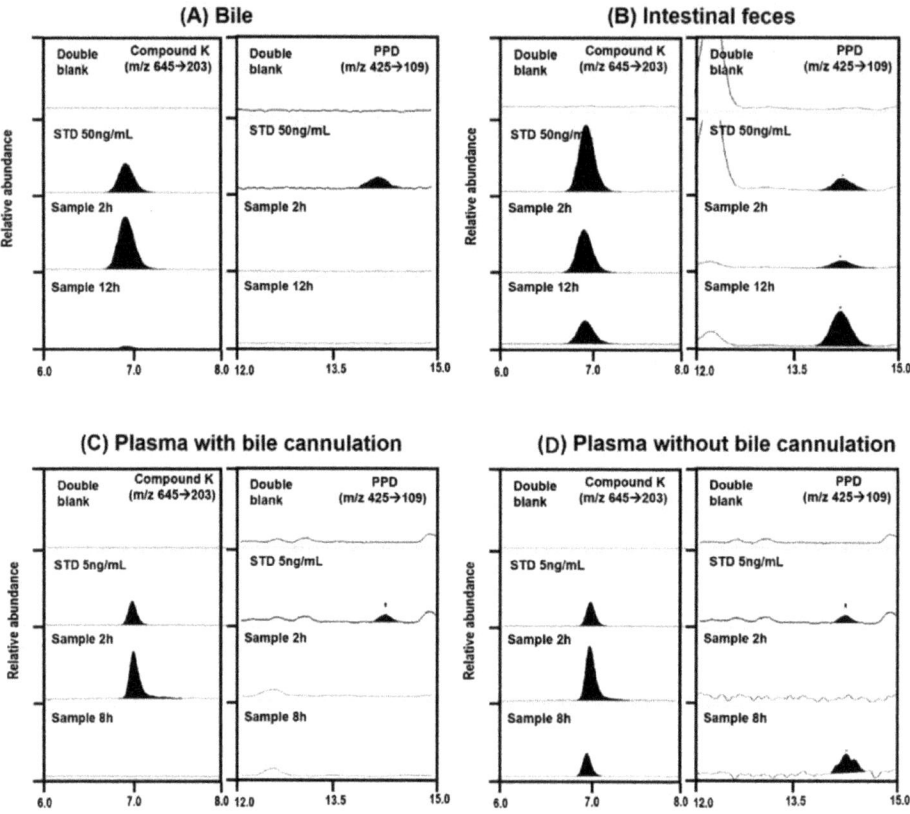

Figure 9. Representative multiple reaction monitoring chromatogram of compound K and PPD in (**A**) bile collected for 0–2 h and 2–12 h from bile cannulated rats, (**B**) intestinal feces samples collected from rats of non-bile cannulation at 2 or 12 h, (**C**) plasma samples taken at 2 and 8 h from bile cannulated rats, and (**D**) plasma samples taken at 2 and 8 h from rats of non-bile cannulation following intravenous injection of compound K (2 mg/kg).

We compared the compound K and PPD levels in the plasma and bile or intestinal feces samples in the bile duct cannulated rats and the control rats (without bile duct cannulation) to determine whether biotransformation from compound K to PPD occurred in the intestine or the plasma. For this, bile samples were collected for 0–2 h and 2–12 h period after administration of compound K from the rats with bile duct cannulation. Since these bile samples were collected directly from the bile duct, the compound K in the sample was distributed to the liver and excreted through the biliary route and, therefore, did not reach the intestinal microbiota. In control group, however, the compound K in the bile sample was excreted via the bile duct, so it reached the intestine and was subjected to further metabolism to PPD. As shown in Figure 8, all of the bile samples collected over a 12 h period from the bile-cannulated rats contained only compound K without PPD (Figure 9A), suggesting no further metabolism of compound K to PPD occurred in the rat plasma, liver, and bile. However, the intestinal fecal samples collected from rats without bile cannulation at 2 and 12 h following intravenous injection of compound K showed peaks for both compound K and PPD, and the amount of PPD was greater in the 12 h samples compared to the 2 h samples (Figure 9B). In addition, PPD was detected in the plasma samples at 8 h in the control rats (Figure 9D), suggesting that the PPD detected in the 8 h sample (which was not present in the 2 h plasma sample) was absorbed from the intestine after metabolism of compound K occurred. These results were consistent with the results from Figure 7A. Contrary to the control group, PPD was not detected in any of the plasma samples collected from bile-cannulated rats (Figure 9C). Taken together, the results suggest slow biotransformation of compound K to PPD in the rat intestine followed by the reabsorption of PPD into the systemic circulation.

4. Discussion

Although much is known about the pharmacological effects of compound K from in vitro studies and in vivo disease models, research on the pharmacokinetics as well as the relationship between the pharmacokinetics and drug response of compound K has been limited. This study aimed to understand the pharmacokinetic features of compound K and to compare its pharmacokinetic behavior in rats and mice, which are often used for disease models. Our study found that biliary excretion of compound K is a major elimination pathway, and fast and extensive liver distribution of compound K was demonstrated in both rats and mice. Oatp transporter-mediated hepatic uptake could be a possible mechanism for the dominant liver distribution compared to other tissues such as kidney, brain, spleen, and testis in both species (Figures 2 and 3), as the hepatic uptake of compound K was significantly inhibited by the pretreatment of rifampin, an Oatp inhibitor (Figure 4). Our results indicate that biotransformation of compound K to PPD occurs in the intestine rather than in the plasma or the liver, based on the comparison between the non-bile-cannulated rats and the bile-cannulated rats (Figure 9). The plasma PPD in rats and mice was then be reabsorbed from the intestine after the metabolism of the excreted compound K (Figures 1 and 9). In addition, the higher plasma AUC and $T_{1/2}$ of compound K in the non-bile cannulated rats compared with those in bile cannulated rats (Table 5) suggests that the excreted compound K was reabsorbed from the intestinal lumen. The $T_{1/2}$ of compound K in non-bile cannulated rats was significantly greater (2.40 ± 0.61 h) than in the bile-cannulated rats (0.78 ± 0.11 h). In addition, the $T_{1/2}$ of compound K in the control rats calculated from the plasma concentration profiles for 48 h was 7.3 ± 0.4 h (Table 3), which is much longer than the $T_{1/2}$ calculated from the plasma concentration profiles for 12 h. Also, the compound K plasma concentrations in the bile-cannulated rats could be fitted to a 1-compartment model while the plasma concentrations in the non-bile cannulated control rats showed 2-exponential decay (Figure 8A). Moreover, the compound K plasma concentrations increased or maintained at 2–4 h after sharply decreasing in the 0–2 h period, and then showed a slow decrease over the 4–48 h time period in both rats and mice (Figure 7A,B). This pattern could be attributable to the continuous reabsorption of compound K. The lipophilicity (LogP value 3.85 for compound K; 5.53 for PPD) and moderate permeability (0.5–2 × 10^{-6} cm/s for compound K; 1.15 × 10^{-6} cm/s for PPD) of compound K and PPD in Caco-2 cells also support the possibility of compound K and PPD reabsorption [3,7,14,15].

The features that differed most significantly between the rats and the mice were the higher plasma concentration (C_0 and AUC) of compound K in mice and the greater fecal recovery of PPD in rats. The percent recovery of the parent form (compound K) in mouse feces was much higher than in rat feces (13.8% in rats vs. 28.4% in mice), while the total fecal recovery (sum of compound K and PPD) was similar for both mice and rats (60.4% in rats vs. 62.8% in mice), suggesting that the elimination process of compound K could differ between rats and mice in addition to the difference in Vd between rats and mice. Multiple previous studies have shown that the tri- or four-glycosylated PPD-type ginsenosides (major components in red ginseng; Rb1, Rb2, Rc, and Rd) have been metabolized to compound K (monoglycosylated PPD-type ginsenoside) and further hydrolyzed to PPD, the final metabolite of the PPD-type ginsenosides, in the presence of lactic acid bacteria and gut microbiota [13,16]. Previous studies have reported that Bacteroides sp., Eubacterium sp., and Bifidobacterium sp. could potentially be involved in compound K metabolism and that subjects who have a higher composition of Bacteroides sp., Eubacterium sp., and Bifidobacterium sp. strains showed higher metabolism of Rb1 to compound K [1,10]. Similarly, differences in the composition of the intestinal microbiota in rats and mice could lead to the different rates of metabolism of compound K to PPD. Wang et al. identified the predominant bacterium in human and animal fecal samples [17]. In human fecal samples, 55% of colonies were identified as Bacteroides sp. but Eubacterium sp. and Bifidobacterium sp. were also present in smaller proportions. In mice and rat fecal samples, Bacteroides sp. showed relatively low expression compared to the human samples. Eubacterium sp. and Bifidobacterium sp. also showed lower expression than other species (Clostridium, Fusobacterium, and Peptosreptococcus sp.). The data suggests that there are species-dependent factors that play a role in the gut metabolism of ginsenosides in mice, rats, and humans. Kim et al. [10] reported that human subjects who have a higher proportion Bacteroides sp. in their fecal microbiota showed 6-fold higher metabolic activity of compound K than the subject group that had a smaller proportion of Bacteroides sp. Choi et al. [7] reported that inter-subject variability in gut metabolism of compound K rather than the intestinal absorption of compound K may contribute to the large inter-individual variations in plasma compound K concentrations. Therefore, differences in the gut metabolism of compound K could also explain the variability of the compound K pharmacokinetics between species. In addition, cytochrome P450 3A-mediated metabolism of PPD has been reported in human plasma and urine samples. Multiple oxidized PPD metabolites were identified from human plasma and urine samples, and cytochrome P450 3A is thought to be involved in this process [18,19]. This metabolism of PPD in the liver microsomes could explain the unrecovered portion of compound K and PPD at 48 h following intravenous administration of compound K in this study.

Collectively, the proposed enterohepatic circulation of compound K and PPD (Figure 10) could explain how compound K shows efficacy in vivo despite its fast and exclusive biliary excretion. The distribution of compound K into the liver could be a possible link to the hepatoprotective effect of compound K. However, the therapeutic use of compound K in other tissues and the oral administration of compound K and PPD may be limited because of poor aqueous solubility (33 µg/mL for compound K; <50 ng/mL for PPD) and P-gp-mediated efflux [4,14,15]. The use of nanocrystals for PPD formulation improved oral bioavailability and brain delivery [15]. The use of the metabolism inhibitor piperine [20] in the formulation of PPD and the use of P-gp inhibitor, α-Tocopheryl polyethylene glycol 1000 succinate (TPGS) [21], in the formulation of PPD and compound K enhanced oral absorption and anticancer efficacy of these PPD and compound K [22,23]. These approaches may provide a strategy for developing formulations for compound K and PPD by modulating their pharmacokinetic features.

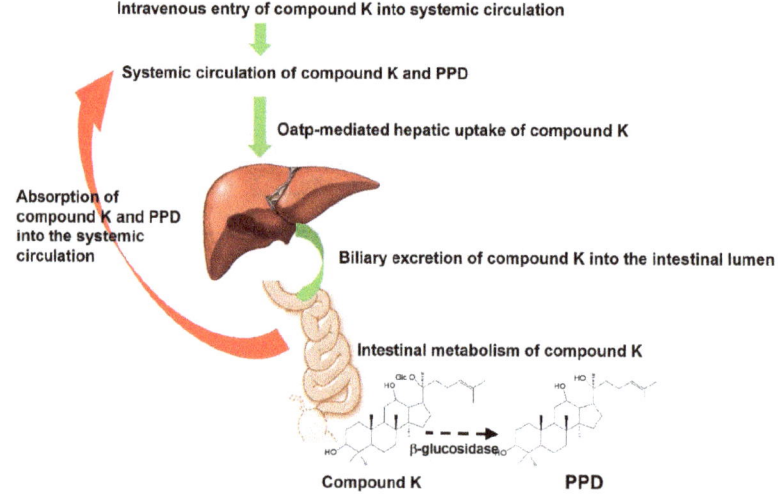

Figure 10. Proposed pharmacokinetic pathway of compound K following intravenous injection. Compound K underwent several steps: (i) intravenous entry of compound K into systemic circulation, (ii) Oatp-mediated hepatic uptake of compound K, (iii) biliary excretion of compound K into the intestinal lumen, (iv) metabolism of compound K into PPD in intestine, and (v) the absorption of compound K and PPD from intestine in blood.

5. Conclusions

This comparative pharmacokinetic and tissue distribution study of compound K in rats and mice demonstrated the following processes (Figure 10). First, the plasma concentration of compound K in mice was significantly greater than that in rats and the fecal recovery of PPD over 48 h in rats was greater than that in mice although the differences in elimination and metabolism between the two species need further investigation. Second, the plasma compound K was quickly distributed into the liver and underwent biliary excretion rather than renal elimination. The distribution of compound K into other major organs (kidney, heart, lung, pancreas, and testis) was much lower than in the liver for both rats and mice. Third, compound K was metabolized into PPD by the intestinal microbiota and the intestinal PPD metabolite was reabsorbed in the systemic circulation of both rats and mice.

Author Contributions: Conceptualization, M.-K.C. and I.-S.S.; Investigation, J.-H.J., B.K., S.L., M.-K.C., S.J. and I.-S.S.; Writing—Original Draft Preparation, J.-H.J. and B.K.; Supervision, M.-K.C. and I.-S.S.; Writing—Review & Editing, M.-K.C. and I.-S.S. All authors have read and agreed to the published version of the manuscript.

Funding: This research received no external funding.

Conflicts of Interest: The authors declare no conflict of interest.

References

1. Yang, X.D.; Yang, Y.Y.; Ouyang, D.S.; Yang, G.P. A review of biotransformation and pharmacology of ginsenoside compound K. *Fitoterapia* **2015**, *100*, 208–220. [CrossRef]
2. Choi, I.D.; Ryu, J.H.; Lee, D.E.; Lee, M.H.; Shim, J.J.; Ahn, Y.T.; Sim, J.H.; Huh, C.S.; Shim, W.S.; Yim, S.V.; et al. Enhanced absorption study of ginsenoside Compound K (20-O-beta-(D-Glucopyranosyl)-20(S)-protopanaxadiol) after oral administration of fermented red ginseng extract (HYFRG) in healthy Korean volunteers and rats. *Evid. Based Complement. Alternat. Med.* **2016**, *2016*, 3908142. [CrossRef] [PubMed]
3. Paek, I.B.; Moon, Y.; Kim, J.; Ji, H.Y.; Kim, S.A.; Sohn, D.H.; Kim, J.B.; Lee, H.S. Pharmacokinetics of a ginseng saponin metabolite compound K in rats. *Biopharm. Drug Dispos.* **2006**, *27*, 39–45. [CrossRef] [PubMed]
4. Yang, Z.; Wang, J.R.; Niu, T.; Gao, S.; Yin, T.J.; You, M.; Jiang, Z.H.; Hu, M. Inhibition of P-glycoprotein leads to improved oral bioavailability of compound K, an anticancer metabolite of red ginseng extract produced by gut microflora. *Drug Metab. Dispos.* **2012**, *40*, 1538–1544. [CrossRef] [PubMed]
5. Chen, L.L.; Zhou, L.P.; Wang, Y.Q.; Yang, G.P.; Huang, J.; Tan, Z.R.; Wang, Y.C.; Zhou, G.; Liao, J.W.; Ouyang, D.S. Food and sex-related impacts on the pharmacokinetics of a single-dose of ginsenoside compound K in healthy subjects. *Front. Pharmacol.* **2017**, *8*, 636. [CrossRef]
6. Fukami, H.; Ueda, T.; Matsuoka, N. Pharmacokinetic study of compound K in Japanese subjects after ingestion of Panax ginseng fermented by Lactobacillus paracasei A221 reveals significant increase of absorption into blood. *J. Med. Food* **2019**, *22*, 257–263. [CrossRef]
7. Choi, M.K.; Jin, S.; Jeon, J.H.; Kang, W.Y.; Seong, S.J.; Yoon, Y.R.; Han, Y.H.; Song, I.S. Tolerability and pharmacokinetics of ginsenosides Rb1, Rb2, Rc, Rd, and compound K after single or multiple administration of red ginseng extract in human beings. *J. Ginseng Res.* **2018**. [CrossRef]
8. Jin, S.; Jeon, J.H.; Lee, S.; Kang, W.Y.; Seong, S.J.; Yoon, Y.R.; Choi, M.K.; Song, I.S. Detection of 13 ginsenosides (Rb1, Rb2, Rc, Rd, Re, Rf, Rg1, Rg3, Rh2, F1, Compound K, 20(S)-Protopanaxadiol, and 20(S)-Protopanaxatriol) in human plasma and application of the analytical method to human pharmacokinetic studies following two week-repeated administration of red ginseng extract. *Molecules* **2019**, *24*, 2618.
9. Kim, H.K. Pharmacokinetics of ginsenoside Rb1 and its metabolite compound K after oral administration of Korean Red Ginseng extract. *J. Ginseng Res.* **2013**, *37*, 451–456. [CrossRef]
10. Kim, K.A.; Jung, I.H.; Park, S.H.; Ahn, Y.T.; Huh, C.S.; Kim, D.H. Comparative analysis of the gut microbiota in people with different levels of ginsenoside Rb1 degradation to compound K. *PLoS ONE* **2013**, *8*, e62409. [CrossRef]
11. Jeong, H.U.; Kwon, M.; Lee, Y.; Yoo, J.S.; Shin, D.H.; Song, I.S.; Lee, H.S. Organic anion transporter 3- and organic anion transporting polypeptides 1B1- and 1B3-mediated transport of catalposide. *Drug Des. Dev. Ther.* **2015**, *9*, 643–653.

12. Jiang, R.; Dong, J.; Li, X.; Du, F.; Jia, W.; Xu, F.; Wang, F.; Yang, J.; Niu, W.; Li, C. Molecular mechanisms governing different pharmacokinetics of ginsenosides and potential for ginsenoside-perpetrated herb-drug interactions on OATP1B3. *Br. J. Pharmacol.* **2015**, *172*, 1059–1073. [CrossRef] [PubMed]
13. Park, S.E.; Na, C.S.; Yoo, S.A.; Seo, S.H.; Son, H.S. Biotransformation of major ginsenosides in ginsenoside model culture by lactic acid bacteria. *J. Ginseng Res.* **2017**, *41*, 36–42. [CrossRef] [PubMed]
14. Jin, X.; Yang, Q.; Cai, N. Preparation of ginsenoside compound-K mixed micelles with improved retention and antitumor efficacy. *Int. J. Nanomed.* **2018**, *13*, 3827–3838. [CrossRef] [PubMed]
15. Chen, C.; Wang, L.S.; Cao, F.R.; Miao, X.Q.; Chen, T.K.; Chang, Q.; Zheng, Y. Formulation of 20(S)-protopanaxadiol nanocrystals to improve oral bioavailability and brain delivery. *Int. J. Pharm.* **2016**, *497*, 239–247. [CrossRef] [PubMed]
16. Kim, D.H. Gut microbiota-mediated pharmacokinetics of ginseng saponins. *J. Ginseng Res.* **2018**, *42*, 255–263. [CrossRef] [PubMed]
17. Wang, R.F.; Cao, W.W.; Cerniglia, C.E. PCR detection and quantitation of predominant anaerobic bacteria in human and animal fecal samples. *Appl. Environ. Microbiol.* **1996**, *62*, 1242–1247. [CrossRef]
18. Ling, J.; Yu, Y.; Long, J.; Li, Y.; Jiang, J.; Wang, L.; Xu, C.; Duan, G. Tentative identification of 20(S)-protopanaxadiol metabolites in human plasma and urine using ultra-performance liquid chromatography coupled with triple quadrupole time-of-flight mass spectrometry. *J. Ginseng Res.* **2019**, *43*, 539–549. [CrossRef]
19. Hu, Z.; Yang, J.; Cheng, C.; Huang, Y.; Du, F.; Wang, F.; Niu, W.; Xu, F.; Jiang, R.; Gao, X.; et al. Combinatorial metabolism notably affects human systemic exposure to ginsenosides from orally administered extract of Panax notoginseng roots (Sanqi). *Drug Metab. Dispos.* **2013**, *41*, 1457–1469. [CrossRef]
20. Atal, C.K.; Dubey, R.K.; Singh, J. Biochemical basis of enhanced drug bioavailability by piperine: Evidence that piperine is a potent inhibitor of drug metabolism. *J. Pharmacol. Exp. Ther.* **1985**, *232*, 258–262.
21. Song, I.S.; Cha, J.S.; Choi, M.K. Characterization, in vivo and in vitro evaluation of solid dispersion of curcumin containing d-alpha-tocopheryl polyethylene glycol 1000 succinate and mannitol. *Molecules* **2016**, *21*, 31386. [CrossRef] [PubMed]
22. Jin, X.; Zhang, Z.H.; Sun, E.; Tan, X.B.; Li, S.L.; Cheng, X.D.; You, M.; Jia, X.B. Enhanced oral absorption of 20(S)-protopanaxadiol by self-assembled liquid crystalline nanoparticles containing piperine: In vitro and in vivo studies. *Int. J. Nanomed.* **2013**, *8*, 641–652.
23. Yang, L.; Zhang, Z.H.; Hou, J.; Jin, X.; Ke, Z.C.; Liu, D.; Du, M.; Jia, X.B.; Lv, H.X. Targeted delivery of ginsenoside compound K using TPGS/PEG-PCL mixed micelles for effective treatment of lung cancer. *Int. J. Nanomed.* **2017**, *12*, 7653–7667. [CrossRef] [PubMed]

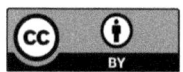 © 2020 by the authors. Licensee MDPI, Basel, Switzerland. This article is an open access article distributed under the terms and conditions of the Creative Commons Attribution (CC BY) license (http://creativecommons.org/licenses/by/4.0/).

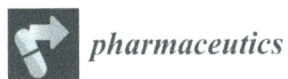

Article

Species Differences in Stereoselective Pharmacokinetics of HSG4112, A New Anti-Obesity Agent

In Yong Bae [1,†], Min Sun Choi [1,†], Young Seok Ji [1], Sang-Ku Yoo [2], Kyungil Kim [2] and Hye Hyun Yoo [1,*]

1. Institute of Pharmaceutical Science and Technology and College of Pharmacy, Hanyang University, Ansan, Gyeonggi-do 15588, Korea; iybae722@naver.com (I.Y.B.); chm2456@hanyang.ac.kr (M.S.C.); wldudtjr23@hanyang.ac.kr (Y.S.J.)
2. Glaceum Inc., Yeongtong-gu, Suwon, Gyeonggi-do 16675, Korea; skyoo@glaceum.com (S.-K.Y.); kikim@glaceum.com (K.K.)
* Correspondence: yoohh@hanyang.ac.kr; Tel.: +82-10-400-5804
† These authors contributed equally to this work.

Received: 29 November 2019; Accepted: 28 January 2020; Published: 3 February 2020

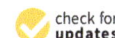

Abstract: HSG4112, a racemic drug, is a new anti-obesity agent. In this study, the stereoselective pharmacokinetics of HSG4112 were investigated in rats and dogs, and the underlying mechanism was investigated. The plasma concentrations of HSG4112(S) and HSG4112(R) were quantitated in plasma from rats and beagle dogs after IV and/or oral administration of racemic HSG4112. The concentration of HSG4112(S) was significantly higher than that of HSG4112(R) in rat plasma. Contrarily, the concentration of HSG4112(R) was significantly higher than HSG4112(S) in dog plasma. A metabolic stability test with liver microsomes showed that HSG4112(S) was more stable than HSG4112(R) in rat liver microsomes, but the difference between stereoisomers did not appear in dog liver microsomes. However, the stereoselectivity was observed in dog liver and intestinal microsomes after uridine 5′-diphospho-glucuronic acid was added. Thus, stereoselective metabolism by uridine 5′-diphospho-glucuronosyltransferases is mainly responsible for the stereoselective pharmacokinetics in dogs. These results suggest that the species difference in the stereoselective plasma pharmacokinetics of HSG4112 is due to the stereoselective metabolism.

Keywords: HSG4112; anti-obesity agent; stereoselectivity; pharmacokinetics

1. Introduction

HSG4112 is a new drug candidate which has been developed as a treatment for obesity. Its chemical structure is derived from glabridin. Glabridin is an isoflavane, which is found in *Glycyrrhiza glabra* extract [1–3]. It is known to have whitening activity by suppressing the activity of tyrosinase during the synthesis of melanin and to help alleviate gastroenteric disorders. Recently, it was confirmed that glabridin is effective in metabolic syndromes, including hyperlipidemia, fatty liver, impaired glucose metabolism, diabetes, and obesity and has anti-inflammatory actions, anticancer actions, and the like [4]. However, in spite of useful medicinal efficacy, glabridin is easily broken down by sunlight, moisture, acidity, basicity, oxygen, heat, and the like due to low chemical stability, so it is very difficult to develop a product actually utilizing glabridin [4]. For these reasons, we synthesized a new pyranochromenylphenol derivative, HSG4112, by modifying the structure of glabridin. HSG4112 is stable under various physical conditions, while maintaining or improving its medicinal efficacy [4]. HSG4112 is a racemic compound with a chiral carbon. Thus, glabridin has the structure of R-enantiomer whereas HSG4112 is a mixture of S and R enantiomers (Figure 1).

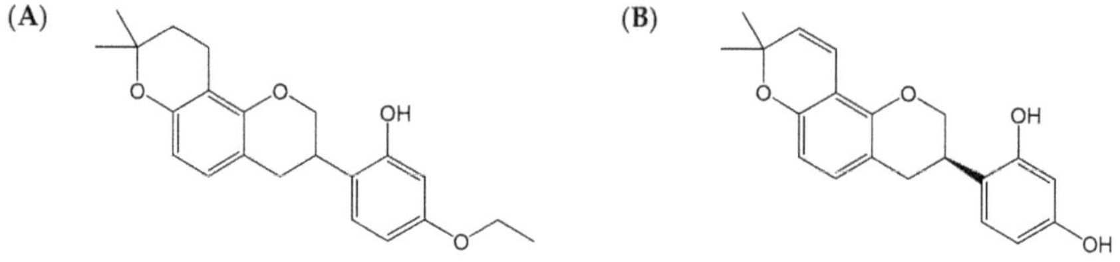

Figure 1. Chemical structures of (**A**) HSG4112 and (**B**) glabridin.

In many cases with chiral drugs, one of the two enantiomers is active and the other is either non-active or even harmful [5–7]. This is because the interaction between a drug molecule and its target is dependent on its three-dimensional environment. The most famous example is thalidomide, which was sold in the 1950s; the drug was introduced as a racemic mixture for use as a sedative but was later withdrawn from the market following the occurrence of birth defects in the children of mothers who took it to treat morning sickness. It was later found that the inactive enantiomer was the cause of the teratogenicity. This disaster was a driving force behind the requirement to strictly test drugs before making them available to the public [8]. In particular, for racemate candidates, both enantiomers should be studied separately as early as possible to assess the relevance of stereoisomerism to effects and fate. Accordingly, a pharmacokinetic evaluation should be provided for each enantiomer [9,10].

In this study, the stereoselective pharmacokinetics of HSG4112 were investigated in rats and beagle dogs. In addition, the metabolic stability was investigated in liver and intestinal microsomes from five different species (rat, mouse, dog, monkey, and human) to evaluate the role of metabolism in the species differences in its stereoselective pharmacokinetic behavior.

2. Materials and Methods

2.1. Chemicals and Materials

HSG4112(S) and HSG4112(R) were given from Glaceum Incorporation (Suwon, Korea). Pooled rat liver microsome (RLM), mouse liver microsome (MLM), dog liver microsome (DLM), and human liver microsome (HLM) were obtained from Gentest (Woburn, MA, USA). Pooled rat intestinal microsome (RIM), mouse intestinal microsome (MIM), dog intestinal microsome (DIM), and human intestinal microsome (HIM) were obtained from Sekisui Xenotech (Kansas City, KS, USA). Glucose 6-phosphate, β-NADP+, glucose 6-phosphate dehydrogenase and alamethicin were obtained from Sigma-Aldrich (St. Louis, MO, USA). HPLC-grade acetonitrile (ACN) and formic acid were purchased from J.T. Baker (Phillipsburg, NJ, USA). Distilled water (DW) was prepared using a Milli-Q purification system (Millipore, Bedford, MA, USA).

2.2. Preparation of Calibration and Quality Control (QC) Standards

HSG4112(S) 10 mg, HSG4112(R) 10 mg, and HSG4112-d5 (internal standard; IS) 5 mg were weighted and transferred to a 10 mL volumetric flask and ACN was added to the marking line to completely dissolve and store in a refrigerator (4 °C). The standard stock solutions of HSG4112(S) and HSG4112(R) were serially diluted to the designated concentrations to prepare the working standard solutions. The IS stock solution was diluted to 100 ng/mL with ACN and used for plasma sample preparation. Working standard solutions (5 μL) were added to plasma (95 μL) to yield calibration standards of 5, 20, 50, 100, 500, 1000, 2000, and 5000 ng/mL. QC samples were prepared at final concentrations of 5(LOQ), 15(low), 400(mid), and 4000(high) ng/mL in the same manner as the calibration standards.

2.3. Animal Plasma Samples

Rat and dog plasma samples were obtained from Biotoxtech Co. Ltd. (Cheongju, Korea). Plasma samples for oral pharmacokinetic study were obtained from the 4-week repeated oral toxicity study. The information on the plasma samples were provided in the Supplementary data. Briefly, for the pharmacokinetic analysis in rats, HSG4112 was orally administered HSG4112 at a dose of 100 mg/kg/day for 4 weeks and the plasma samples were collected on the 28th day. The blood drain time point was 0, 0.5, 1, 2, 4, 6, 10, and 24 h ($n = 3$; Table S1). In addition, rats were intravenously administered HSG4112 at a dose of 10 mg/kg and blood was collected at 0, 0.083, 0.25, 0.5, 0.75, 1, 2, 3, 6, 12, and 24 h ($n = 3$). For the pharmacokinetic analysis in dogs, HSG4112 was orally administered at a dose of 100 mg/kg/day for 4 weeks ($n = 3$), and the plasma samples were collected on the 28th day. Blood samples were taken at 0, 1, 2, 4, 6, 10, 12, and 24 h. In addition, dogs were administered HSG4112 intravenously at a dose of 2 mg/kg ($n = 2$) and blood was collected at 0, 0.083, 0.25, 0.5, 1, 2, 3, 4, 6, 12, and 24 h. All animal studies were performed according to the guidelines of the Ethics Committee for Use of Experimental Animals and approved by the Institutional Animal Care and Use Committee of Biotoxtech Co. Ltd. (Approval ID and date: 2016-05-160252, 2016-05-160276).

2.4. Sample Preparation

The plasma (30 µL) sample was put into a 1.5 mL tube and added with 60 µL IS solution. The tube was vortexed and centrifuged at 13,200 rpm for 5 min at room temperature. The supernatant was transferred to an LC vial for LC-MS/MS analysis.

2.5. In Vitro Metabolic Stability

Incubation mixture containing liver or intestinal microsomes (1 mg/mL), and HSG4112 (10 µM) in potassium phosphate buffer (0.1 M, pH 7.4) were preincubated at 37 °C for 5 min. The reactions were initiated by the addition of an NADPH-generation solution in a final incubation volume of 100 µL ($n = 3$). For glucuronide conjugate formation, incubation mixture containing microsomes (1 mg/mL), magnesium chloride (2.5 mM), UDPGA (2 mM), alamethicin (25 µg/mL), and drug (10 µM) in potassium phosphate buffer (0.1 M, pH 7.4) were preincubated at 37 °C for 5 min. The reactions were initiated by the addition of the NADPH-generation solution in a final incubation volume of 200 µL ($n = 3$). After the incubation for 0, 30, 60, and 120 min, the reaction was stopped by the addition of 200 µL ACN with IS. The samples were vortex-mixed and centrifuged at 13,200 rpm for 5 min. The supernatant (5 µL) was injected on to ultra-performance liquid chromatographic (UPLC) column for LC-MS/MS analysis. The experiment was performed in triplicate.

2.6. LC-MS/MS

In order to quantify HSG4112(S) and HSG4112(R), the Acquity UPLC-MS/MS system (Waters, Milford, MA, USA) was used with an electrospray ionization source. Mass detection was performed in the negative ion mode, and the column temperature was maintained at 40 °C using a thermostatically controlled column oven. The column used for the separation was a CHIRALPAK® IC-U (1.6 µm, 3.0 × 100 mm; DAICEL, New York, NY, USA). The mobile phases consisted of D.W (solvent A) and ACN (solvent B). For quantification of the analytes, isocratic elution was performed at a flow rate of 0.5 mL/min. Solvent B was maintained at 60%. For multiple reaction monitoring (MRM) analyses, the target ions used were m/z 353.3→137.1 for HSG4112(S) and HSG4112(R) and m/z 358.3→142.0 for HSG4112-d5. The capillary voltage was 3 kV and cone voltage was 50 V. Collision energy was 23 V. Nitrogen was used as the desolvation gas at a flow rate of 650 L/h and at 450 °C. The representative chromatograms of HSG4112(S) and HSG4112(R) in rat and dog plasma are provided in Supplementary data (Figure S1). The validation for the quantitation method was conducted and the resulting data were satisfactory (Supplementary data). For metabolite profiling, an ACQUITY UPLC BEH C18 column (2.1 × 150 mm, 1.7 µm; Waters, Milford, MA, USA) was used and a gradient elution program was used as follows: 30%B to 75% B at 10 min, to 30% B at 10.1 min, and held at 30% B for 3 min. The metabolite levels were measured using selected ion monitoring based on the *m/z* values of the deprotonated ions of metabolites. Other mass spectrometer conditions were the same as above.

2.7. LC-QTOF/MS for Metabolite Analysis

The high performance liquid chromatography quadruple time of the flight mass spectrometer (LC-QTOF/MS) system consisted of an Agilent 1260 series binary pump HPLC system and an Agilent 6530 Q-TOF/MS/MS equipped with an electrospray ionization source (Agilent Technologies, Palo Alto, CA, USA). The column used for the separation was a Thermo Hypersil Gold column (2.1 × 150 mm, 3 μm; Thermo Fisher Scientific Inc., Waltham, MA, USA). Column temperature was maintained at 40 °C using a thermostatically controlled column oven. The HPLC mobile phases consisted of 0.1% formic acid in distilled water (A) and 90% acetonitrile in 0.1% formic acid (B). A gradient program was used for the HPLC separation with a flow rate of 0.2 mL/min. The initial composition of the mobile phase was 30% B and it was changed to 90% B over 13 min and followed by a 7 min re-equilibration to the initial condition. The entire column eluent was directly introduced into the mass spectrometer. Nitrogen was used both as the nebulizing gas at 20 psi and as the drying gas at a flow rate of 10 L/min at 300 °C. The mass spectrometer was operated in the negative ion mode in *m/z* 50–400.

2.8. Pharmacokinetic and Data Analysis

All data were expressed as mean ± SD. Pharmacokinetic parameters were calculated by non-compartmental analysis using Pheonix WinNonlin (Ver. 6.2, Pharsight-A Certara Company, USA). The area under the concentration–time curve from time zero to the last measurable concentration (AUC_{last}), area under the plasma concentration–time curve to the infinite time (AUC_{inf}), maximum plasma concentration (C_{max}), time to reach C_{max} (T_{max}), terminal elimination half-life ($t_{1/2}$), total body clearance (C_l), apparent volume of distribution (V_z), apparent volume of distribution at steady state (V_{ss}), and equation for the mean residence time (MRT) were estimated by non-compartmental analysis of the plasma concentration versus time. The significance of the pharmacokinetic parameters was assessed using the paired Student's *t*-test. The analysis was performed on log-transformed data. When *p* value was less than 0.05, it was judged to be significant.

3. Results

3.1. Analysis of HSG4112(S) and HSG4112(R) in Rat Plasma

The time–plasma concentration plots of HSG4112(S) and HSG4112(R) are presented in Figure 2A, and the pharmacokinetic parameters are described in Table 1. The plasma concentration levels of HSG4112(S) were significantly higher than those of HSG4112(R) throughout all time points. The C_{max} of HSG4112(S) and HSG4112(R) were 2904.9 ng·h/mL and 984.6 ng/mL, respectively. The area under the curve (AUC) of HSG4112(S) and HSG4112(R) were 45,733.3 and 12,190.6 ng·h/mL, respectively. The pharmacokinetics of HSG4112(S) and HSG4112(R) after IV administration of HSG4112 were also investigated. The plasma concentration profiles of HSG4112(S) and HSG4112(R) after IV injection of HSG4112 at a dose of 10 mg/kg are presented in Figure 2B, and the pharmacokinetic parameters are described in Table 2. The stereoselective differences in plasma concentration were also observed in the IV administration. The AUC of HSG4112(S) and HSG4112(R) were 3806.7 ± 894.6 ng·h/mL and 1390.4 ± 92.7 ng·h/mL, respectively. Validation Data are presented in Tables S2–S5.

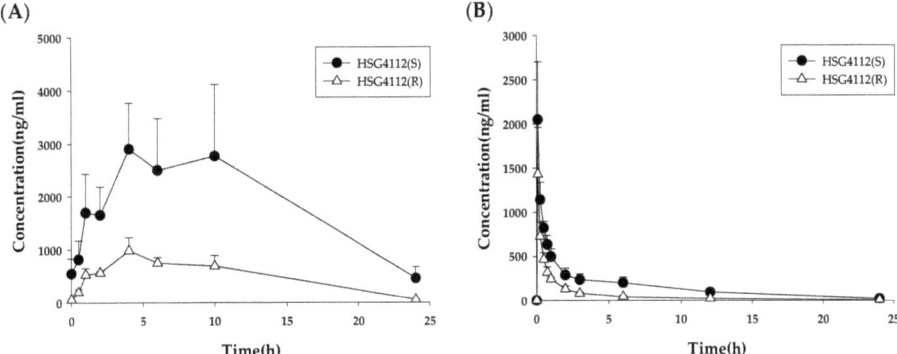

Figure 2. Plot for time-plasma concentration of HSG4112 after (**A**) oral (100 mg/kg/day, 28th day, $n = 3$) and (**B**) iv (10 mg/kg, single dose, $n = 3$) administration in rats.

Table 1. Pharmacokinetic parameters of HSG4112(S) and HSG4112(R) after PO administration at a repeated dose of 100 mg/kg/day to rats.

PK Parameter [a]	Rat 100 mg/kg (PO, 28th Day)	
	HSG4112(S)	HSG4112(R)
T_{max} (h)	4	4
C_{max} (ng/mL)	2904.9	984.6
AUC_{last} (ng·h/mL)	45,733.3	12,190.6
$T_{1/2}$ (h)	7.3	4.7
AUC_{inf} (ng·h/mL)	50,555.8	12,558.1
MRT (h)	8.8	7.8

[a] The blood samples were collected by a sparse sampling method from six rats (Table S1). Accordingly, the pharmacokinetic parameters were calculated from the mean plasma concentration data.

Table 2. Pharmacokinetic parameters of HSG4112(S) and HSG4112(R) after IV administration at a single dose of 10 mg/kg to rats.

PK Parameter	Rat 10 mg/kg (IV, $n = 3$)	
	HSG4112(S)	HSG4112(R)
C_{max} (ng/mL)	2049.7 ± 654.0	1431.7 ± 530.5 ***
AUC_{last} (ng·h/mL)	3806.7 ± 894.6	1390.4 ± 92.7 **
$T_{1/2}$ (h)	5.3 ± 1.0	5.9 ± 0.4
AUC_{inf} (ng·h/mL)	3976.5 ± 1027.7	1436 ± 98.7 **
V_z (mL/kg)	9667.6 ± 697.8	29,483.8 ± 393.6 ***
C_l (mL/h/kg)	1318.8 ± 360.1	3493.4 ± 247.2 **
MRT (h)	5.4 ± 0.9	3.9 ± 0.4 *
V_{ss} (mL/kg)	16374 ± 1281	33,462 ± 4228 ***

*: $p < 0.05$, **: $p < 0.01$, ***: $p < 0.005$ versus HSG4112(S).

3.2. Analysis of HSG4112(S) and HSG4112(R) in Dog Plasma

The time–plasma concentration plots of HSG4112(S) and HSG4112(R) are presented in Figure 3A, and the pharmacokinetic parameters are described in Table 3. The C_{max} of HSG4112(S) and HSG4112(R) were 102.6 ± 69.6 and 707.6 ± 442.7, respectively. The AUC of HSG4112(S) and HSG4112(R) were 1408.4 ± 1418.0 and 12,324.8 ± 9715.7, respectively. The plasma concentration profiles of HSG4112(S) and HSG4112(R) after IV injection of HSG4112 at a dose of 2 mg/kg are presented in Figure 3B, and the pharmacokinetic parameters are described in Table 4. After IV injection of 2 mg/kg to beagle dogs, the AUC of HSG4112(S) and HSG4112(R) were 1002.6 ± 163.6 and 1837.4 ± 20.4 ng·h/mL, respectively. Validation Data are presented in Tables S6–S9.

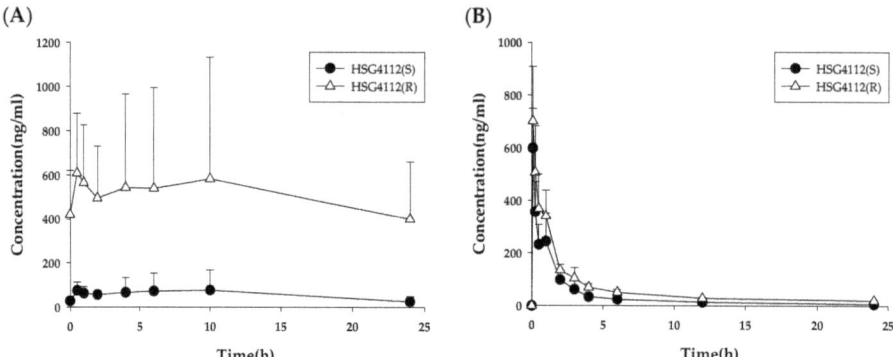

Figure 3. Plot for time–plasma concentration of HSG4112 after (**A**) oral (100 mg/kg/day, 28th day, n = 3) and (**B**) iv (2 mg/kg, single dose, n = 2) administration in dogs.

Table 3. Pharmacokinetic parameters of HSG4112(S) and HSG4112(R) after PO administration at a repeated dose of 100 mg/kg/day to dogs.

PK Parameter	Dog 100 mg/kg (PO, 28th day, n = 3)	
	HSG4112(S)	HSG4112(R)
T_{max} (h)	4.2 ± 5.1	3.7 ± 5.5
C_{max} (ng/mL)	102.6 ± 69.6	707.6 ± 442.7 ***
AUC_{last} (ng·h/mL)	1408.4 ± 1418.0	12324.8 ± 9715.7 ***
$T_{1/2}$ (h)	17.5 ± 4.5	49.4 ± 19.1
AUC_{inf} (ng·h/mL)	NA	24329.9 ± 6226.4 **
MRT (h)	9.2 ± 0.4	11.1 ± 0.2 *

*: $p < 0.05$, **: $p < 0.01$, ***: $p < 0.005$ versus HSG4112(S). NA: not available.

Table 4. Pharmacokinetic parameters of HSG4112(S) and HSG4112(R) after IV administration at a single dose of 2 mg/kg to dogs.

PK Parameter	Dog 2 mg/kg (IV, n = 2)	
	HSG4112(S)	HSG4112(R)
C_{max} (ng/mL)	598.8 ± 149.2	700.9 ± 208.7
AUC_{last} (ng·h/mL)	902.7 ± 165.2	1519.0 ± 95.1
$T_{1/2}$ (h)	10.3 ± 1.5	12.0 ± 1.6
AUC_{inf} (ng·h/mL)	1002.6 ± 163.6	1837.4 ± 20.4
V_z (mL/kg)	15180.7 ± 4635.6	9437.1 ± 1333.6
C_l (mL/h/kg)	1008.6 ± 164.5	533.1 ± 5.2
MRT (h)	4.4 ± 0.3	5.7 ± 0.1
V_{ss} (mL/kg)	8047.5 ± 1885.4	6500.5 ± 1157.4

3.3. Metabolic Stability

The results for the metabolic stability of HSG4112(S) and HSG4112(R) in rat (RLM), mouse (MLM), dog (DLM), and human liver microsomes (HLM) is shown in Figure 4 (left). The remaining amounts of HSG4112(S) at 120 min were 9.1 ± 3.2%, 6.9 ± 1.5%, 84.1 ± 6%, and 78.4 ± 0.5% in the RLM, MLM, DLM, and HLM, respectively. The half-life of HSG4112(S) was 15.5, 14.2, 664.8, and 424.6 min in the RLM, MLM, DLM, and HLM, respectively. The remaining amounts of HSG4112(R) at 120 min were 4.9 ± 3%,

23.9 ± 1.1%, 77.9 ± 2.9%, and 54.5 ± 1.1% in the RLM, MLM, DLM, and HLM, respectively. The half-life of HSG4112(R) was 8.2, 28.0, 376.8, and 133.9 min in the RLM, MLM, DLM, and HLM, respectively.

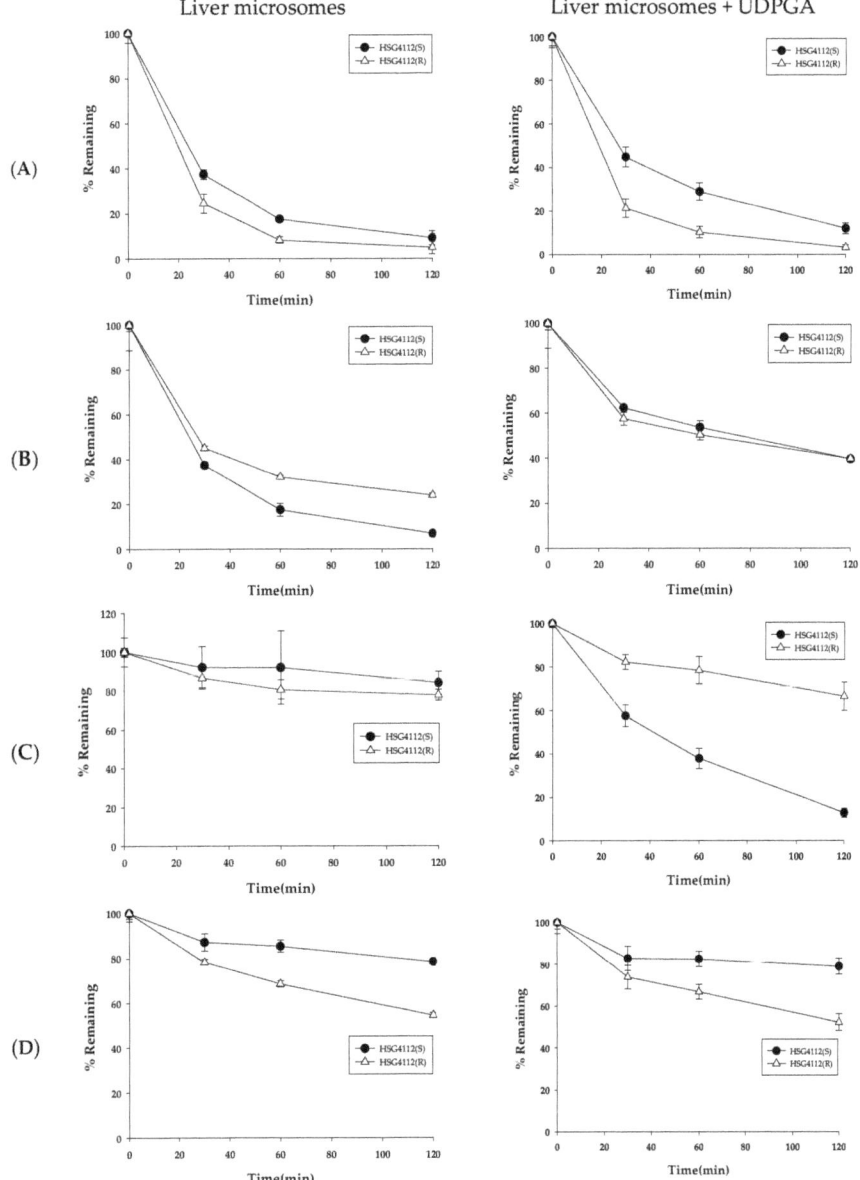

Figure 4. Metabolic stability of HSG4112 in (**A**) rat, (**B**) mouse, (**C**) dog, and (**D**) human liver microsomes (n = 3). UDPGA, uridine 5′-diphosphoglucuronic acid.

To investigate the effects of the phase II metabolism by glucuronidation, metabolic stability was tested after adding the glucuronidation cofactor, UDPGA. The results for the metabolic stability of HSG4112(S) and HSG4112(R) in rat, mouse, dog, and human liver microsomes with UDPGA are shown in Figure 4 (right). The remaining amounts of HSG4112(S) at 120 min were 11.9 ± 2.5%, 39.6 ± 1.5%,

12.8 ± 2%, and 78.9 ± 3.8% in the RLM, MLM, DLM, and HLM, respectively. The half-life of HSG4112(S) was 25.6, 64.3, 40.0, and 419.6 min in the RLM, MLM, DLM, and HLM, respectively. The remaining amounts of HSG4112(R) at 120 min were 3.2 ± 1.1%, 39.7 ± 0.9%, 66.5 ± 6.6%, and 52.2 ± 4% in the RLM, MLM, DLM, and HLM, respectively. The half-life values of HSG4112(R) were 9.1, 52.4, 226.8, and 150.5 min in the RLM, MLM, DLM, and HLM, respectively.

As glucuronidases are also predominantly distributed in the intestine, HSG4112 was tested in intestinal microsomes to confirm the metabolic stability results while considering glucuronidation. The results for the metabolic stability of HSG4112(S) and HSG4112(R) in rat (RIM), mouse (MIM), dog (DIM), and human intestinal microsomes (HIM) with UDPGA are shown in Figure 5. The remaining amounts of HSG4112(S) at 120 min were 87.9 ± 2.3%, 70.1 ± 6.1%, 37.9 ± 1.8%, and 76.7 ± 2.1% in RIM, MIM, DIM, and HIM, respectively. The half-life values of HSG4112(S) were 733.9, 247.9, 78.1, and 368.1 min in the RIM, MIM, DIM, and HIM, respectively. The remaining amounts of HSG4112(R) at 120 min were 95.8 ± 5.6%, 59.4 ± 6.3%, 65.9 ± 1.8%, and 75.5 ± 3.6% in RIM, MIM, DIM, and HIM, respectively. The half-life of HSG4112(R) was 1943.9, 136.7, 215.3, and 351.1 min in RIM, MIM, DIM, and HIM, respectively.

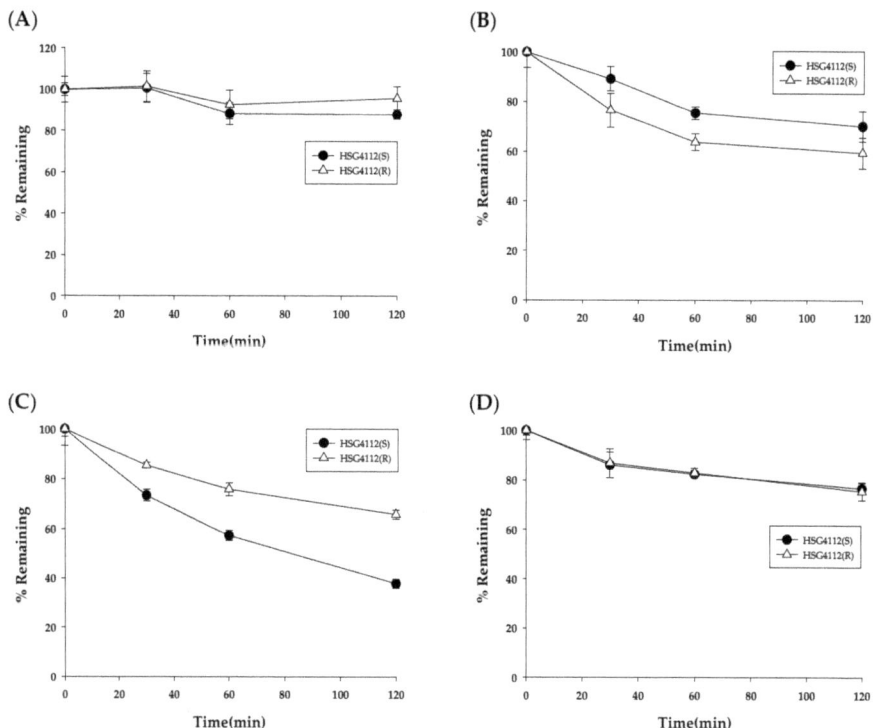

Figure 5. Metabolic stability of HSG4112 in (**A**) rat, (**B**) mouse, (**C**) dog, and (**D**) human intestinal microsomes ($n = 3$).

3.4. Metabolite Profile

To elucidate the main factor responsible for the stereospecific pharmacokinetic properties in rats, the metabolite profiles of HSG4112(S) and HSG4112(R) were investigated. When HSG4112(S) and HSG4112(R) were incubated in the rat liver microsomes for 60 min, the remaining amounts of HSG4112(S) and HSG4112(R) were 36.2% and 17.6%, respectively (Figure 6A). HSG4112(S) and HSG4112(R) were metabolized to yield metabolites by oxidation (M1a ~ M2b). M1c-1 and M1c-2 were detected as one peak on a general C18 column but they were separated on a chiral column. Thus, M1c-1 and M1c-2 were supposed to be stereoisomers. The types of metabolites produced from the two isomers were similar, but the amounts produced were different. The predominant metabolites of HSG4112(S) were M1a and M2b, whereas those of HSG4112(R) were M1c-2 and M1a (Figure 6B). Subsequently, the metabolite profile was investigated in the rat plasma samples (on the 28th day of an oral dose of 100 mg/kg/day). A total of seven metabolites were detected (Figure 7); a metabolite with hydroxyl and carbonyl groups (M3a) and glucuronide conjugate (M4) were additionally detected besides the metabolites observed in liver microsomes. Their peak area values were plotted according to the time (Figure 8A), and the concentration of the parent (as racemate), M1c-1, and M1c-2 were quantitated (Figure 8B). M1c-2 was shown to be the predominant metabolite (Figure 8C). The accurate mass data for each postulated metabolite is tabulated in Table 5. The tentative structures of HSG4112 metabolites are provided as Supplementary data (Figure S2).

Table 5. Accurate mass data for HSG4112 and its postulated metabolites in rats.

Metabolites	ΔM	Theoretical Mass [M-H]$^-$	Measured Mass [M-H]$^-$	Error (ppm)
HSG4112	-	353.1758	353.1756	−0.57
M1a	+16	369.1707	369.1712	1.35
M1c-1	+16	369.1707	369.1718	2.98
M1c-2	+16	369.1707	369.1718	2.98
M2a	+30	383.1500	383.1499	−0.26
M2b	+30	383.1500	383.1531	8.09
M3a	+30	385.1657	385.1662	1.30
M4	+30	529.2079	529.2071	−1.51

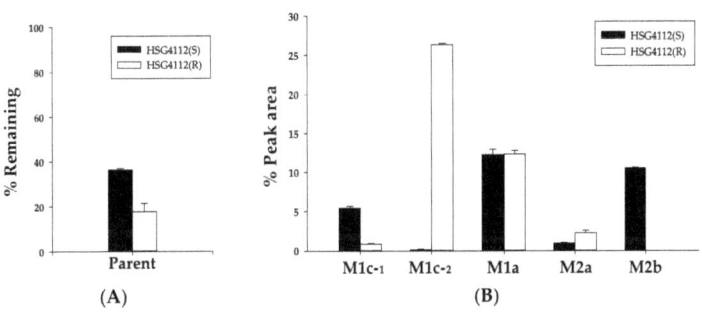

Figure 6. Metabolic profiles of HSG4112(S) and HSG4112(R) in rat liver microsomes. (A) Percent remaining amounts of HSG4112(S) and HSG4112(R). (B) Relative peak areas of the metabolites generated from HSG4112(S) and HSG4112(R). HSG4112(S) and HSG4112(R) were incubated separately in rat liver microsomes for 60 min and the resulting amount of the parent drug and its metabolites was measured based on peak area.

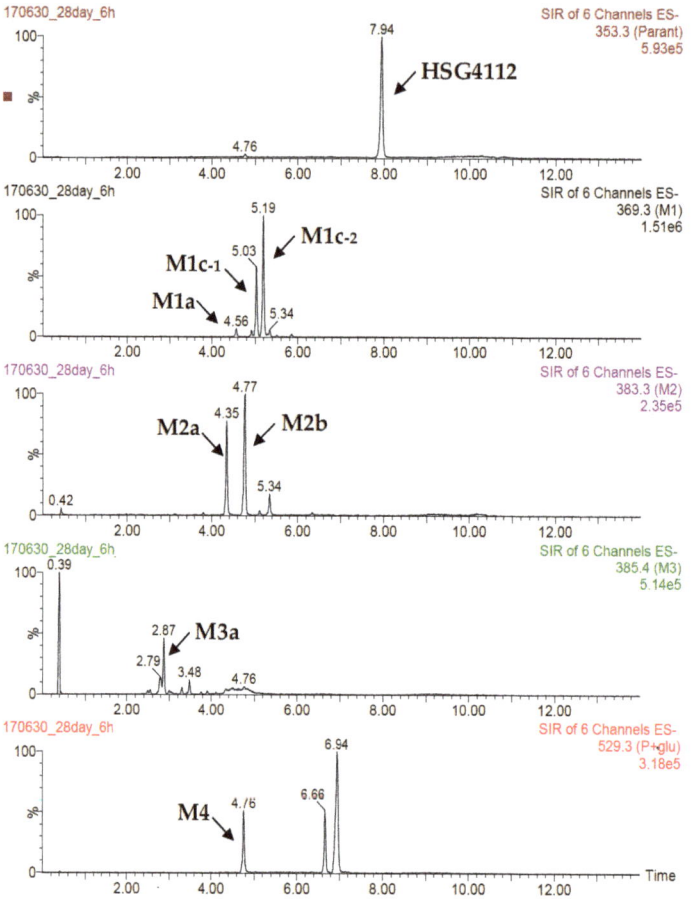

Figure 7. Representative extracted ion chromatograms of HSG4112 and its metabolites in rat plasma.

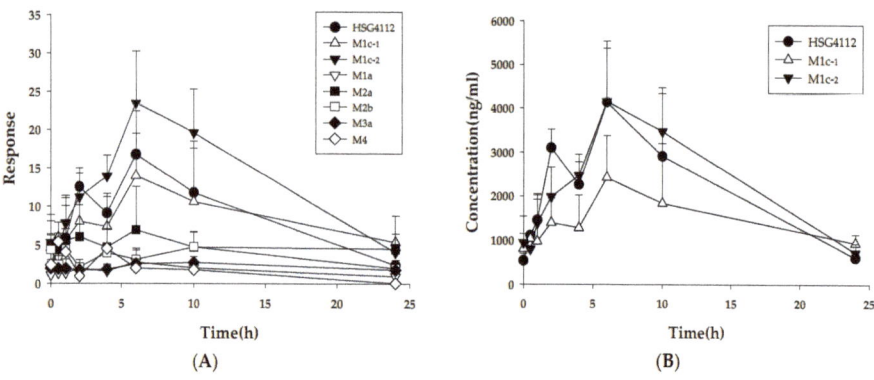

Figure 8. *Cont.*

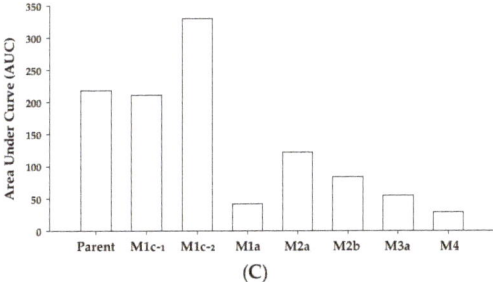

(C)

Figure 8. Metabolic profiles of HSG4112 in rat plasma after oral administration (100 mg/kg/day, 28th day, $n = 3$). (**A**) Plot for time-peak area of HSG4112 and its metabolites. (**B**) Plot for time-plasma concentration of HSG4112, M1c-1 and M1c-2. (**C**) Area under curve values of HSG4112 and its metabolites calculated from (**A**).

Meanwhile, the dog plasma sample showed only two metabolites (M1d and M4); M4, the glucuronide metabolite, was the predominant metabolite (Figure 9). Due to the unavailability of the sample and reference standards, the time–plasma concentration profile could not be obtained.

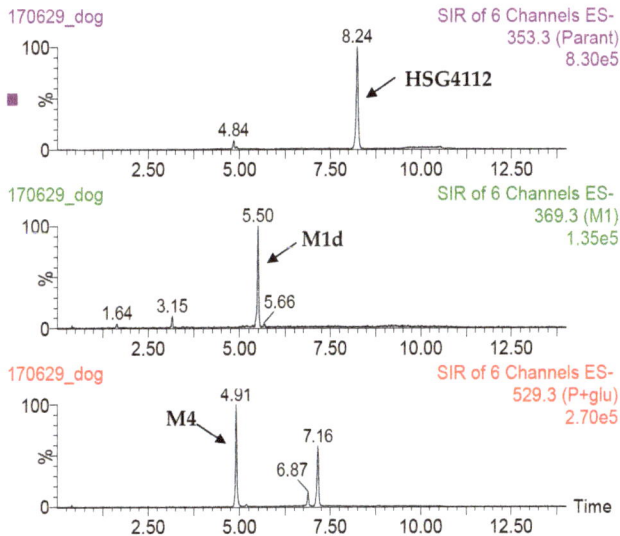

Figure 9. Representative extracted ion chromatograms of HSG4112 and its metabolites in dog plasma.

4. Discussion

In this study, concentration profiles of HSG4112(S) and HSG4112(R) after intravenous and/or oral administration of HSG4112 were investigated in rats and dogs, and the stereoselectivity in the metabolism of HSG4112 was investigated in vitro and in vivo. The resulting data showed a characteristic stereoselective pharmacokinetic pattern depending on the species.

When HSG4112(S) and HSG4112(R) were quantified in rat plasma, the concentration of HSG4112(S) generally measured higher, and, consequently, the AUC of HSG4112(S) was 4.9–7.8 times higher than that of HSG4112(R). This trend was also observed in the plasma samples from rats administered intravenously; the concentration ratio (S/R) over time was 1.4–4.8, and the AUC of HSG4112(S) was 2.7 times higher than that of HSG4112(R). Therefore, the systemic exposure of HSG4112(S) was significantly higher than that of HSG4112(R) in rats, indicating stereospecificity in the pharmacokinetics.

This stereoselective pharmacokinetic property in rats is supposedly due to the stereoselective metabolism of HSG4112. The possible metabolic pathways of HSG4112 isomers in rats are presented in Figure S3. The metabolic stability data and the metabolite profiles in rat plasma showed that HSG4112(R) is metabolized more extensively than HSG4112(S), and their main metabolic pathways are different. The metabolic profile data suggested that the formation of M1c is predominantly responsible for the stereoselective pharmacokinetics of HSG4112.

When HSG4112 was orally administered to beagle dogs, the concentration ratio (S/R) over time was 0.06–0.24, and the concentration of HSG4112(R) measured at a much higher level. The AUC ratio of HSG4112(S) and HSG4112(R) was 0.12–0.13 in the oral administration group. In addition, when HSG4112 was intravenously administered to beagle dogs, the concentration ratio (S/R) over time was 0.3–0.9, and the AUC ratio of HSG4112(S) and HSG4112(R) was 0.5. Therefore, the systemic exposure of HSG4112(R) was significantly higher than HSG4112(S) in beagle dogs, indicating stereospecificity in the pharmacokinetics. Interestingly, the predominant isomer form in dogs was opposite to that of rats. The metabolic stability data for phase I metabolism did not exhibit any difference between HSG4112(S) and HSG4112(R). However, the metabolic stability data including glucuronide formation showed significant differences between HSG4112(S) and HSG4112(R); the metabolic rate of HSG4112(S) was much higher than that of HSG4112(R). This metabolism pattern was also obviously observed in dog intestinal microsomes, which also have high glucuronidase activities. This revealed that the stereoselective glucuronide formation is mainly responsible for the stereoselective pharmacokinetics of HSG4112 in dogs. This was also supported by the in vivo metabolism profile data of dog plasma; the glucuronide metabolite (M4) was found to be the predominant metabolite in dog plasma. Notably, the longer terminal half-life was observed after oral administration compared with IV injection in dogs. Thus, it is supposed that HSG4112 has a general-case pharmacokinetic property in rats but a flip-flop pharmacokinetic property in dogs. This phenomenon occurs when the absorption rate of drugs is much slower than the elimination rate [11,12]. In this case, bioavailability factors such as the absorption rate and extent mainly affect the terminal slope of oral administration than clearance and volume of distribution.

Glabridin, the motive compound of HSG4112, has the R configuration at carbon C-3. According to the previous report, the systemic bioavailability of glabridin was very low (about 7.5% in rats). Glabridin is mainly metabolized by glucuronidases in the intestine and liver, and the first-pass effects of glucuronidation are one of the main factors responsible for the low oral bioavailability of glabridin. Guo et al. investigated the tissue and species differences in the glucuronidation of glabridin. In their study, glabridin was metabolized to yield two glucuronide metabolites: M1 and M2. M2 formation was predominant whereas the formation of M1 was negligible in most species tested. The authors could not determine the exact position of glucuronidation for M1 and M2, but they suggested that M2 might have a glucuronide moiety at the C-4 hydroxyl group in the B ring based on the earlier reports. The C-4 hydroxyl group of HSG4112 is masked by an alkyl chain. This is the reason why the glucuronidation was not the main metabolic pathway in humans and rats in our study with HSG4112. It is notable that dog liver microsomes showed the highest value of the intrinsic clearance by M1 formation (glucuronidation at the C-2 hydroxyl group) in glabridin. This result agrees with our finding that the formation of the glucuronide metabolite predominantly occurred in dog liver and intestinal microsomes. The results by Guo et al. showed that the metabolic clearance by glucuronidation both for M1 and M2 was negligible in humans. This is also consistent with our data that the contribution of glucuronidation to the metabolic clearance of HSG4112 was minimal.

Stereoselectivity for HSG 4112 metabolism was also shown in human liver microsomes. The metabolism pattern in human liver microsomes is somewhat close to that in rat liver microsomes. Thus, this is supposedly due to CYP-mediated metabolism rather than glucuronidation. Although the metabolic rate in humans is lower than that in other species, the present data suggests that stereoselective pharmacokinetics by stereoselective metabolism (i.e., higher exposure of the (S)-isomer) could be shown in the clinical trial of HSG4112. Another factor that should be considered regarding stereoselective pharmacokinetics is the possibility of interconversion between the isomers. To address this issue, HSG4112 isomers were analyzed after oral administration of each isomer to rats. When one isomer was administered, the other isomer was not detected (data not shown). This suggests that interconversion between isomers does not occur at least in rats. Further investigation should be followed in humans.

In conclusion, the present study demonstrates that HSG4112 showed species-specific stereoselective pharmacokinetics. Notably, the pharmacokinetic stereoselectivity of HSG4112 isomers showed opposing patterns between rats and dogs. This is because the major metabolic pathways involved in the clearance of HSG4112 are different in rats and dogs. Each metabolic enzyme may have different stereoselectivity. We presented the possible mechanisms for these stereoselective pharmacokinetic patterns by the metabolite profiling data in vitro and in vivo. These results will provide helpful information for understanding the pharmacological and toxicological effects of HSG4112, depending on its configurations. In addition, caution should be taken in extrapolating preclinical data with different experimental animal models to clinical data for humans.

Supplementary Materials: The following are available online at http://www.mdpi.com/1999-4923/12/2/127/s1, Figure S1: Representative chromatograms of HSG4112(S) and HSG4112(R) in (A) rat (oral, 100 mg/kg, 6h) and (B) dog (oral, 100 mg/kg, 6h) plasma, Figure S2: Proposed chemical structures of HSG4112 metabolites, Figure S3: Postulated metabolic pathways of HSG4112 isomers, Table S1: Blood drain time points for oral pharmacokinetic analysis in rats (repeated dose, 100 mg/kg/day, 28th day), Table S2: Linearity of HSG4112(S) and HSG4112(R) in rat plasma ($n = 3$), Table S3: Intra-day and inter-day accuracy and coefficient of variation for determination of HSG4112(S) and HSG4112(R) in rat plasma, Table S4: Matrix effect, recovery and process efficiency data for HSG4112(S) and HSG4112(R) in rat plasma ($n = 3$), Table S5: Stability of HSG4112(S) and HSG4112(R) in rat plasma, Table S6: Linearity of HSG4112(S) and HSG4112(R) in dog plasma, Table S7: Intra-day and inter-day accuracy and coefficient of variation for determination of HSG4112(S) and HSG4112(R) in dog plasma, Table S8: Matrix effect, recovery and process efficiency data for HSG4112(S) and HSG4112(R) in dog plasma ($n = 3$), Table S9: Stability of HSG4112(S) and HSG4112(R) in dog plasma.

Author Contributions: Contributed to the research design: H.H.Y., S.-K.Y., K.K.; Conducted experiments: I.Y.B., Y.S.J.; Contributed to data analysis and interpretation: M.S.C.; Contributed to the preparation of the manuscript: I.Y.B., M.S.C., H.H.Y. All authors have read and agreed to the published version of the manuscript.

Funding: This research was supported by the National Research Foundation of Korea funded by the Korea government (NRF-2017R1A2B4001814).

Conflicts of Interest: The authors declare no conflict of interest. S.K.Y. and K.K. are from Glaceum Inc., the company had no role in the design of the study; in the collection, analyses, or interpretation of data; in the writing of the manuscript, and in the decision to publish the results.

References

1. Simmler, C.; Pauli, G.F.; Chen, S.N. Phytochemistry and biological properties of glabridin. *Fitoterapia* **2013**, *90*, 160–184. [CrossRef] [PubMed]
2. Cui, Y.M.; Ao, M.Z.; Li, W.; Yu, L.J. Effect of glabridin from Glycyrrhiza glabra on learning and memory in mice. *Planta Med.* **2008**, *74*, 377–380. [CrossRef] [PubMed]
3. Ito, C.; Oi, N.; Hashimoto, T.; Nakabayashi, H.; Aoki, F.; Tominaga, Y.; Yokota, S.; Hosoe, K.; Kanazawa, K. Absorption of dietary licorice isoflavan glabridin to blood circulation in rats. *J. Nutr. Sci. Vitaminol. (Tokyo)* **2007**, *53*, 358–365. [CrossRef] [PubMed]
4. Guo, B.; Fang, Z.; Yang, L.; Xiao, L.; Xia, Y.; Gonzalez, F.J.; Zhu, L.; Cao, Y.; Ge, G.; Yang, L.; et al. Tissue and species differences in the glucuronidation of glabridin with UDP-glucuronosyltransferases. *Chem. Biol. Interact.* **2015**, *231*, 90–97. [CrossRef] [PubMed]
5. Kasprzyk-Hordern, B. Pharmacologically active compounds in the environment and their chirality. *Chem. Soc. Rev.* **2010**, *39*, 4466–4503. [CrossRef] [PubMed]
6. Eriksson, T.; Bjorkman, S.; Roth, B.; Fyge, A.; Hoglund, P. Stereospecific determination, chiral inversion in vitro and pharmacokinetics in humans of the enantiomers of thalidomide. *Chirality* **1995**, *7*, 44–52. [CrossRef] [PubMed]
7. Agranat, I.; Wainschtein, S.R. The strategy of enantiomer patents of drugs. *Drug Discov. Today* **2010**, *15*, 163–170. [CrossRef] [PubMed]

8. Stephens, T.D.; Bunde, C.J.; Fillmore, B.J. Mechanism of action in thalidomide teratogenesis. *Biochem. Pharmacol.* **2000**, *59*, 1489–1499. [CrossRef]
9. Williams, K.; Lee, E. Importance of drug enantiomers in clinical pharmacology. *Drugs* **1985**, *30*, 333–354. [CrossRef] [PubMed]
10. Chu, D.T.; Nordeen, C.W.; Hardy, D.J.; Swanson, R.N.; Giardina, W.J.; Pernet, A.G.; Plattner, J.J. Synthesis, antibacterial activities, and pharmacological properties of enantiomers of temafloxacin hydrochloride. *J. Med. Chem.* **1991**, *34*, 168–174. [CrossRef] [PubMed]
11. Toutain, P.L.; Bousquet-Mélou, A. Plasma terminal half-life. *J. Vet. Pharmacol. Ther.* **2004**, *27*, 427–439. [CrossRef] [PubMed]
12. Kim, H.; Ji, Y.S.; Rehman, S.U.; Choi, M.S.; Gye, M.C.; Yoo, H.H. Pharmacokinetics and Metabolism of Acetyl Triethyl Citrate, a Water-Soluble Plasticizer for Pharmaceutical Polymers in Rats. *Pharmaceutics* **2019**, *11*, 162. [CrossRef] [PubMed]

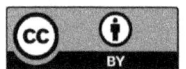

© 2020 by the authors. Licensee MDPI, Basel, Switzerland. This article is an open access article distributed under the terms and conditions of the Creative Commons Attribution (CC BY) license (http://creativecommons.org/licenses/by/4.0/).

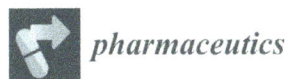

Article

Slower Elimination of Tofacitinib in Acute Renal Failure Rat Models: Contribution of Hepatic Metabolism and Renal Excretion

Sung Hun Bae, Sun-Young Chang and So Hee Kim *

Department of Pharmacy, College of Pharmacy and Research Institute of Pharmaceutical Science and Technology, Ajou University, 206 Worldcup-ro, Yeongtong-gu, Suwon 16499, Korea; baezzam@ajou.ac.kr (S.H.B.); sychang@ajou.ac.kr (S.-Y.C.)
* Correspondence: shkim67@ajou.ac.kr; Tel.: +82-31-219-3451; Fax: +82-31-219-3435

Received: 29 June 2020; Accepted: 27 July 2020; Published: 30 July 2020

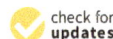

Abstract: Tofacitinib is a Jak inhibitor developed as a treatment for rheumatoid arthritis. Tofacitinib is metabolized mainly through hepatic CYP3A1/2, followed by CYP2C11. Rheumatoid arthritis tends to increase renal toxicity due to drugs used for long-term treatment. In this study, pharmacokinetic changes of tofacitinib were evaluated in rats with gentamicin (G-ARF) and cisplatin-induced acute renal failure (C-ARF). The time-averaged total body clearance (CL) of tofacitinib in G-ARF and C-ARF rats after 1-min intravenous infusion of 10 mg/kg was significantly decreased by 37.7 and 62.3%, respectively, compared to in control rats. This seems to be because the time-averaged renal clearance (CL_R) was significantly lower by 69.5 and 98.6%, respectively, due to decreased creatinine clearance (CL_{CR}). In addition, the time-averaged nonrenal clearance (CL_{NR}) was also significantly lower by 33.2 and 57.4%, respectively, due to reduction in the hepatic CYP3A1/2 and CYP2C11 subfamily in G-ARF and C-ARF rats. After oral administration of tofacitinib (20 mg/kg) to G-ARF and C-ARF rats, both CL_R and CL_{NR} were also significantly decreased. In conclusion, an increase in area under plasma concentration-time curves from time zero to time infinity (AUC) of tofacitinib in G-ARF and C-ARF rats was due to the significantly slower elimination of tofacitinib contributed by slower hepatic metabolism and urinary excretion of the drug.

Keywords: tofacitinib; acute renal failure; gentamicin; cisplatin; pharmacokinetics; hepatic CYP3A1(23); creatinine clearance; renal clearance; nonrenal clearance

1. Introduction

Tofacitinib (Figure 1) was developed as a Jak inhibitor for the treatment of rheumatoid arthritis and is particularly effective when methotrexate is poorly treated [1]. Recently, tofacitinib was approved in 2018 for chronic use to treat moderate to severe ulcerative colitis [2], making it the first Food and Drug Administration (FDA)-approved oral Jak inhibitor [3]. Tofacitinib is currently under clinical trials for various diseases, such as psoriasis [4,5], alopecia [6], atopic dermatitis [7], and ankylosing spondylitis [8].

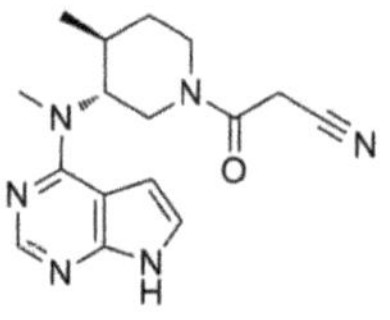

Figure 1. Chemical structure of tofacitinib.

Pharmacokinetic analysis following oral administration of tofacitinib (10 mg) to healthy volunteers showed a half-life of 3.2 h and a volume of distribution of 87 L [9–11]. Approximately 40% of the oral dose bound to plasma protein, 30% of the dose was excreted in the urine as an unmetabolized form, and 70% was metabolized and excreted in the urine as metabolized forms [9–11]. Absolute oral bioavailability (F) of tofacitinib was found to be approximately 74% [11]. Tofacitinib is primarily metabolized by oxidation and N-demethylation in the liver through cytochrome P450 (CYP) 3A4 and CYP2C19 and is further metabolized into glucuronide conjugates [9]. According to a report by Lee and Kim [12], following intravenous, oral, intraportal, intragastric, and intraduodenal administration of 10 mg/kg tofacitinib in male Sprague–Dawley rats, the F value was 29.1%, the unabsorbed fraction up to 24 h was 3.16% of the oral dose, the gastric first-pass effect was not significant after intragastric administration of tofacitinib, and 46.1% of the dose administered intraduodenally was metabolized before entering the portal vein. The hepatic first-pass effect was 42% after absorption into the portal vein.

Kidney disease has clinically important significance for patients with rheumatoid arthritis. Kidney disease is correlated with mortality in patients with rheumatoid arthritis [13,14]; therefore, renal impairment can be seen as a predictor of high mortality in patients with rheumatoid arthritis [15]. In addition, rheumatoid arthritis requires long-term treatment, and thus, the possibility of kidney damage is high due to long-term administration of drugs with renal toxicity, such as methotrexate or nonsteroidal anti-inflammatory drugs. Therefore, it is important to accurately measure kidney function in patients with rheumatoid arthritis and necessary to adjust the dose according to the kidney function of the patient. Approximately 36–38% of drugs prescribed in patients with glomerular filtration rate (GFR) < 60 mL/min require dosage adjustment due to pharmacokinetic changes of these drugs [16]. It is known that renal failure occurs in 5–50% of patients with rheumatoid arthritis [17]. Krishnaswami et al. [18] reported that, relative to patients with normal renal function, the mean AUC ratio of tofacitinib for rheumatoid arthritis patients increased progressively with deterioration of renal function. However, no mechanisms for increase of tofacitinib AUC in patients with renal impairment were proposed. There were no reports of tofacitinib showing pharmacokinetic changes associated with hepatic and/or intestinal metabolism, such as CYP protein expression, CYP enzyme activity, or renal function in the acute renal failure model. Since 70% of the dose is metabolized and 30% is excreted in the urine [9–11], renal failure seems to significantly impact the metabolism and excretion of tofacitinib as well as its absorption and distribution.

The aim of this study was to evaluate the effects of renal failure on the pharmacokinetics of tofacitinib using gentamicin (G-ARF) and cisplatin-induced acute renal failure (C-ARF) rat models and to report that the increase in AUC of tofacitinib is attributed to the decreases in renal and nonrenal clearances following intravenous and oral administration of tofacitinib to G-ARF and C-ARF rats.

2. Materials and Methods

2.1. Chemicals

Tofacitinib citrate and hydrocortisone (an internal standard) were obtained from Sigma Aldrich (St. Louis, MO, USA), and ethyl acetate for high-performance liquid chromatography (HPLC) analysis was purchased from J.T. Baker (Phillipsburg, NJ, USA). Gentamicin and cisplatin were obtained from Shin Poong Pharmaceutical (Seoul, Korea) and Tokyo Chemical Industry (Tokyo, Japan), respectively.

Heparin and 0.9% NaCl-injectable solution were purchased from JW Pharmaceutical Corporation (Seoul, Korea), and β-cyclodextrin is a product of Wako (Osaka, Japan). Primary antibodies to CYP2B1/2, CYP1A1/2, CYP2D1, CYP2C11, CYP2E1, and CYP3A1/2 were produced by Detroit R&D Inc. (Detroit, MI, USA). β-actin was purchased from Cell Signaling Technology (Beverly, MA, USA). Secondary goat, rabbit, and mouse antibodies were purchased from Bio-Rad (Hercules, CA, USA). All other chemicals and reagents were analysis- or HPLC-grade and used without further purification.

2.2. Animals

Sprague–Dawley rats (male, 7 weeks old, weight 200–230 g) were purchased from OrientBio Korea (Seongnam, Korea) and individually managed in a clean room maintained under 12-h light (07:00–19:00)/12-h dark (19:00–07:00) cycles at 22 ± 1 °C with a relative humidity of $50 \pm 5\%$ through air purification (Laboratory Animal Research Center of Ajou University Medical Center, Suwon, Korea). All rats were fed with food and water as desired without any restriction. All experimental methods and protocols were carried out according to standard operating procedures with approval by Institutional Animal Care and Use Committee (IACUC No. 2017-0074, 2018) of Laboratory Animal Research Center of Ajou University Medical Center.

2.3. Induction of Acute Renal Failure

Rats were randomly divided into three groups: control, G-ARF, and C-ARF rats. Acute renal failure was induced in rats by intraperitoneal injection of gentamicin (100 mg/kg, dissolved in 0.9% NaCl-injectable solution) daily for 8 days [19] or by a single intraperitoneal injection of cisplatin (7.5 mg/kg, dissolved in 0.9% NaCl-injectable solution) [20], while control rats were injected with 0.9% NaCl-injectable solution only. The end times of renal failure induction for pharmcokinetic study of tofacitinib were the next day from the last administration of gentamicin and the sixth day from a single intraperitoneal injection of cisplatin. BUN (Blood urea nitrogen) levels were measured in rats on the last day of induction using a BUN detection kit (Asan Pharmaceutical, Seoul, Korea). Rats with a urea nitrogen level of 36 mg/dL or higher were considered to be acute renal failure-induced [21] and were selected for the study.

2.4. Preliminary Study

For preliminary study, plasma samples were collected from control, G-ARF, and C-ARF rats ($n = 3$ per group) to measure total protein, albumin, creatinine, glutamate pyruvate transaminase (GPT), and glutamate oxaloacetate transaminase (GOT) levels (Green Cross Reference Lab, Seoul, Korea). Urine samples were collected for 24 h, and urine volumes and creatinine levels were also measured to estimate the creatinine clearance (CL_{CR}). CL_{CR} was calculated by dividing the total amount of creatinine excreted in urine for 24 h by area under the plasma concentration-time curve of creatinine from 0 to 24 h ($AUC_{0-24\,h}$), assuming that renal function was stable during the experiment. Whole liver and kidneys were removed from each rat, weighed, partially excised, and soaked in 10% formalin to fix for tissue biopsies.

2.5. Intravenous and Oral Administration of Tofacitinib

For oral and intravenous administration, pretreatment and surgical procedures were performed as previously reported [12]. For oral study, the rats were restricted from eating food overnight but water was freely accessible. The next day, after anesthesia with ketamine at a dose of 100 mg/kg, polyethylene 50 tubes (Clay Adams, Parsippany, NJ, USA) was cannulated into the carotid artery for blood collection. For intravenous study, polyethylene 50 tubes were cannulated into the carotid artery and jugular vein for blood collection and drug administration, respectively. After surgery, rats were allowed to rest for 2–3 h to recover from anesthesia and were free in the individual metabolic cage during the experiment.

For intravenous administration, tofacitinib (dissolved in 0.9% NaCl-injectable solution containing 0.5% β-cyclodextrin) was infused for 1 min at a dose of 10 mg/kg via the jugular veins of control ($n = 6$), G-ARF ($n = 8$), and C-ARF ($n = 7$) rats. Blood samples (110 µL) were collected through the carotid artery at 0 (prior to drug infusion), 1 (at the end of drug infusion), 5, 15, 30, 45, 60, 90, 120, 180, 240, 360, 480, 600, and 720 min and were centrifuged at 8000 × g for 1 min. Plasma samples were collected and immediately stored in a −80 °C freezer until HPLC analysis of tofacitinib could be performed [22]. After collecting each blood sample, 0.3 mL of heparinized 0.9% NaCl-injectable solution (10 IU/mL) was immediately administered to the carotid artery to prevent blood clotting. At 24 h, the rat's abdomen was open and the entire gastrointestinal tract was removed, transferred to a beaker with 50 mL of methanol, and cut into small pieces. After mixing the contents in the beaker thoroughly, two 100 µL aliquots of supernatant were taken and stored at −80 °C until HPLC analysis of tofacitinib could be performed [22].

At 24 h after drug administration, urine samples were also collected. The metabolic cage was rinsed with 20 mL of distilled water, which was combined with the 24-h urine sample. The volume of combined urine sample was measured and two 100 µL aliquots of each combined sample were taken and stored in the −80 °C freezer until tofacitinib analysis by HPLC could be performed [22].

For oral administration, tofacitinib at a dose of 20 mg/kg was administered to control ($n = 8$), G-ARF ($n = 6$), and C-ARF ($n = 8$) rats. Blood samples (110 µL) were collected through the carotid artery at 0 (prior to drug administration), 5, 15, 30, 45, 60, 90, 120, 180, 240, 360, 480, 600, and 720 min. At 24 h after drug administration, urine and gastrointestinal tract samples were collected and handled similarly to those in the intravenous study.

2.6. Measurement of V_{max}, K_m, and CL_{int}

For preparation of hepatic and intestinal microsomes, the experimental processes were similar to a previously reported method [23,24]. Protein concentration in the hepatic and intestinal microsomes was measured using the bicinchoninic acid (BCA) assay. The in vitro metabolic system consisted of microsomes (equivalent to 1 mg protein); 5 µL dimethylsulfoxide containing final tofacitinib concentrations of 1, 2, 5, 10, 20, 50, 100, 200, 300, and 400 µM; and an nicotinamide adenine dinucleotide phosphate hydrogen (NADPH)-generating system (Corning Inc., Corning, NY, USA). The volume of the system was adjusted to 1 mL by adding 0.1 M phosphate buffer (pH 7.4), and the components were incubated in a water-bath shaker at 37 °C with 50 oscillations per min (opm) for 15 min. After this incubation, the reaction was terminated by adding two volumes of acetonitrile. Subsequently, two 50-µL aliquots of each reaction mixture were collected. The kinetic constants, maximum velocity (V_{max}) and apparent Michaelis–Menten constant (K_m; the concentration at which the rate is one-half of V_{max} for the metabolism of tofacitinib) were determined using the Lineweaver–Burk plot [24,25]. The intrinsic clearance (CL_{int}) for the metabolism of tofacitinib was determined by dividing V_{max} by K_m [24,25].

2.7. Immunoblot Analysis

For immunoblot analysis, microsomal protein samples (20–40 µg protein per lane) were resolved by 10% sodium dodecyl sulfate polyacrylamide gel electrophoresis (SDS-PAGE) gel and the loaded gel was transferred onto a nitrocellulose membrane for 1 h. For immunodetection, blots were incubated overnight with a primary antibody diluted in Tris-buffered saline (TBS) with 0.1% Tween 20 (TBS-T) containing 5% bovine serum albumin (1:2000) at 4 °C with gentle shaking. Subsequently, blots were incubated with secondary antibody conjugated to horseradish peroxide diluted at 1:10,000 with TBS-T containing 5% skim milk for 1 h at room temperature. Protein expression was measured by enhanced chemiluminescence (Bio-Rad) using an Image Quant LAS 4000 Mini (GE Healthcare Life Sciences, Piscataway, NJ, USA). β-actin was used as the internal standard [26]. The density of bands was quantified using ImageJ 1.45s software (NIH, Bethesda, MA, USA).

2.8. HPLC Analysis

A 50-μL aliquot of biological sample was mixed with 1 μL hydrocortisone (5 mg/mL); then, 20 μL of 20% ammonia solution was added, mixed with a vortex-mixer (Scientific Industries, Bohemia, NY, USA) for 30 s, and extracted with 750 μL ethyl acetate. The organic layer was collected, evaporated on a thermobath (Eyela, Tokyo, Japan) under a gentle stream of nitrogen gas at 40 °C and redissolved by adding 130 μL 20% acetonitrile, and 50 μL of each reconstituted sample was analyzed by HPLC [12,22].

The concentration of tofacitinib in the biological sample was measured using a Prominence LC-20A HPLC system (Shimadzu, Kyoto, Japan). The reconstituted biological samples were filtered through a 0.45-μm filter (Millipore, Billerica, MA, USA) and analyzed with a reversed-phase column (C_{18}; 25 cm × 4.6 mm, 5 μm; Young Jin Biochrom, Seongnam, Korea) using a UV detector at 287 nm. The mobile phase consisted of 10 mM ammonium acetate buffer (pH 5.0) and acetonitrile at a ratio of 69.5:30.5 (v/v) with a flow rate of 1.0 mL/min. Tofacitinib and the internal standard were separated at approximately 7.21 and 11.3 min, respectively. The lower limits of quantitation of tofacitinib in rat plasma and urine were 0.01 and 0.1 μg/mL, respectively, and the intraday assay precisions (coefficients of variation) were 3.69–5.88% and 4.21–6.18%, respectively. In addition, interday assay precisions in rat plasma and urine were 5.06% and 5.46%, respectively [22].

2.9. Pharmacokinetic Analysis

To estimate pharmacokinetic parameters such as terminal half-life, the apparent volume of distribution at steady state (V_{ss}), area under plasma concentration-time curves from time zero to time infinity (AUC), mean residence time (MRT), and time-averaged total body (CL), and renal (CL_R) and nonrenal (CL_{NR}) clearances, standard methods [27] were applied using noncompartmental analysis (WinNonlin, Pharsight Corporation, Mountain View, CA, USA). AUCs were calculated using the trapezoidal rule-extrapolation method [28]. The peak plasma concentration (C_{max}) and time that the plasma concentration was peak (T_{max}) were directly confirmed from plasma concentration-time curves. To calculate the average values of clearances [29], terminal half-life [30], and V_{ss} [31], the harmonic mean method was applied.

2.10. Statistical Analysis

The p values were estimated using Tukey's posttest for comparison among three means after analysis of variance (ANOVA) and were considered significant when less than 0.05. All data are expressed as mean ± standard deviation, and a median (ranges) value is used for T_{max}.

3. Results

3.1. Induction of Acute Renal Failure

Renal dysfunction was observed in G-ARF and C-ARF rats. Urea nitrogen (898% and 3449% increase, respectively) and creatinine level (111% and 768% increase, respectively) in the blood showed a significant increase and kidney weight (% of body weight) (58.4% and 59.9% increase, respectively) and urine output (172% and 436% increase, respectively) also showed a significant increase, but CL_{CR} was significantly decreased by 39.7% and 95.3% in G-ARF and C-ARF rats, respectively, than in control rats (Figure 2A). A decrease in renal function was also confirmed by kidney microscopy; severe renal damage including tubular necrosis and inflammation was observed in G-ARF and C-ARF rats (Figure 2B). Liver function also appeared to be impaired in G-ARF and C-ARF rats. GOT was significantly increased by 66.2 and 69.0%, respectively; however, no considerable tissue alterations were found in liver microscopy (Figure 2B). In terms of weight gain changes, the body weight gains significantly decreased in G-ARF (8.24% decrease) and C-ARF (23.0% decrease) rats compared to that in control rats (5.75% increase) (Figure 2A). Comparing the two ARF rat models, the C-ARF model showed more severe renal impairment based on urea nitrogen, creatinine, CL_{CR}, urine output, kidney weight (% of body weight), and kidney microscopy (Figure 2A,B).

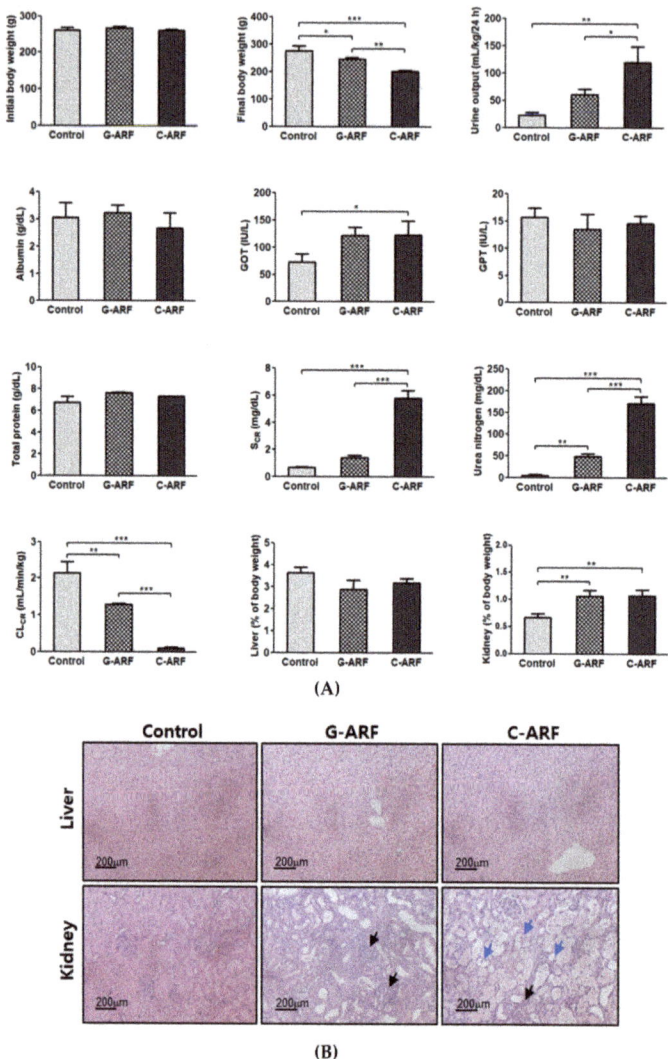

Figure 2. (**A**) The mean values (± standard deviation) of initial and final body weights, 24-h urine output, plasma concentrations of albumin, glutamate oxaloacetate transaminase (GOT), glutamate pyruvate transaminase (GPT), total protein, S_{CR}, urea nitrogen, CL_{CR}, and relative liver and kidney weights in control, gentamicin (G-ARF) and cisplatin-induced acute renal failure (C-ARF) rats: Bars mean standard deviation. * $p < 0.05$, ** $p < 0.01$, and *** $p < 0.001$; (**B**) Liver and kidney biopsies in control, G-ARF, and C-ARF rats. Black arrows indicate infiltration with immune cells. Blue arrows indicate the tissue damages including tubular necrosis and massive cell death. CL_{CR}: creatinine clearance; S_{CR}: serum creatinine.

3.2. Pharmacokinetics of Tofacitinib After Intravenous Administration

After intravenous administration of 10 mg/kg tofacitinib to control, G-ARF, and C-ARF rats, the mean arterial plasma concentration-time curves of tofacitinib declined in a polyexponential fashion for the three groups, with significantly higher plasma levels in rats with G-ARF and C-ARF than in control rats (Figure 3). This resulted in a significantly higher AUC of tofacitinib (64.0 and 163% increase, respectively) than that in control rats (Table 1). The higher AUC of tofacitinib could be due to the significantly lower CL of tofacitinib by 37.7 and 62.3% in rats with G-ARF and C-ARF, respectively (Table 1). A significantly longer terminal half-life (78.7 and 240% increase, respectively) and MRT (96.7 and 154% increase, respectively) of tofacitinib in rats with G-ARF and C-ARF also supports the lower CL of tofacitinib in rats with G-ARF and C-ARF. Lower CL of tofacitinib was due to the slower metabolism of tofacitinib; CL_{NR}s of tofacitinib in rats with G-ARF and C-ARF were significantly lower by 33.2 and 57.4%, respectively (Table 1). Tofacitinib excreted in urine as unchanged for 24 h ($Ae_{0-24\,h}$) was significantly lower by 37.7 and 95.2% in rats with G-ARF and C-ARF, respectively, than that in control rats (Table 1), perhaps due to significantly impaired kidney function in rats with G-ARF and C-ARF. Thus, CL_Rs of tofacitinib were significantly lower by 69.5 and 98.6% in rats with G-ARF and C-ARF, respectively, compared to that in control rats (Table 1). The percentage of dose remaining in the gastrointestinal tract at 24 h ($GI_{24\,h}$) was 0.00919–0.195% of the intravenous dose and did not significantly differ among the three groups of rats, suggesting that the contribution of gastrointestinal excretion (including biliary excretion) of tofacitinib to CL_{NR} of tofacitinib was not significant. The V_{ss} values were comparable among the three groups (Table 1). Therefore, the significantly lower CL of tofacitinib in rats with G-ARF and C-ARF may be due to slower metabolism and lower renal excretion of tofacitinib than control rats. Plasma concentration and pharmacokinetic parameters of tofacitinib in C-ARF rats were significantly different from those in G-ARF rats (Table 1 and Figure 3) due to more severe renal impairment in C-ARF rats (Figure 2).

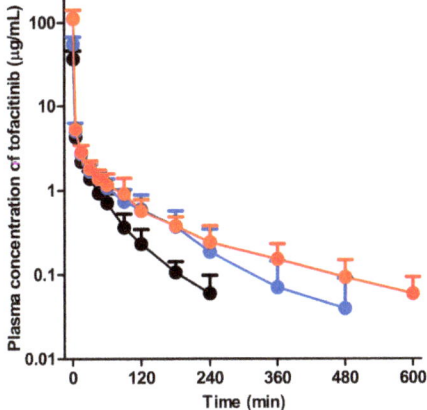

Figure 3. Mean arterial plasma concentration-time curves of tofacitinib after 1-min intravenous infusion at a dose of 10 mg/kg to control (black; $n = 6$), G-ARF (blue; $n = 8$) and C-ARF (red; $n = 7$) rats: Bars represent standard deviation. G-ARF: gentamicin-induced acute renal failure; C-ARF: cisplatin-induced acute renal failure.

Table 1. Mean (±standard deviation) pharmacokinetic parameters of tofacitinib after 1-min intravenous infusion at a dose of 10 mg/kg to control, G-ARF, and C-ARF rats.

Parameters	Control ($n = 6$)	G-ARF ($n = 8$)	C-ARF ($n = 7$)
Body weight (g) [a]	280 ± 19.0	251 ± 21.3	188 ± 10.2
Terminal half-life (min) [b]	39.4 ± 11.3	70.4 ± 29.6	134 ± 40.9
AUC (μg·min/mL) [a]	264 ± 45.4	433 ± 90.0	693 ± 105
MRT (min) [c]	27.2 ± 10.4	53.5 ± 30.2	69.1 ± 39.6
CL (mL/min/kg) [d]	39.0 ± 7.97	24.3 ± 6.95	14.7 ± 2.29
CL_R (mL/min/kg) [e]	4.75 ± 1.28	1.45 ± 1.54	0.0679 ± 0.0917
CL_{NR} (mL/min/kg) [f]	34.3 ± 6.77	22.9 ± 5.54	14.6 ± 2.26
V_{ss} (mL/kg)	1042 ± 402	1174 ± 519	1002 ± 558
$Ae_{0-24\,h}$ (% of dose) [a]	9.51 ± 0.879	5.92 ± 2.76	0.458 ± 0.626
$GI_{24\,h}$ (% of dose)	0.153 ± 0.306	0.00919 ± 0.0225	0.195 ± 0.157

$Ae_{0-24\,h}$: percentage of the dose excreted in the 24-h urine; AUC: total area under the plasma concentration–time curve from time zero to time infinity; C-ARF: cisplatin-induced acute renal failure; CL: time-averaged total body clearance; CL_{NR}: time-averaged nonrenal clearance; CL_R: time-averaged renal clearance; G-ARF: gentamicin-induced acute renal failure; $GI_{24\,h}$: percentage of the dose remaining in the gastrointestinal tract (including its contents and feces) at 24 h; MRT: mean residence time; V_{ss}: apparent volume of distribution at steady state. [a] Control is significantly different ($p < 0.01$) from C-ARF and G-ARF. [b] Control is significantly different from C-ARF ($p < 0.001$) and G-ARF ($p < 0.01$). [c] Control is significantly different from G-ARF ($p < 0.05$). [d] Control is significantly different from G-ARF and C-ARF ($p < 0.001$). G-ARF and C-ARF were significantly different ($p < 0.05$). [e] Control is significantly different from G-ARF and C-ARF ($p < 0.001$). [f] Control is significantly different from G-ARF ($p < 0.01$) and C-ARF ($p < 0.001$). G-ARF and C-ARF were significantly different ($p < 0.01$).

3.3. Pharmacokinetics of Tofacitinib After Oral Administration

After oral administration of 20 mg/kg tofacitinib to control, G-ARF, and C-ARF rats, the mean arterial plasma concentration-time profiles of tofacitinib were created and are shown in Figure 4. Relevant pharmacokinetic parameters of tofacitinib were summarized in Table 2.

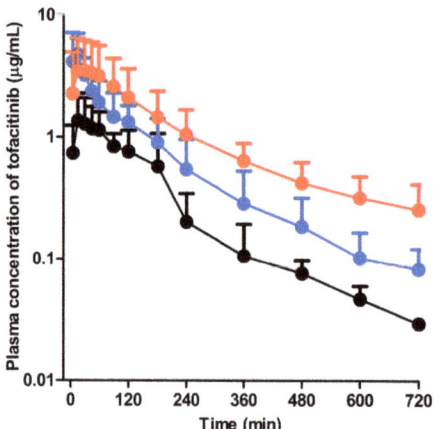

Figure 4. Mean arterial plasma concentration–time curves of tofacitinib after oral administration at a dose of 20 mg/kg to control (black; $n = 8$), G-ARF (blue; $n = 6$), and C-ARF (red; $n = 8$) rats: Bars represent standard deviation. G-ARF: gentamicin-induced acute renal failure; C-ARF: cisplatin-induced acute renal failure.

Table 2. Mean (±standard deviation) pharmacokinetic parameters of tofacitinib after oral administration at a dose of 20 mg/kg to control, G-ARF, and C-ARF rats.

Parameters	Control ($n = 8$)	G-ARF ($n = 6$)	C-ARF ($n = 8$)
Body weight (g) [a]	264 ± 26.3	206 ± 14.9	174 ± 11.7
AUC (µg·min/mL) [b]	217 ± 22.3	525 ± 178	752 ± 420
C_{max} (µg/mL) [c]	1.74 ± 0.606	5.18 ± 2.59	4.20 ± 3.03
T_{max} (min)	71.9 ± 64.7	30.8 ± 43.9	41.3 ± 36.5
CL_R (mL/min/kg) [a]	5.66 ± 1.03	1.71 ± 0.871	0.300 ± 0.495
$Ae_{0-24\,h}$ (% of dose) [d]	6.21 ± 1.12	4.82 ± 3.06	1.16 ± 1.37
$GI_{24\,h}$ (% of dose)	0.231 ± 0.235	1.27 ± 1.72	0.505 ± 0.535

$Ae_{0-24\,h}$: percentage of the dose excreted in the 24-h urine; AUC: total area under the plasma concentration–time curve from time zero to last time; C-ARF: cisplatin-induced acute renal failure; CL_R: time-averaged renal clearance; C_{max}: peak plasma concentration; G-ARF: gentamicin-induced acute renal failure; $GI_{24\,h}$: percentage of the dose remaining in the gastrointestinal tract (including its contents and feces) at 24 h; T_{max}: time that the plasma concentration was peak. [a] Control is significantly different from G-ARF and C-ARF ($p < 0.001$). G-ARF and C-ARF were significantly different ($p < 0.05$). [b] Control is significantly different from C-ARF ($p < 0.01$). [c] Control is significantly different from G-ARF ($p < 0.05$). [d] C-ARF is significantly different from control ($p < 0.001$) and G-ARF ($p < 0.05$).

Absorption of tofacitinib from the gastrointestinal tract occurred rapidly; the plasma concentration of tofacitinib was found at 5 min, the first blood collection time after oral administration in all three groups. Compared to the control rats, G-ARF and C-ARF rats showed higher mean arterial plasma concentration of tofacitinib, resulting in a significant increase in AUC (142 and 247% increase, respectively) and C_{max} (198 and 141% increase, respectively) (Table 2). However, the CL_R values significantly decreased by 69.8 and 94.0% in G-ARF and C-ARF rats, respectively, due to the significant increase in AUC and a significant decrease in $Ae_{0-24\,h}$ (22.4 and 81.3% decrease, respectively) in G-ARF and C-ARF rats (Table 2). $GI_{24\,h}$ values were 0.231, 1.27, and 0.505% of the oral dose in control, G-ARF, and C-ARF rats, respectively, indicating that absorption of tofacitinib from the gastrointestinal tract was almost complete with no significant difference among the three groups (Table 2). The T_{max} values were likewise not significantly different among the three groups. After oral administration, F values of tofacitinib were 41.3, 60.7, and 54.3% in control, G-ARF, and C-ARF rats, respectively (Table 2). Plasma concentration and pharmacokinetic parameters of tofacitinib in C-ARF rats, such as AUC, CL_R, and $Ae_{0-24\,h}$, were significantly different from those in G-ARF rats due to severe renal impairment in C-ARF rats (Table 2 and Figure 4); this was similar to the results produced by the intravenous study.

3.4. Effect of Acute Renal Failure on CYP Enzyme Expression

In rats with G-ARF and C-ARF, hepatic and intestinal expression of CYP2B1/2, CYP1A1/2, CYP2D1, CYP2C11, CYP2E1, and CYP3A1/2 were monitored (Figure 5). Immunoblot analysis showed that hepatic expression of CYP2C11 in rats with G-ARF and C-ARF decreased to 53.1 and 49.2% of the level in control rats, respectively, and CYP3A1/2 expression in rats with G-ARF and C-ARF also decreased by 14.6 and 60.8%, respectively, compared to that in control rats. However, CYP2E1 expression in rats with G-ARF and C-ARF increased by 1.33 and 1.73 times, respectively, compared to that in control rats. Expression of CYP1A1/2 and CYP2D1 was comparable among the three groups of rats. Interestingly, protein expression in the intestine showed the opposite trend (Figure 5). The intestinal expression of CYP3A1/2 in rats with G-ARF and C-ARF increased 5.30 and 7.97 times, respectively, and CYP2C11 expression also increased by 3.30 and 3.27 times, respectively, compared to those in control rats. Other CYP protein expressions except CYP2E1 also increased in the intestine of G-ARF and C-ARF rats.

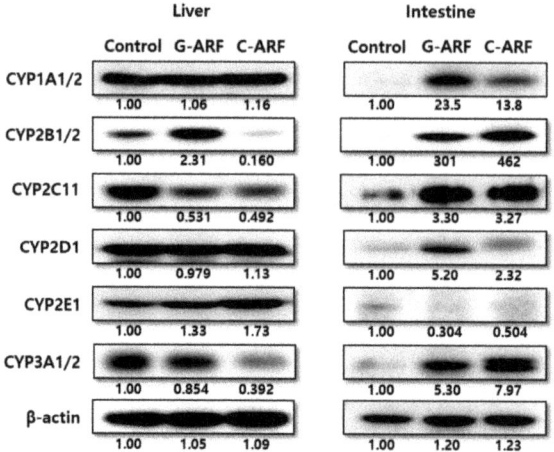

Figure 5. Protein expression of CYP450 isozymes in hepatic and intestinal microsomes in control, G-ARF, and C-ARF rats by immunoblot analyses: ß-actin was used as a loading control. This experiment was performed three times. Band density was measured using ImageJ1.45s software (NIH). G-ARF: gentamicin-induced acute renal failure; C-ARF: cisplatin-induced acute renal failure.

3.5. Measurement of V_{max}, K_m, and CL_{int} of Tofacitinib in Hepatic Microsomes

In rats with G-ARF and C-ARF, the V_{max} values for the disappearance of tofacitinib in the hepatic microsomal protein decreased by 9.52 and 28.7%, respectively, but were not significantly different compared to that in control rats (Figure 6). K_m values were comparable among the three groups (Figure 6). However, CL_{int} for the disappearance of tofacitinib in the hepatic microsomal protein was significantly lower (54.4% decrease) in rats with C-ARF compared to that in control rats (Figure 6), suggesting that disappearance of tofacitinib could be slower in C-ARF rats. CL_{int} was also lower (31.1% decrease) but not significantly different in G-ARF rats compared to that in control rats. Taken together, our data indicate that G-ARF or C-ARF affect hepatic function to inhibit the expression of CYP3A1/2 and CYP2C11, resulting in slower metabolism of tofacitinib.

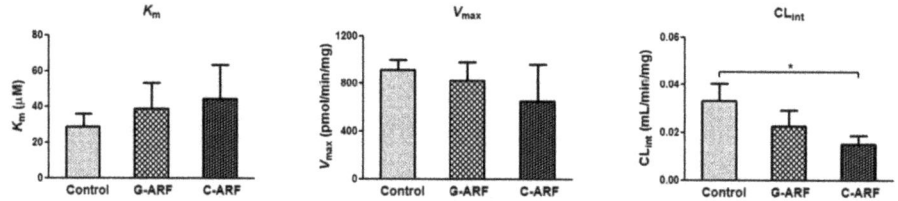

Figure 6. Measurement of V_{max}, K_m, and CL_{int} for the disappearance of tofacitinib in hepatic microsomes of control, G-ARF, and C-ARF rats (n = 3 per group): This experiment was performed three times, and data are expressed as mean ± standard deviation. Bars represent standard deviation. * $p < 0.05$. V_{max}: maximum velocity; K_m: apparent Michaelis–Menten constant, the concentration at which the rate is one-half of V_{max} for the metabolism of tofacitinib; CL_{int}: intrinsic clearance; G-ARF: gentamicin-induced acute renal failure; C-ARF: cisplatin-induced acute renal failure.

4. Discussion

To establish acute renal failure, gentamicin and cisplatin were chosen. Gentamicin, a representative aminoglycoside antibiotic, induces moderate and reversible acute renal failure [32], while cisplatin, a chemotherapeutic drug, causes more severe and irreversible acute renal failure [33]. Both drugs accumulate in the renal tubule; produce reactive oxygen species (ROS) such as superoxide anion, hydrogen peroxide, and hydroxyl radical; and result in the induction of tubular necrosis and/or apoptosis [34–36]. The impaired renal function caused by these drugs was fully demonstrated, but liver damage did not seem to be serious in our preliminary study. Induction of acute renal failure by gentamicin and cisplatin was confirmed not only by a significant decrease in weight gain and CL_{CR} but also by significant increases in 24-h urine output and plasma levels of urea nitrogen and creatinine than those in control rats. Renal biopsy also demonstrated the induction of acute renal failure.

The contribution of gastrointestinal excretion (including biliary excretion) as unchanged tofacitinib to CL_{NR} of the drug seems to be nearly negligible. The GI_{24h} values were negligible in control, G-ARF, and C-ARF rats, i.e., less than 0.195% of the intravenous dose in the three groups (Table 1). This lower GI_{24h} did not appear to be caused by chemical or enzymatic degradation of tofacitinib in the rat's gastrointestinal tract; tofacitinib was stable when incubated for 24 h in various buffers of pH 2–10 [22] and in the gastric juice of rats (pH 3.5) (data not shown). Furthermore, according to a report by Lee and Kim [12], when 10 mg/kg tofacitinib was intravenously administered to rats ($n = 3$) after bile duct cannulation, biliary excretion of unchanged tofacitinib for 24 h was 0.703% of the intravenous dose, a nearly negligible contribution to CL_{NR} of tofacitinib. Therefore, the CL_{NR} value shown in Table 1 may represent the metabolic clearance of tofacitinib.

The AUCs of tofacitinib were not dose proportional after intravenous doses over 20 mg/kg and oral doses over 50 mg/kg were administered [12]. A dose of 10 mg/kg of tofacitinib was chosen for the intravenous study, and 20 mg/kg of tofacitinib was selected for the oral study. After intravenous administration of tofacitinib to G-ARF and C-ARF rats, its AUCs were significantly higher, possibly as a result of significantly slower CL than in control rats. The lower CL of tofacitinib was attributable to significantly decreased CL_R and CL_{NR} of the drug in rats with G-ARF and C-ARF than in controls. The lower CL_R may have been due to both significantly lower Ae_{0-24h} and higher AUCs in G-ARF and C-ARF rats. The higher AUC in rats with G-ARF and C-ARF was due to lower Ae_{0-24h} and lower CL_{NR} than those in control rats. The lower Ae_{0-24h} in G-ARF and C-ARF rats could have been due to impaired kidney function. Tofacitinib did not show a urine flow rate-dependent timed-interval CL_R in rats; a straight line was not found between 1/timed-interval CL_R of tofacitinib and 1/urine flow rate among the three groups [37]. Greater urine output did not result in higher Ae_{0-24h} of tofacitinib, indicating that tofacitinib was not predominantly reabsorbed in the renal tubule. The significantly greater urine output in rats with G-ARF and C-ARF was because reabsorption of water was decreased in the renal tubule due to decrease in protein expression of aquaporins caused by gentamicin and cisplatin [38]. However, Ae_{0-24h} of some drugs showed a urine flow rate-dependent timed-interval CL_R in rats; the lower the urine output, the lower the Ae_{0-24h} [37], which resulted in a straight line between 1/timed-interval CL_R and 1/urine flow rate in both control and uranyl nitrate-induced acute renal failure (U-ARF) rats [23,39].

The CL_R values of tofacitinib were estimated from free (unbound to plasma proteins) fractions in plasma; the values thus estimated were 5.99, 1.83, and 0.0856 mL/min/kg for control, G-ARF, and C-ARF rats, respectively, based on 20.7% plasma protein binding of tofacitinib measured by equilibrium dialysis [22]. The CL_R values of tofacitinib were faster than their respective CL_{CR}s in control and G-ARF rats, but CL_Rs of tofacitinib and CL_{CR} in C-ARF rats were comparable each other, suggesting that tofacitinib is mainly excreted in urine via active secretion for control and G-ARF-rats [12,18,24] and in glomerular filtration for C-ARF rats. This was also supported by control and U-ARF rats; CL_R of metformin and chlorzoxazone were faster than CL_{CR} in control rats, but CL_R of both drugs and CL_{CR} were comparable in U-ARF rats, and thus both drugs were mainly excreted in urine via active secretion for control rats and glomerular filtration for U-ARF rat [23,39]. As shown in the results, both gentamicin and cisplatin induced acute renal failure by tubular necrosis through ROS production, but cisplatin induced more severe renal failure and seemed to completely inhibit the function of active secretion [40].

Based on the AUC difference between intravenous and intraportal administration of tofacitinib to rats, the first-pass metabolism of tofacitinib by the liver after reaching the portal vein was approximately 42.0% [12]. Therefore, tofacitinib has a characteristic with an intermediate hepatic extraction ratio and its hepatic clearance could be changed by both the hepatic CL_{int} and the hepatic blood flow rates [41]. Thus, a significantly lower CL_{NR} of tofacitinib when administered intravenously to rats with G-ARF and C-ARF could have been due to a significantly lower CL_{int} for the elimination of tofacitinib in the liver. The reduced protein expressions and activities of the hepatic CYP3A1/2 and CYP2C11 subfamily could have been responsible for the lower hepatic CL_{int} in G-ARF and C-ARF rats. Similar results with regard to changes in hepatic CYP3A1/2 and/or CYP2C11 isozymes have been reported in acute renal failure rats induced by glycerol, bilateral ureter ligation, and nephrectomy [42]. Surgically induced chronic kidney disease rat models also showed lower levels of hepatic CYP3A and CYP2C subfamilies compared to sham-operated control rats [43]. Consistent with our result in renal failure rat models, the CYP3A subfamily also decreased in patients with end-stage renal failure [44].

After intravenous administration of tofacitinib to control, G-ARF, and C-ARF rats, its V_{ss} values were not significantly different among the three groups of rats, since the free fractions of tofacitinib in the plasma from control, G-ARF and C-ARF rats were comparable (data not shown). Similar results were also reported for cyclosporin [45] in G-ARF rats and tacrolimus [46] in C-ARF rats, whereas the V_{ss} of metformin [23]; omeprazole [26]; and DA-1131, a new carbapenem [47] in U-ARF rats, significantly increased compared to that in control rats, which was due to the increase in free fraction of the drugs.

After oral administration of tofacitinib to rats with G-ARF and C-ARF, the AUC values were also significantly higher than in control rats. The absorption of tofacitinib from the gastrointestinal tract was almost complete among all three groups; GI_{24h} values were less than 1.27% of oral dose for control, G-ARF, and C-ARF rats. Therefore, absorption is not a factor for the higher AUCs in rats with G-ARF and C-ARF. However, decreased absorption after oral administration of azosemide [48]; oltipraz [49]; and YJA-20379-8, a new proton pump inhibitor [50], to rats with U-ARF has been reported. Although the expression of CYP3A1/2 and CYP2C11 in the intestine markedly increased in rats with G-ARF and C-ARF compared to those in control rats, AUC of tofacitinib increased in rats with G-ARF and C-ARF. The CL_{int} for the disappearance of tofacitinib in the intestinal microsome was not measured in this study because the active site of CYP3A1/2 and CYP2C11 in the intestine was sensitive and very unstable [51]. It has been reported that CYP3A activity in the intestine was increased in renal failure models induced by cisplatin, glycerol, bilateral ligation, or nephrectomy [42]. The AUC increase in rats with G-ARF and C-ARF might be because active secretion of tofacitinib was reduced by tubular necrosis caused by gentamicin and cisplatin. Thus, tofacitinib accumulated in the body, resulting in significantly lower Ae_{0-24h} of oral dose and significantly lower CL_R along with increased AUCs in rats with G-ARF and C-ARF than in control rats (Table 2). In addition, considering that approximately 21.3% of the oral dose was metabolized in the liver of control rats after oral administration of tofacitinib [12], the hepatic first-pass effect seemed to decrease in rats with G-ARF and C-ARF after absorption of tofacitinib into the portal vein. This was likely due to decreased hepatic enzyme activity, and protein expression of CYP3A1/2 and CYP2C11 in rats with G-ARF and C-ARF, which also contributed to the increase in AUC of tofacitinib after oral administration of the drug.

Consistent with our data in renal-failure rat models, results of a previous study showed that CYP3A subfamily decreased in patients with end-stage renal failure [44]. In patients with severe renal impairment, the plasma concentration of tofacitinib was significantly increased and, thus, the AUC of tofacitinib in these patients was higher than twice that in normal healthy subjects, suggesting that the reduction of tofacitinib dosage is recommended in patients with severe renal failure [18]. Because the renal excretion of tofacitinib was different between human and rats (approximately 30% of oral tofacitinib in human [9] and 6.21% of oral dose in rats), it is difficult to clearly conclude the clinical significance of the rat's results, but it seems clear that the increase of AUC in the renal failure state was due to slower hepatic metabolism and smaller urinary excretion of the drug. Our study could be applied to drug–drug interactions in clinical practice when administered in combination with CYP3A4 and CYP2C19 inhibitors, such as itraconazole and erythromycin, which may result in an increase in plasma concentration of tofacitinib by reduced nonrenal elimination of tofacitinib. Therefore, it is necessary to consider the dose reduction of tofacitinib when AUC increases twice or more.

5. Conclusions

After intravenous administration of tofacitinib to G-ARF and C-ARF rats, its AUC was significantly higher than that in control rats due to a significantly lower CL_{NR} (due to a decrease in the protein expressions of the hepatic CYP3A1/2 and CYP2C11 subfamily) and CL_R (due to a significantly lower CL_{CR} by an impaired kidney function) than in control rats. A reduced dosage of tofacitinib could be considered in patients with renal impairment based on their level of renal dysfunction.

Author Contributions: S.H.B. performed all of the animal experiments and the HPLC analysis of tofacitinib in the biological samples and estimated the pharmacokinetic parameters. S.-Y.C. performed the liver and kidney biopsies and interpreted the results. S.H.K. designed the experiments, performed the statistical analysis and graphics work, and drafted the manuscript. All authors have read and approved the final manuscript.

Funding: This work was supported by the Korea Health Technology R&D Project (HI16C0992) through the Korea Health Industry Development Institute (KHIDI) funded by the Ministry of Health and Welfare and the Basic Science Research Program (NRF-2018R1A2B6004895) through the National Research Foundation of Korea (NRF) grant funded by the Ministry of Science and ICT (MSIT), Republic of Korea.

Conflicts of Interest: The authors declare no competing financial interests.

References

1. Claxton, L.; Taylor, M.; Soonasra, A.; Bourret, J.A.; Gerber, R.A. An economic evaluation of tofacitinib treatment in rheumatoid arthritis after methotrexate or after 1 or 2 TNF inhibitors from a U.S. payer perspective. *J. Manag. Care Spec. Pharm.* **2018**, *24*, 1010–1017. [CrossRef] [PubMed]
2. Fukuda, T.; Naganuma, M.; Kanai, T. Current new challenges in the management of ulcerative colitis. *Intest. Res.* **2019**, *17*, 36–44. [CrossRef] [PubMed]
3. Antonelli, E.; Villanacci, V.; Bassotti, G. Novel oral-targeted therapies for mucosal healing in ulcerative colitis. *World J. Gastroenterol.* **2018**, *24*, 5322–5330. [CrossRef]
4. Bachelez, H.; Van de Kerkhof, P.C.; Strohal, R.; Kubanov, A.; Valenzuela, F.; Lee, J.H.; Gupta, P. Tofacitinib versus etanercept or placebo in moderate-to-severe chronic plaque psoriasis: A phase 3 randomised non-inferiority trial. *Lancet* **2015**, *386*, 552–561. [CrossRef]
5. Papp, K.A.; Menter, M.A.; Abe, M.; Elewski, B.; Feldman, S.R.; Gottlieb, A.B.; Langley, R.; Luger, T.; Thaci, D.; Buonanno, M.; et al. OPT Pivotal 1 and OPT Pivotal 2 investigators. Tofacitinib, an oral Janus kinase inhibitor, for the treatment of chronic plaque psoriasis: Results from two randomized, placebo-controlled, phase III trials. *Br. J. Dermatol.* **2015**, *173*, 949–961. [CrossRef] [PubMed]
6. Kennedy Crispin, M.; Ko, J.M.; Craiglow, B.G.; Li, S.; Shankar, G.; Urban, J.R.; Marinkovich, M.P. Safety and efficacy of the JAK inhibitor tofacitinib citrate in patients with alopecia areata. *JCI Insight* **2016**, *1*, e89776. [CrossRef]
7. Levy, L.L.; Urban, J.; King, B.A. Treatment of recalcitrant atopic dematitis with the oral Janus kinase inhibitor tofacitinib citrate. *J. Am. Acad. Dermatol.* **2015**, *73*, 395–399. [CrossRef] [PubMed]
8. Tahir, H. Therapies in ankylosing spondylitis-from clinical trials to clinical practice. *Rheumatology* **2018**, *57*, vi23–vi28. [CrossRef]
9. Dowty, M.E.; Lin, J.; Ryder, T.F.; Wang, W.; Walker, G.S.; Vaz, A.; Prakash, C. The pharmacokinetics, metabolism, and clearancemechanisms of tofacitinib, a janus kinase inhibitor, in humans. *Drug Metab. Dispos.* **2014**, *42*, 759–773. [CrossRef]
10. Cada, D.J.; Demaris, K.; Levien, T.L.; Baker, D.E. Tofacitinib. *Hosp. Pharm.* **2013**, *48*, 413–424. [CrossRef] [PubMed]
11. Scott, L.J. Tofacitinib: A review of its use in adult patients with rheumatoid arthritis. *Drugs* **2013**, *73*, 857–874. [CrossRef] [PubMed]
12. Lee, J.S.; Kim, S.H. Dose-dependent pharmacokinetics of tofacitinib in rats: Influence of hepatic and intestinal first-pass metabolism. *Pharmaceutics* **2019**, *11*, e318. [CrossRef]

13. Koivuniemi, R.; Paimela, L.; Suomalainen, R.; Leirisalo-Repo, M. Amyloidosis as a cause of death in patients with rheumatoid arthritis. *Clin. Exp. Rheumatol.* **2008**, *26*, 408–413. [PubMed]
14. Thomas, E.; Symmons, D.P.; Brewster, D.H.; Black, R.J.; Macfarlane, G.J. National study of cause-specific mortality in rheumatoid arthritis, juvenile chronic arthritis, and other rheumatic conditions: A 20 year followup study. *J. Rheumatol.* **2003**, *30*, 958–965. [PubMed]
15. Sihvonen, S.; Korpela, M.; Mustonen, J.; Laippala, P.; Pasternack, A. Renal disease as a predictor of increased mortality among patients with rheumatoid arthritis. *Nephron Clin. Pract.* **2004**, *96*, c107–c114. [CrossRef]
16. Karie, S.; Gandjbakhch, F.; Janus, N.; Launay-Vacher, V.; Rozenberg, S.; Mai Ba, C.U.; Bourgeois, P.; Deray, G. Kidney disease in RA patients: Prevalence and implication on RA-related drugs management: The MATRIX study. *Rheumatology* **2008**, *47*, 350–354. [CrossRef]
17. Karstila, K.; Korpela, M.; Sihvonen, S.; Mustonen, J. Prognosis of clinical renal disease and incidence of new renal findings in patients with rheumatoid arthritis: Follow-up of a population-based study. *Clin. Rheumatol.* **2007**, *26*, 2089–2095. [CrossRef]
18. Krishnaswami, S.; Chow, V.; Boy, M.; Wang, C.; Chan, G. Pharmacokinetics of tofacitinib, a Janus kinase inhibitor, in patients with impaired renal function and end-stage renal disease. *J. Clin. Pharmacol.* **2014**, *54*, 46–52. [CrossRef]
19. Erdem, A.; Gündoğan, N.U.; Usubütün, A.; Kilinç, K.; Erdem, S.R.; Kara, A.; Bozkurt, A. The protective effect of taurine against gentamicin-induced acute tubular necrosis in rats. *Nephrol. Dial. Transplant.* **2000**, *15*, 1175–1182. [CrossRef]
20. Abd El-Kader, M.; Taha, R.I. Comparative nephroprotective effects of curcumin and etoricoxib against cisplatin-induced acute kidney injury in rats. *Acta. Histochem.* **2020**, *122*, 151534. [CrossRef]
21. Feng, Y.; Liu, Y.; Wang, L.; Cai, X.; Wang, D.; Wu, K.; Chen, H.; Li, J.; Lei, W. Sustained oxidative stress causes late acute renal failure via duplex regulation on p38 MAPK and Akt phosphorylation in severely burned rats. *PLoS ONE* **2013**, *8*, e54593. [CrossRef] [PubMed]
22. Kim, J.E.; Park, M.Y.; Kim, S.H. Simple determination and quantification of tofacitinib, a JAK inhibitor, in rat plasma, urine and tissue homogenates by HPLC and its application to a pharmacokinetic study. *J. Pharm. Investig.* **2020**. [CrossRef]
23. Choi, Y.H.; Lee, I.; Lee, M.G. Slower clearance of intravenous metformin in rats with acute renal failure induced by uranyl nitrate: Contribution of slower renal and non-renal clearance. *Eur. J. Pharm. Sci.* **2010**, *39*, 1–7. [CrossRef] [PubMed]
24. Gwak, E.H.; Yoo, H.Y.; Kim, S.H. Effects of diabetes mellitus on the disposition of tofacitinib, a Janus kinase inhibitor, in rats. *Biomol. Ther.* **2020**, *28*, 361–369. [CrossRef]
25. Duggleby, R.G. Analysis of enzyme progress curves by nonlinear regression. *Methods Enzymol.* **1995**, *249*, 61–90.
26. Lee, D.Y.; Jung, Y.S.; Shin, H.S.; Lee, I.; Kim, Y.C.; Lee, M.G. Faster clearance of omeprazole in rats with acute renal failure induced by uranyl nitrate: Contribution of increased expression of hepatic cytochrome P450 (CYP) 3A1 and intestinal CYP1A and 3A subfamilies. *J. Pharm. Pharmacol.* **2008**, *60*, 843–851. [CrossRef]
27. Gibaldi, M.; Perrier, D. *Pharmacokinetics*, 2nd ed.; Marcel-Dekker: New York, NY, USA, 1982.
28. Chiou, W.L. Critical evaluation of the potential error in pharmacokinetic studies of using the linear trapezoidal rule method for the calculation of the area under the plasma level-time curve. *J. Pharmacokinet. Biopharm.* **1978**, *6*, 539–546. [CrossRef]
29. Chiou, W.L. New calculation method of mean total body clearance of drugs and its application to dosage regimens. *J. Pharm. Sci.* **1980**, *69*, 90–91. [CrossRef]
30. Eatman, F.B.; Colburn, W.A.; Boxenbaum, H.G.; Posmanter, H.N.; Weinfeld, R.E.; Ronfeld, R.; Kaplan, S.A. Pharmacokinetics of diazepam following multiple-dose oral administration to healthy human subjects. *J. Pharmacokinet. Biopharm.* **1977**, *5*, 481–494. [CrossRef]
31. Chiou, W.L. New calculation method for mean apparent drug volume of distribution and application to rational dosage regimens. *J. Pharm. Sci.* **1979**, *68*, 1067–1069. [CrossRef]
32. Ozer, J.S.; Dieterle, F.; Troth, S.; Perentes, E.; Cordier, A.; Verdes, P.; Staedtler, F.; Mahl, A.; Grenet, O.; Roth, D.R.; et al. A panel of urinary biomarkers to monitor reversibility of renal injury and a serum marker with improved potential to assess renal function. *Nat. Biotechnol.* **2010**, *28*, 486–494. [CrossRef] [PubMed]
33. Siddik, Z.H.; Newell, D.R.; Boxall, F.E.; Harrap, K.R. The comparative pharmacokinetics of carboplatin and cisplatin in mice and rats. *Biochem. Pharmacol.* **1987**, *36*, 1925–1932. [CrossRef]

34. Martínez-Salgado, C.; López-Hernández, F.J.; López-Novoa, J.M. Glomerular nephrotoxicity of aminoglycosides. *Toxicol. Appl. Pharmacol.* **2007**, *223*, 86–98. [CrossRef]
35. Arjumand, W.; Seth, A.; Sultana, S. Rutin attenuates cisplatin induced renal inflammation and apoptosis by reducing NFκB, TNF-α and caspase-3 expression in wistar rats. *Food Chem. Toxicol.* **2011**, *49*, 2013–2021. [CrossRef] [PubMed]
36. Malik, S.; Suchal, K.; Bhatia, J.; Gamad, N.; Dinda, A.K.; Gupta, Y.K.; Arya, D.S. Molecular mechanisms underlying attenuation of cisplatin-induced acute kidney injury by epicatechin gallate. *Lab. Invest.* **2016**, *96*, 853–861. [CrossRef] [PubMed]
37. Chiou, W.L. A new simple approach to study the effect of changes in urine flow and/or urine pH on renal clearance and its applications. *Int. J. Clin. Pharmacol. Ther. Toxicol.* **1986**, *24*, 519–527.
38. Bae, E.H.; Lee, J.; Ma, S.K.; Kim, I.J.; Frøkiaer, J.; Nielsen, S.; Kim, S.Y.; Kim, S.W. Alpha-lipoic acid prevents cisplatin-induced acute kidney injury in rats. *Nephrol. Dial. Transplant.* **2009**, *24*, 2692–2700. [CrossRef] [PubMed]
39. Moon, Y.J.; Lee, A.K.; Chung, H.C.; Kim, E.J.; Kim, S.H.; Lee, D.C.; Lee, I.; Kim, S.G.; Lee, M.G. Effects of acute renal failure on the pharmacokinetics of chlorzoxazone in rats. *Drug Metab. Dispos.* **2003**, *31*, 776–784. [CrossRef]
40. Peyrou, M.; Hanna, P.E.; Cribb, A.E. Cisplatin, gentamicin, and p-aminophenol induce markers of endoplasmic reticulum stress in the rat kidneys. *Toxicol. Sci.* **2007**, *99*, 346–353. [CrossRef]
41. Wilkinson, G.R.; Shand, D.G. A physiological approach to hepatic drug clearance. *Clin. Pharmacol. Ther.* **1975**, *18*, 377–390. [CrossRef]
42. Okabe, H.; Hasunuma, M.; Hashimoto, Y. The hepatic and intestinal metabolic activities of P450 in rats with surgery- and drug-induced renal dysfunction. *Pharm. Res.* **2003**, *20*, 1591–1594. [CrossRef] [PubMed]
43. Velenosi, T.J.; Fu, A.Y.; Luo, S.; Wang, H.; Urquhart, B.L. Down-regulation of hepatic CYP3A and CYP2C mediated metabolism in rats with moderate chronic kidney disease. *Drug Metab. Dispos.* **2012**, *40*, 1508–1514. [CrossRef] [PubMed]
44. Dowling, T.C.; Briglia, A.E.; Fink, J.C.; Hanes, D.S.; Light, P.D.; Stackiewicz, L.; Karyekar, C.S.; Eddington, N.D.; Weir, M.R.; Henrich, W.L. Characterization of hepaticcytochrome P4503A activity in patients with end-stage renal disease. *Clin. Pharmacol. Ther.* **2003**, *73*, 427–434. [CrossRef]
45. Shibata, N.; Morimoto, J.; Hoshino, N.; Minouchi, T.; Yamaji, A. Factors that affect absorption behavior of cyclosporin a in gentamicin-induced acute renal failure in rats. *Ren. Fail.* **2000**, *22*, 181–194. [CrossRef]
46. Okabe, H.; Hashimoto, T.; Inui, K.I. Pharmacokinetics and bioavailability of tacrolimus in rats with experimental renal dysfunction. *J. Pharm. Pharmacol.* **2000**, *52*, 1467–1472. [CrossRef] [PubMed]
47. Kim, S.H.; Shim, H.J.; Lee, M.G. Pharmacokinetics of a new carbapenem, DA-1131, after intravenous administration to rats with uranyl nitrate-induced acute renal failure. *Antimicrob. Agents Chemother.* **1998**, *42*, 1217–1221. [CrossRef]
48. Park, K.J.; Yoon, W.H.; Kim, S.H.; Shin, W.G.; Lee, M.G. Pharmacokinetic and pharmacodynamic changes of azosemide after intravenous and oral administration of azosemide to uranyl nitrate-induced acute renal failure rats. *Biopharm. Drug Dispos.* **1998**, *19*, 141–146. [CrossRef]
49. Bae, S.K.; Lee, S.J.; Kim, J.W.; Kim, Y.H.; Kim, S.G.; Lee, M.G. Effects of acute renal failure on the pharmacokinetics of oltipraz in rats. *J. Pharm. Sci.* **2004**, *93*, 2353–2363. [CrossRef]
50. Kim, H.J.; Han, K.S.; Chung, Y.K.; Chang, M.S.; Lee, M.G. Pharmacokinetic changes of a new proton pump inhibitor, YJA-20379-8, after intravenous and oral administration to rats with uranyl nitrate-induced acute renal failure. *Res. Commun. Mol. Pathol. Pharmacol.* **1998**, *102*, 43–56.
51. Bruyère, A.; Declèves, X.; Bouzom, F.; Proust, L.; Martinet, M.; Walther, B.; Parmentier, Y. Development of an optimized procedure for the preparation of rat intestinal microsomes: Comparison of hepatic and intestinal microsomal cytochrome P450 enzyme activities in two rat strains. *Xenobiotica* **2009**, *39*, 22–32. [CrossRef]

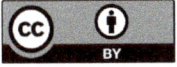

© 2020 by the authors. Licensee MDPI, Basel, Switzerland. This article is an open access article distributed under the terms and conditions of the Creative Commons Attribution (CC BY) license (http://creativecommons.org/licenses/by/4.0/).

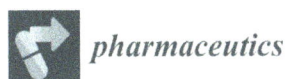

Article

Comparative Pharmacokinetics and Pharmacodynamics of a Novel Sodium-Glucose Cotransporter 2 Inhibitor, DWP16001, with Dapagliflozin and Ipragliflozin

Min-Koo Choi [1], So Jeong Nam [2], Hye-Young Ji [3], Mi Jie Park [3], Ji-Soo Choi [3] and Im-Sook Song [2],*

1. College of Pharmacy, Dankook University, Cheon-an 31116, Korea; minkoochoi@dankook.ac.kr
2. College of Pharmacy and Research Institute of Pharmaceutical Sciences, Kyungpook National University, Daegu 41566, Korea; goddns159@nate.com
3. Life Science Institute, Daewoong Pharmaceutical, Yongin, Gyeonggido 17028, Korea; hychi138@daewoong.co.kr (H.-Y.J.); mjpark201@daewoong.co.kr (M.J.P.); jschoi172@daewoong.co.kr (J.-S.C.)
* Correspondence: isssong@knu.ac.kr; Tel.: +82-53-950-8575

Received: 21 February 2020; Accepted: 12 March 2020; Published: 15 March 2020

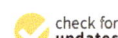

Abstract: Since sodium-glucose cotransporter 2 (SGLT2) inhibitors reduced blood glucose level by inhibiting renal tubular glucose reabsorption mediated by SGLT2, we aimed to investigate the pharmacokinetics and kidney distribution of DWP16001, a novel SGLT2 inhibitor, and to compare these properties with those of dapagliflozin and ipragliflozin, representative SGLT2 inhibitors. The plasma exposure of DWP16001 was comparable with that of ipragliflozin but higher than that of dapagliflozin. DWP16001 showed the highest kidney distribution among three SGLT2 inhibitors when expressed as an area under curve (AUC) ratio of kidney to plasma (85.0 ± 16.1 for DWP16001, 64.6 ± 31.8 for dapagliflozin and 38.4 ± 5.3 for ipragliflozin). The organic anion transporter-mediated kidney uptake of DWP16001 could be partly attributed to the highest kidney uptake. Additionally, DWP16001 had the lowest half-maximal inhibitory concentration (IC_{50}) to SGLT2, a target transporter (0.8 ± 0.3 nM for DWP16001, 1.6 ± 0.3 nM for dapagliflozin, and 8.9 ± 1.7 nM for ipragliflozin). The inhibition mode of DWP16001 on SGLT2 was reversible and competitive, but the recovery of the SGLT2 inhibition after the removal of SGLT2 inhibitors in CHO cells overexpressing SGLT2 was retained with DWP16001, which is not the case with dapagliflozin and ipragliflozin. In conclusion, selective and competitive SGLT2 inhibition of DWP16001 could potentiate the efficacy of DWP16001 in coordination with the higher kidney distribution and retained SGLT2 inhibition of DWP16001 relative to dapagliflozin and ipragliflozin.

Keywords: sodium-glucose cotransporter 2 (SGLT2) inhibitors; DWP16001; kidney distribution; inhibition mode

1. Introduction

Achieving appropriate glycemic control for type 2 diabetes patients is a prerequisite for preventing cardiovascular and microvascular complications, and this can be guided by a combination of antidiabetic drugs with different modes of action [1].

Sodium-glucose cotransporter 2 (SGLT2) inhibitors are the latest class of antidiabetic drugs that act through the inhibition of renal tubular glucose reabsorption and a reduction of blood glucose levels without stimulating insulin release [2]. SGLT2 is expressed in the S1 segment of proximal kidney tubules and is responsible for roughly 90% of the reabsorption of filtered glucose [3]. Additionally, SGLT2 inhibitors exhibit low hypoglycemia risk and have been associated with a significant reduction in major adverse cardiovascular events in clinical trials [4], garnering SGLT2 inhibitors increased attention.

Several SGLT2 inhibitors have been approved for the treatment of type 2 diabetes, including canagliflozin (Invokana®), dapagliflozin (Farxiga®), empagliflozin (Jardiance®), ipragliflozin (Suglat®), and tofogliflozin (Apleway®) [3,5].

Additionally, there are several other similar compounds in the pipeline that may be approved in the near future. DWP16001 (Figure 1), a selective SGLT2 inhibitor, is under development by Daewoong Pharmaceutical Co. Ltd. (Yongin, Korea) and is currently undergoing phase 2 clinical trials (Registration No. NCT04014023).

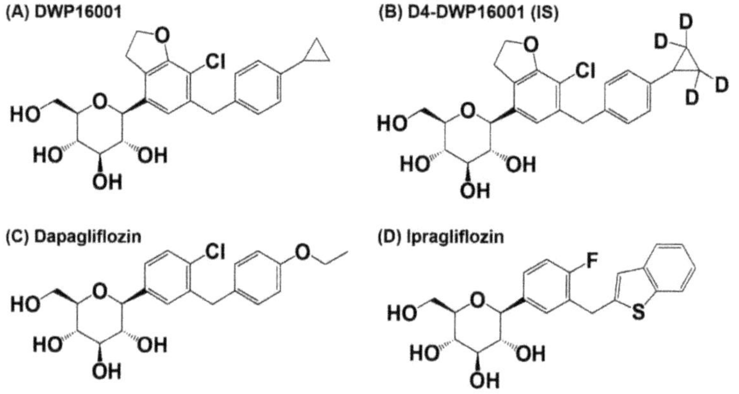

Figure 1. Structure of (**A**) DWP16001, (**B**) D4-DWP16001 (IS), (**C**) dapagliflozin, and (**D**) ipragliflozin.

Recently, Tahara et al. [5] compared the pharmacokinetics, pharmacodynamics, and pharmacological characteristics of six SGLT2 inhibitors, such as ipragliflozin, dapagliflozin, tofogliflozin, canagliflozin, empagliflozin, and luseogliflozin. The study showed that all the SGLT2 inhibitors induced urinary glucose excretion in a dose-dependent manner but the duration of action differed among the six drugs. Ipragliflozin and dapagliflozin showed persistent duration of action; these two drugs exhibited increased urinary glucose excretion even 18 h post dose but the others showed about 12 h of duration. In addition, ipragliflozin and dapagliflozind showed the lowest blood glucose and insulin level following the same daily dose (3 mg/kg) in diabetic mice. The long duration of action and glucose lowering efficacy of these two drugs closely correlated with the drug distribution and retention in the kidney and elimination half-life [5], suggesting the importance of kidney distribution and elimination profile is prerequisite in the efficacy of SGLT2 inhibitors, as well as the potent SGLT2 inhibition. Therefore, this study aimed to compare the pharmacokinetic properties and kidney distribution of DWP16001 with those of dapagliflozin and ipragliflozin, representative SGLT2 inhibitors that showed potent and long duration efficacy [5] and to compare the selectivity and mode of inhibition of DWP16001 on SGLT2 with dapagliflozin and ipragliflozin to evaluate the potency of DWP16001 over other SGLT2 inhibitors.

2. Materials and Methods

2.1. Materials

DWP16001 and D4-DWP16001 (for internal standard (IS)), were obtained from Daewoong Pharmaceutical Co. Ltd. (Yongin, Korea). Dapagliflozin and ipragliflozin were obtained from Toronto Research Chemicals Inc. (North York, ON, Canada) (Figure 1).

Para-aminohipuric acid (PAH), methyl α-D-glucopyranoside (AMG), sodium dodecyl sulfate (SDS), G418, non-essential amino acids, 4-(2-hydroxyethyl)-1-piperazineethanesulfonic acid (HEPES), and Hank's balances salts solution (HBSS, pH 7.4) were purchased from Sigma–Aldrich Chemical Co. (St. Louis, MO, USA). [^{14}C]Methyl-α-D-glucopyranoside (AMG) (290 mCi/mmol) was purchased from

Moravek (Brea, CA, USA). [^{3}H]Estrone-3-sulfate (ES) (2.12 TBq/mmol) and [^{3}H]para-aminohipuric acid (PAH) (0.13 TBq/mmol) were purchased from Perkin Elmer Inc. (Boston, MA, USA). Dulbecco's modified Eagle's medium (DMEM), RPMI1640 medium, fetal bovine serum (FBS), and poly-D-lysine-coated 24-well plates were purchased from Corning (Tewksbury, MA, USA). All other chemicals and solvents were reagent or analytical grade.

CHO cells overexpressing SGLT1 and SGLT2 (CHO-SGLT1 and -SGLT2, respectively) and CHO-mock cells were obtained from Daewoong Pharmaceutical Co. Ltd. (Yongin, Korea). HEK293 cells overexpressing organic anion transporter 1 (OAT1) and OAT3 (HEK293-OAT1 and -OAT3, respectively) and HEK293-mock cells were purchased from Corning (Tewksbury, MA, USA).

2.2. Animals and Ethical Approval

Male Institute of Cancer Research (ICR) mice (7–8-weeks-year-old, 30–35 g) were purchased from Samtako Co. (Osan, Korea). Animals were acclimatized for 1 week in an animal facility at Kyungpook National University. Food and water were available ad libitum. All animal procedures were approved by the Animal Care and Use Committee of Kyungpook National University (Approval No. 2016-0138) and carried out in accordance with the National Institutes of Health guidance for the care and use of laboratory animals.

2.3. Pharmacokinetic Study

ICR mice were randomly divided into three groups and were fasted for at least 12 h before the oral administration of DWP16001, dapagliflozin, and ipragliflozin but had free access to water. On the day of pharmacokinetic study, the mice received DWP16001, dapagliflozin, or ipragliflozin solution at a dose of 1 mg/kg (dissolved in a mixture of 10% DMSO and 90% saline) using oral gavage. Blood samples were collected at 0.5, 1, 2, 4, 8, 24, 48, and 72 h following the oral administration (1 mg/kg each) of DWP16001, dapagliflozin, or ipragliflozin and centrifuged at 12,000× g for 1 min to separate the plasma. An aliquot (30 µL) of each plasma sample was stored at −80 °C until the analysis. Kidney samples were also isolated at 8, 24, 48, and 72 h following the oral administration of DWP16001, dapagliflozin, or ipragliflozin, minced thoroughly, and homogenized with four volumes of saline using tissue grinder. An aliquot (50 µL) of each kidney homogenate sample was stored at −80 °C until the analysis.

For the analysis of SGLT2 inhibitors, aliquots of plasma (30 µL) and kidney homogenate (50 µL) were added to 100 µL of aqueous solution of D4-DWP16001 (IS, 20 ng/mL), and vigorously mixed with 500 µL methyl tert-butyl ether (MTBE) for 15 min. After centrifugation at 16,000 g for 5 min, samples were kept for 1 h at −80 °C to make an aqueous layer freeze. An organic upper layer was transferred to a clean tube and evaporated to dryness under a gentle stream of nitrogen. Then, the dried extract was reconstituted in 150 µL of mobile phase, and a 3 µL aliquot of the reconstituent was injected into a liquid chromatography–tandem mass spectrometry (LC–MS/MS) system.

Pharmacokinetic parameters, such as the area under plasma concentration-time curve from zero to infinity (AUC), were calculated from plasma concentration vs time curves using non-compartment analysis with WinNonlin (version 5.1; Pharsights, Cary, NC, USA). The AUC ratios (i.e., ratios of kidney AUC to plasma AUC) were calculated by dividing the AUC of the three SGLT2 inhibitors in the kidney by the plasma AUC values of the three SGLT2 inhibitors.

2.4. Protein Binding

The protein binding of DWP16001, dapagliflozin, and ipragliflozin (1000 ng/mL) in mouse plasma and 20% kidney homogenate was determined using a rapid equilibrium dialysis kit (ThermoFisher Scientific Korea, Seoul, Korea) according to the manufacturer's instructions. Briefly, 100 µL of mouse plasma and 20% kidney homogenate samples containing 1000 ng/mL of DWP16001, dapagliflozin, or ipragliflozin were added to the sample chamber of a semipermeable membrane (molecular weight cut-off 8000 Da) and 300 µL of phosphate buffered saline (PBS) was added to the outer buffer chamber.

Four hours after incubation at 37 °C on a shaking incubator at 300 rpm, aliquots (50 µL) were collected from both the sample and buffer chambers and treated with equal volumes of fresh PBS and blank plasma or blank kidney homogenate, respectively, to match the sample matrices. The matrix-matched sample (100 µL) was added 100 µL of aqueous solution of D4-DWP16001 (IS, 20 ng/mL), and vigorously mixed with 1000 µL MTBE for 15 min. After centrifugation at 16,000 g for 5 min, samples were kept for 1 h at −80 °C. An organic upper layer was transferred to a clean tube and evaporated to dryness under a gentle stream of nitrogen. Then, the dried extract was reconstituted in 300 µL of mobile phase and a 3 µL aliquot of the reconstituent was injected into the LC-MS/MS system.

Plasma protein binding was calculated using the following Equation (1) [6,7].

$$\text{Undiluted free drug fraction (fu)} = \frac{\text{Drug concentration in buffer chamber}}{\text{Drug concentration in plasma sample chamber}} \quad (1)$$

Kidney protein binding was calculated using the following equations, Equations (2) and (3), and a dilution factor (D as a value of 5) for tissue homogenates was used since we used 20% kidney homogenates [6,7].

$$\text{Diluted free drug fraction (fu\prime)} = \frac{\text{Drug concentration in buffer chamber}}{\text{Drug concentration in kidney homogenate chamber}}, \quad (2)$$

$$\text{Undiluted free drug fraction (fu)} = \frac{1/D}{\left(\frac{1}{fu\prime} - 1\right) + 1/D} = \frac{fu\prime \times 0.2}{1 - fu\prime \times 0.8}. \quad (3)$$

2.5. Substrate Specificity of DWP16001, Dapagliflozin, and Ipragliflozin for OAT1 and OAT3

HEK293-mock cells and HEK293 cells overexpressing OAT1 and OAT3 transporters (HEK293-OAT1 and -OAT3, respectively) were seeded in poly-D-lysine-coated 24-well plates at a density of 4×10^5 cells/well and cultured for 24 h in DMEM supplemented with 10% FBS and 5 mM non-essential amino acids at 37 °C in 8% CO_2 condition.

For each experiment, the growth medium was discarded after 24 h, and the attached cells were washed with pre-warmed HBSS and incubated with pre-warmed HBSS for 20 min at 37 °C. To confirm the functionality of OAT1 and OAT3, we measured the uptake of 0.1 µM [^{3}H]PAH and 0.1 µM [^{3}H]ES, representative substrates for OAT1 and OAT3, respectively, into in the HEK293-mock cells and HEK293-OAT1 and -OAT3 cells, respectively, for 5 min in the presence and absence of 20 µM probenecid, a typical inhibitor for both OAT1 and OAT3 [8,9]. The cells were then washed three times with 500 µL of ice-cold HBSS immediately after placing the plates on ice. Subsequently, cells were lysed with 10% sodium dodecyl sulfate and mixed with Optiphase cocktail solution overnight. The radioactivity of the cell lysate was measured using a liquid scintillation counter (Microbeta 2; Perkin Elmer Inc., Boston, MA, USA).

The uptake of DWP16001, dapagliflozin, and ipragliflozin (2 µM each) was measured for 5 min at 37 °C in the HEK293-mock cells and HEK293-OAT1 and -OAT3 cells, respectively, in the absence and presence of 20 µM probenecid. For the concentration dependency in the uptake of DWP16001, the uptake of DWP16001 in a concentration range of 0.5–50 µM dissolved in HBSS was measured for 5 min at 37 °C in the mock cells and HEK293-OAT1 and -OAT3 cells, respectively. After 5 min, the cells were washed three times with 500 µL of ice-cold HBSS immediately after placing the plates on ice. Subsequently, the cells were scraped using a cell scraper with 100 µL of PBS, and cell suspensions were transferred to a clean tube, combined with 100 µL of aqueous solution of D4-DWP16001 (IS, 20 ng/mL), and vigorously mixed with 1000 µL MTBE for 15 min. After centrifugation at 16,000 g for 5 min, samples were kept for 1 h at −80 °C. An organic upper layer was transferred to a clean tube and evaporated to dryness under a gentle stream of nitrogen. Then, the dried extract was reconstituted in 300 µL of mobile phase and a 3 µL aliquot of the reconstituent was injected into the LC-MS/MS system.

In the concentration-dependent uptake studies, the transporter-mediated uptake of DWP16001 was calculated by the subtraction of the transport rates of DWP16001 into the mock cells from those of the HEK293-OAT1 and -OAT3 cells. Kinetic parameters for the OAT1- and OAT3-mediated transport of DWP16001 were determined using the Michaelis-Menten equation $[V = V_{max} \cdot S/(K_m + S)]$ [10].

2.6. LC-MS/MS Analysis of DWP16001, Dapagliflozin, and Ipragliflozin

Concentrations of DWP16001, dapagliflozin, and ipragliflozin in plasma and kidney homogenate samples were analyzed using an Agilent 6470 triple quadrupole LC–MS/MS system (Agilent, Wilmington, DE, USA).

DWP16001, dapagliflozin, and ipragliflozin were separated on a Synergi Polar RP column (2.0 × 150 mm, 4 µm particle size; Phenomenex, Torrence, CA) using a mobile phase consisting of water (15%) and methanol (85%) containing 0.1% formic acid at a flow rate of 0.25 mL/min.

Quantification of a separated analyte peak was performed at m/z 464 → 131 for DWP16001 (T_R (retention time) 2.8 min), m/z 422 → 151 for ipragliflozin (T_R 2.5 min), m/z 426 → 167 for dapagliflozin (T_R 2.5 min), m/z 468 → 135 for D4-DWP16001 (T_R 2.8 min), in the positive ionization mode with a collision energy (CE) of 25 eV. The calibration standards of a mixture of DWP16001, dapagliflozin, and ipragliflozin in mouse plasma were 5–1000 ng/mL, and intraday and interday precision and accuracy were less than 14.7% in all samples. The calibration standards of a mixture of DWP16001, dapagliflozin, and ipragliflozin in mouse kidney homogenate were 5–1000 ng/mL, and intraday and interday precision and accuracy were less than 13.8% in all samples.

2.7. Inhibitory Effects of DWP16001, Dapagliflozin, and Ipragliflozin on the SGLT1 and SGLT2 Activities

CHO cells overexpressing SGLT1 and SGLT2 cells (CHO-SGLT1 and -SGLT2) and CHO-mock cells were characterized as previously described [11]. Cells were maintained in RPMI1640 medium supplemented with 10% fetal bovine serum and 200 µg/mL G418 at 37 °C in 5% CO_2 conditions. CHO-SGLT1 and -SGLT2 cells were seeded at a density of 1×10^5 cells/well in 96-well plates. After 24 h, the growth medium was discarded from the cells, and the cells were washed with pre-warmed Na^+-free buffer (10 mM HEPES, 5 mM Tris, 140 mM choline chloride, 2 mM KCl, 1 mM $CaCl_2$, 1 mM $MgCl_2$, pH7.4) and incubated for 1 h in Na^+-free buffer. After replacing Na^+-free buffer with Na^+ gradient buffer (10 mM HEPES, 5 mM Tris, 140 mM NaCl, 2 mM KCl, 1 mM $CaCl_2$, 1 mM $MgCl_2$, pH7.4) containing 10 µM [^{14}C]AMG, the uptake of [^{14}C]AMG into the CHO-mock cells and CHO-SGLT1 and -SLGT2 cells was measured for 0.5, 1, 1.5, 2, and 3 h. After a predetermined incubation time, cells were washed three times with 200 µL of ice-cold Na^+-free buffer immediately after placing the plates on ice. Then, the cells were lysed with 10% SDS, and the cell lysates were mixed with Optiphase cocktail solution. Thereafter, the radioactivity of the cell lysates was measured using a liquid scintillation counter.

The inhibitory effect of known inhibitors, such as dapagliflozin and ipragliflozin, on [^{14}C]AMG uptake in the CHO-mock cells and CHO-SGLT1 and -SLGT2 cells was measured in the presence or absence of dapagliflozin and ipragliflozin (1, 10 µM for SGLT1; 10, 100 nM for SGLT2) for 2 h. For the calculation of IC_{50} values, the uptake of 10 µM [^{14}C]AMG in the CHO-mock cells and CHO-SGLT1 and -SLGT2 cells was measured for 2 h with or without DWP16001, dapagliflozin, or ipragliflozin (1 nM–50 µM for SGLT1; 0.01 nM–1 µM for SGLT2). After 2 h, cells were washed three times with 200 µL of ice-cold Na^+-free buffer and the cells were lysed with 10% SDS (40 µL), followed by adding Optiphase cocktail solution (200 µL). The radioactivity of the cell lysates was measured using a liquid scintillation counter. The SGLT1 or SGLT2-mediated uptake of [^{14}C]AMG was calculated by the subtraction of the uptake rates of [^{14}C]AMG into the mock cells from those of the CHO-SGLT1 and -SLGT2 cells. In the inhibition studies, the percentages of the transport rate of AMG with or without SGLT2 inhibitors were calculated and the data were fitted to an inhibitory effect model. The IC_{50} (the concentration of the inhibitor to show half-maximal inhibition) values were calculated using Sigma Plot ver.10.0 (Systat Software, Inc.; San Jose, CA, USA) [12].

To investigate time dependency in the inhibition of SGLT2, CHO-mock and -SGLT2 cells were seeded at a density of 1×10^5 cells/well in 96-well plates. After 24 h, the growth medium was discarded from the cells, and the cells were washed with pre-warmed Na^+-free buffer and pre-incubated with Na^+-free buffer containing various concentrations of DWP16001, dapagliflozin, or ipragliflozin (0.001 nM–100 nM) for 1 and 2 h. Then, after replacing Na^+-free buffer with Na^+ gradient buffer containing 10 μM [^{14}C]AMG and various concentrations of DWP16001, dapagliflozin, or ipragliflozin (0.001 nM–100 nM), the uptake of [^{14}C]AMG into the CHO-mock and -SGLT2 cells was measured for 2 h. After 2 h of incubation, the radioactivity of the cell lysate was measured following the same sample preparation method described above.

To investigate the mode of inhibition of the three SGLT2 inhibitors, the inhibition experiments were initiated by replacing Na^+-free buffer with Na^+ gradient buffer containing 1, 2.5, 5, and 50 μM [^{14}C]AMG and various concentrations of DWP16001, dapagliflozin, or ipragliflozin (0.001 nM–250 nM) and the uptake of [^{14}C]AMG into the CHO-mock and -SGLT2 cells was measured for 2 h. The radioactivity of the cell lysate was measured following the same sample preparation method described above. Uptake rate of AMG and concentrations of DWP16001, dapagliflozin, or ipragliflozin were plotted to Dixon plots to identify the mode of inhibition [13,14].

To investigate the recovery of SGLT2 activity depending on the washout period after 24 h exposure of DWP16001, dapagliflozin, or ipragliflozin, CHO-SGLT2 cells were seeded at a density of 1×10^5 cells/well in 96-well plates. After 24 h, the growth medium was discarded from the cells, and the cells were treated with RPMI1640 medium containing DWP16001, dapagliflozin, or ipragliflozin (0.2, 2, 20, and 200 nM) for 24 h. After 24 h, the RPMI1640 medium was replaced with pre-warmed fresh RPMI1640 medium and incubated for 1, 2, 3, 5, and 6 h, and proceeded another pre-incubation with Na^+-free buffer for 1 h. Then, after replacing Na^+-free buffer with Na^+ gradient buffer containing 10 μM [^{14}C]AMG, the uptake of [^{14}C]AMG into the CHO-SGLT2 cells was measured for 2 h. After 2 h of incubation, the radioactivity of the cell lysate was measured following the same sample preparation method described above.

2.8. Statistics

The statistical significance was assessed by t-test using SPSS for Windows (version 24.0; IBM Corp., Armonk, NY, USA).

3. Results

3.1. LC-MS/MS Analysis of DWP16001, Dapagliflozin, and Ipragliflozin

To compare the pharmacokinetics and tissue distribution of DWP16001, dapagliflozin, ipragliflozin in mice, analyses of the three SGLT2 inhibitors using LC-MS/MS were applied. Figure 2 shows the selected precursor and product ions of DWP16001, dapagliflozin, ipragliflozin, and D4-DWP16001 (IS). The selected precursor and product ions of dapagliflozin and ipragliflozin were consistent with previously published findings [12,15].

Representative multiple reaction-monitoring (MRM) chromatograms of DWP16001, D4-DWP16001 (IS), dapagliflozin, and ipragliflozin (Figure 3) showed that all the analyte peaks obtained using the liquid-liquid extraction method using MTBE were well separated with no interfering peaks at their respective retention times.

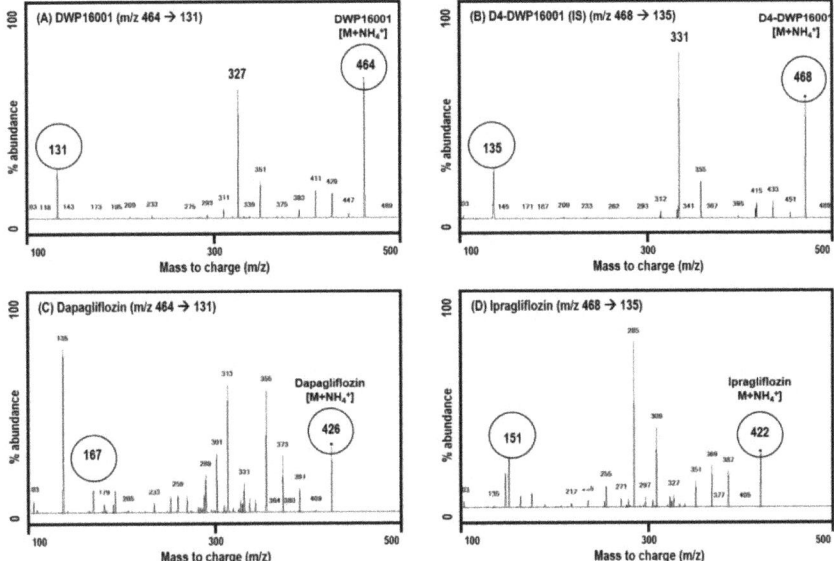

Figure 2. Product ion spectra of (**A**) DWP16001, (**B**) D4-DWP16001 (IS), (**C**) dapagliflozin, and (**D**) ipragliflozin.

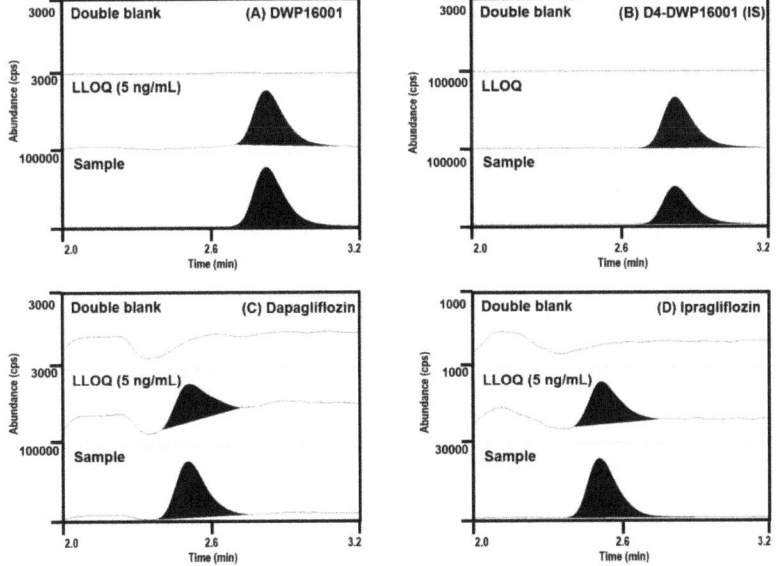

Figure 3. Representative multiple reaction-monitoring (MRM) chromatograms of (**A**) DWP16001, (**B**) D4-DWP16001 (IS), (**C**) dapagliflozin, and (**D**) ipragliflozin in mouse double-blank plasma, blank plasma spiked with DWP16001, dapagliflozin, ipragliflozin at the lower limit of quantification (LLOQ) (5 ng/mL), and plasma samples at 1 h following single oral administration of DWP16001, dapagliflozin, or ipragliflozin at a dose of 1 mg/kg.

3.2. Pharmacokinetics and Kidney Distribution of DWP16001, Dapagliflozin, and Ipragliflozin in Mice

To compare the pharmacokinetic profile of DWP16001 with those of dapagliflozin and ipragliflozin, the same dose of the three SGLT2 inhibitors was orally administered to ICR mice (1 mg/kg each), and the concentrations of DWP16001, dapagliflozin, and ipragliflozin in plasma and kidney samples were analyzed. The PK profiles of DWP16001, dapagliflozin, and ipragliflozin are shown in Figure 4 and the PK parameters were summarized in Table 1.

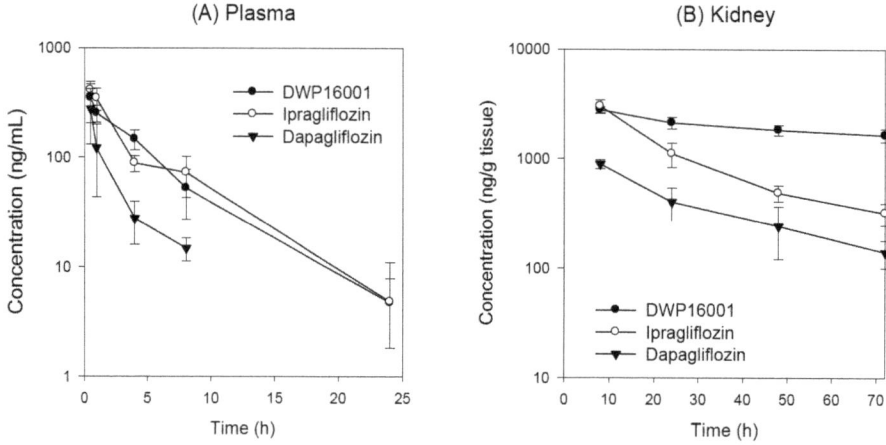

Figure 4. (**A**) Plasma and (**B**) kidney concentration vs. time profile of DWP16001 (●), dapagliflozin (▼), and ipragliflozin (○) after a single oral administrations of DWP16001, dapagliflozin, and ipragliflozin at a dose of 1 mg/kg in Institute of Cancer Research (ICR) mice, respectively. Data are expressed as mean±SD from five mice.

Table 1. Pharmacokinetic parameters of DWP16001, dapagliflozin, and ipragliflozin after a single oral administrations of DWP16001, dapagliflozin, and ipragliflozin at a dose of 1 mg/kg in ICR mice, respectively.

	Parameters	DWP16001	Dapagliflozin	Ipragliflozin
Plasma	C_{max} (ng/mL)	371.4 ± 108.6	274.8 ± 143.6	409.6 ± 59.1
	T_{max} (h)	0.7 ± 0.3	0.5 ± 0.0	0.6 ± 0.2
	AUC_{72h} (µg·h/mL)	1.69 ± 0.34	0.48 ± 0.18 *	1.96 ± 0.41
	AUC_{∞} (µg·h/mL)	1.73 ± 0.34	0.55 ± 143.8 *	1.97 ± 0.41
	$t_{1/2}$ (h)	3.8 ± 1.4	2.1 ± 0.2 *	3.1 ± 0.5
Kidney	AUC_{72h} (µg·h/g tissue)	139.2 ± 5.19	26.30 ± 3.34 *	73.65 ± 7.05 *
	AUC ratio	85.0 ± 16.1	64.6 ± 31.8	38.4 ± 5.3 *
	$t_{1/2}$ (h)	125.5 ± 80.4	24.9 ± 5.4 *	24.3 ± 5.7 *

Area under curve (AUC) ratio: Ratios of Kidney AUC to plasma AUC; Data expressed as mean ± SD from five mice; *: $p < 0.05$, compared with DWP16001 group.

As shown in Figure 4, plasma concentrations of DWP16001 were similar to those of ipragliflozin and greater than those of dapagliflozin. Consequently, the AUC and C_{max} values of DWP16001 were similar to those of ipragliflozin and higher than those of dapagliflozin. However, the concentrations of DWP16001 in the kidney were maintained at higher concentrations for 72 h compared with those of ipragliflozin and dapagliflozin, suggesting the prolonged efficacy of DWP16001 via the inhibition of SGLT2, which is located in the renal proximal tubule [3]. Because of the high and prolonged concentration of DWP16001, the AUC, AUC ratio, and $t_{1/2}$ values of DWP16001 were significantly greater than those of dapagliflozin and ipragliflozin (Table 1).

3.3. Substrate Specificity of DWP16001, Dapagliflozin, and Ipragliflozin for OAT1 and OAT3

The AUC ratios of these three SGLT2 inhibitors were much greater than unity, suggesting that DWP16001, dapagliflozin, and ipragliflozin are distributed in the kidney, in which tissue protein binding ability to the specific protein or drug transporters may be involved. Therefore, firstly, we measured the protein binding of DWP16001, dapagliflozin, and ipragliflozin in the plasma and kidney homogenate.

The plasma and kidney tissue protein binding of DWP16001, dapagliflozin, and ipragliflozin were high and comparable and the logP values of three compound were also comparable (i.e., in the range of 2.27–2.65) (Table 2). It suggests that the large distribution of DWP16001, dapagliflozin, and ipragliflozin in the kidney was not necessarily reliant on plasma/tissue-specific binding ability or lipophilicity of these compounds.

Table 2. Protein binding of DWP16001, dapagliflozin, and ipragliflozin in mouse plasma and kidney homogenates.

Compounds	logP [a]	Protein Binding (% Bound) [b]	
		Plasma	Kidney
DWP16001	2.65	98.50 ± 0.20	97.24 ± 0.08
Dapagliflozin	2.27	94.19 ± 1.07	95.83 ± 0.68
Ipragliflozin	2.56	96.58 ± 0.75	96.50 ± 1.01

[a] logP values were obtained from the partition coefficient of n-octanol/water; [b] Data expressed as mean ± SD of triplicate experiments.

We conducted further investigations into the tissue-specific transport of DWP16001, dapagliflozin, and ipragliflozin by using cell systems overexpressing OAT1 and OAT3 since OAT1 and OAT3 are exclusively distributed in the kidney and contribute to the drug distribution to the kidney [16]. The functionality of the OAT1 and OAT3 transport system was confirmed by the significantly greater uptake rates of the probe substrates in HEK293-OAT1 and -OAT3 cells than that in HEK293-mock cells (i.e., 14.7-fold increase in PAH uptake for OAT1 and 16.4-fold increase in ES uptake for OAT3) and by the decreased uptake rate of each probe substrate by the addition of a representative inhibitor, probenecid (Figure 5A,B) [17]. The uptake of DWP16001 in HEK293-OAT1 and OAT3 cells was significantly higher than that in HEK293-mock cells, and it was significantly decreased by the presence of probenecid (Figure 5C). However, dapagliflozin and ipragliflozin were not substrates for both OAT1 and OAT3 (Figure 5D,E). Next, we investigated the concentration dependency in the OAT1 and OAT3-mediated DWP16001 uptake. As shown in the figure, the OAT1 and OAT3-mediated uptake of DWP16001 showed saturable kinetics, and the kinetic parameters, such as K_m and V_{max}, calculated from the concentration-dependent uptake of DWP16001 in HEK293-OAT1 and –OAT3 cells are shown in Figure 6. Collectively, OAT1 and OAT3-mediated uptake of DWP16001 could contribute to the highest kidney distribution of DWP16001 among three SGLT2 inhibitors. However, these processes were not dominant over the cellular uptake of the three SGLT2 inhibitors into HEK293-mock cells (i.e., passive diffusion), which is evident from two-fold increases in HEK293-OAT1 or -OAT3 cells compared with mock cells (Figure 5C). Therefore, OAT1- and OAT3-mediated active transport and passive diffusion all contributed to the highly permeable absorptive process of DWP16001 in the kidney, and dapagliflozin and ipragliflozin also showed higher uptake levels into HEK293 cells via passive diffusion.

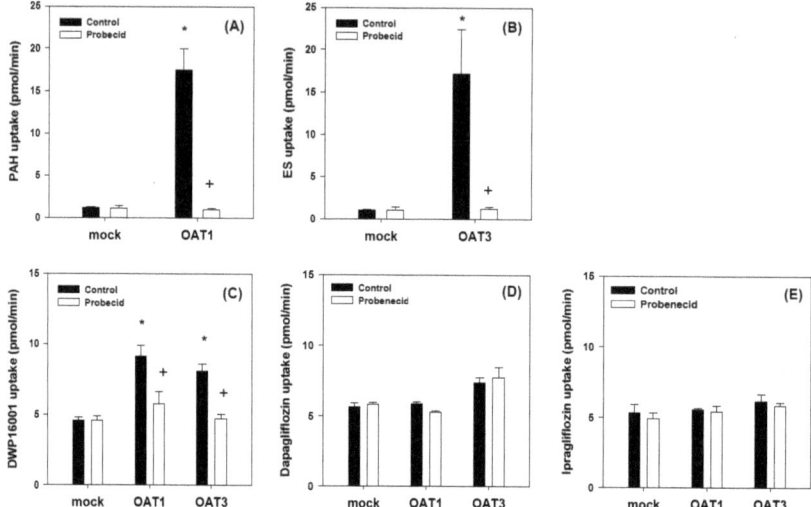

Figure 5. (**A**) Uptake of 0.1 μM [^{3}H]para-aminohippuric acid (PAH) was measured in HEK293-mock and –OAT1 cells in the presence and absence of 20 μM probenecid for 5 min. (**B**) Uptake of 0.1 μM [^{3}H]Estrone-3-sulfate (ES) was measured in HEK293-mock and –OAT3 cells in the presence and absence of 20 μM probenecid. Uptake of (**C**) DWP16001, (**D**) dapagliflozin, and (**E**) ipragliflozin (2 μM each) into HEK293-mock and HEK293 cells expressing OAT1 and OAT3 was measured for 5 min. Each data point represents the mean±standard deviation of triplicate experiments. *: $p < 0.05$, compared with mock cells; +: $p < 0.05$, compared with control group.

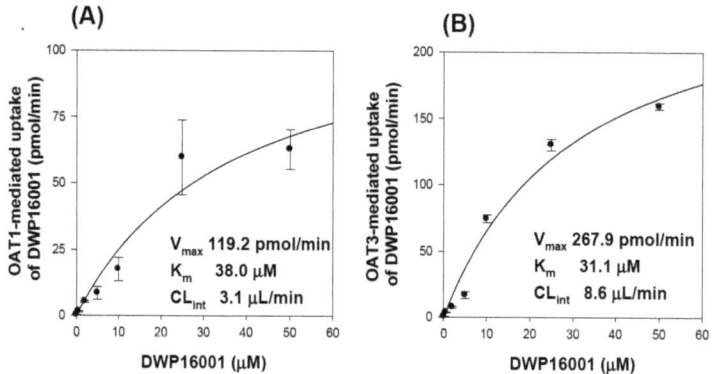

Figure 6. (**A**) OAT1- and (**B**) OAT3-mediated uptake of DWP16001. Concentration dependent uptake of DWP16001 was measured for 5 min into HEK293-mock cells and HEK293 cells expressing OAT1 and OAT3. The transporter-mediated uptake rate was obtained by subtracting the uptake in HEK293-mock cells (passive diffusion) from those in HEK293 cells expressing OAT1 and OAT3 (total uptake). Each data point represents the means ± standard deviation from triplicate experiments.

3.4. Inhibition Potential of DWP16001, Dapagliflozin, Ipragliflozin on SGLT1 and SGLT2 Activities

3.4.1. Comparison of IC$_{50}$ Values of DWP16001, Dapagliflozin, and Ipragliflozin on SGLT1 and SGLT2

To confirm the functionality of CHO-SGLT1 cells, we measured the time-dependent uptake of AMG, a representative substrate for SGLT1 [11,18]. As shown in Figure 7A, AMG uptake was increased with incubation time, and the optimal incubation time was selected as 2 h from the linear phase of the slope. AMG uptake into CHO-SGLT1 cells was 42-fold greater than that into CHO-mock cells and significantly inhibited by the presence of known inhibitors, such as dapagliflozin and ipragliflozin [3,5] (Figure 7B). With the same experimental condition, the inhibitory effect of DWP16001, dapagliflozin, and ipragliflozin on the AMG uptake into CHO-SGLT1 cells was measured in a concentration range of 1–50,000 nM and IC_{50} values were calculated (Figure 7C–E; Table 3).

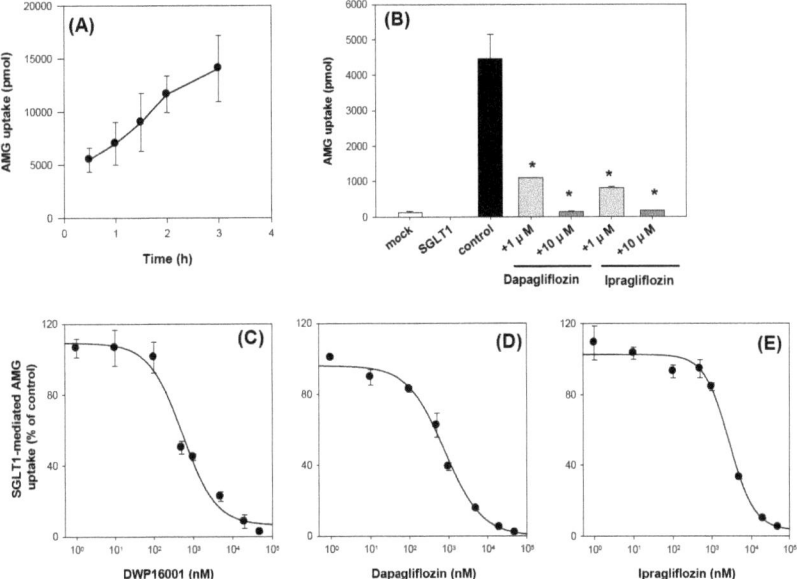

Figure 7. (**A**) Uptake of 10 μM [^{14}C]methyl-a-D-glucopyranoside (AMG) was measured in CHO-sodium-glucose cotransporter 1 (SGLT1) cells with a various incubation time (0.5–3 h). (**B**) Inhibitory effect of dapagliflozin and ipragliflozin (1, 10 μM) on the uptake of 10 μM [^{14}C]AMG in CHO-mock and -SGLT1 cells was measured for 2 h. Concentration dependent inhibition of DWP16001 (**C**), dapagliflozin (**D**), and ipragliflozin (**E**) on the SGLT1-mediated uptake of [^{14}C]AMG. SGLT1-mediated uptake of [^{14}C]AMG was calculated by subtracting the uptake of 10 μM [^{14}C]AMG for 2 h in CHO-mock cells from that in CHO-SGLT1 cells in a concentration range of 1–50,000 nM of DWP16001, dapagliflozin, and ipragliflozin. Each data point represents the mean ± standard deviation of three independent experiments. *: $p < 0.05$, compared with control group.

Table 3. Inhibition potential of DWP16001, dapagliflozin, and ipragliflozin on SGLT1 and SGLT2 activities.

	IC_{50} (nM)		Selectivity
	SGLT1	SGLT2	(IC_{50} Ratio of SGLT1/SGLT2)
DWP16001	549.3 ± 139.6	0.8 ± 0.3	667
Ipragliflozin	2328.7 ± 377.6	8.9 ± 1.7	261
Dapagliflozin	803.0 ± 96.8	1.6 ± 0.3	493

Data were expressed as mean ± SD from triplicate measurement.

Similarly, the functionality of CHO-SGLT2 cells was confirmed from the time-dependent uptake of AMG, a representative substrate for SGLT2 [3,5]. As shown in Figure 8A, AMG uptake was increased with incubation time, and the optimal incubation time was selected as 2 h from the linear phase of the slope. AMG uptake into CHO-SGLT1 cells was 9.8-fold greater than that into CHO-mock cells and significantly inhibited by the presence of known inhibitors, such as dapagliflozin and ipragliflozin [3] (Figure 8B). With the same experimental conditions, the inhibitory effect of DWP16001, dapagliflozin, and ipragliflozin on the AMG uptake into CHO-SGLT2 cells was measured in a concentration range of 0.001–100 nM, and IC_{50} values were calculated (Figure 8C–E; Table 3).

DWP16001 showed greater affinity for SGLT2 compared with dapagliflozin and ipragliflozin. Moreover, the affinity to SGLT1 was also greater with DWP16001 compared with dapagliflozin and ipragliflozin. When compared with selectivity, which was calculated from the SGLT1/SGLT2 IC_{50} ratio, the selectivity of DWP16001 was high relative to that of dapagliflozin and ipragliflozin (Table 3).

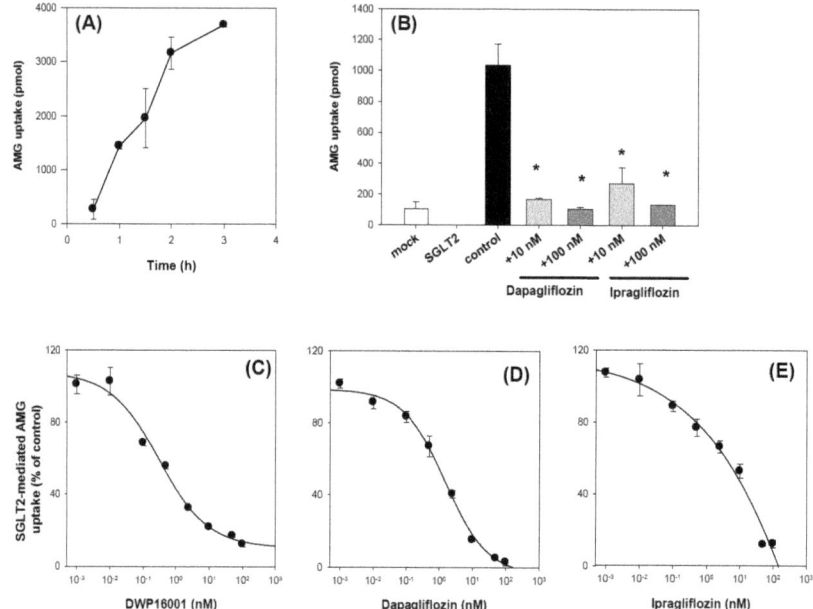

Figure 8. (**A**) The uptake of 10 μM [^{14}C]methyl-a-D-glucopyranoside (AMG) was measured in CHO-SGLT2 cells with a various incubation time (0.5, 1, 1.5, 2, 3 h). (**B**) Inhibitory effect of dapagliflozin and ipragliflozin (10, 100 nM) on the uptake of 10 μM [^{14}C]AMG in CHO-mock and –SGLT2 cells was measured for 2 h. Representative concentration dependent inhibition of DWP16001 (**C**), dapagliflozin (**D**), and ipragliflozin (**E**) on the SGLT2-mediated uptake of [^{14}C]AMG. SGLT2-mediated uptake of [^{14}C]AMG was calculated by subtracting the uptake of 10 μM [^{14}C]AMG for 2 h in CHO-mock cells from that in CHO-SGLT2 cells in a concentration range of 1–100 nM of DWP16001, dapagliflozin, and ipragliflozin. Each data point represents the mean±standard deviation of three independent experiments. *: $p < 0.05$, compared with control group.

3.4.2. Mode of Inhibition

To investigate whether the inhibition of SGLT2 was time-dependent, the inhibitory effects of DWP16001, dapagliflozin, and ipragliflozin on SGLT2-mediated uptake of AMG were measured with or without pretreatment with DWP16001, dapagliflozin, and ipragliflozin, respectively. Figure 9 shows that the inhibitory potential of DWP16001, dapagliflozin, and ipragliflozin on SGLT2 did not change with different pretreatment times, suggesting that all the DWP16001, dapagliflozin, and ipragliflozin inhibited SGLT2 function in a time-independent manner.

To determine the mode of inhibition on SGLT2, the inhibitory effects of DWP16001, dapagliflozin, and ipragliflozin on the AMG uptake into CHO-SGLT2 cells were measured with different substrate concentrations, and the results were expressed as Dixon plots (Figure 10A–C) and a replot of the Dixon slopes (Figure 10D–F) [13,19,20]. Dixon transformation of inhibition profile by DWP16001 (0.001–250 nM) for different concentrations of AMG indicated competitive inhibition of DWP16001 on SGLT2 activity (Figure 10A). A replot of the Dixon slopes vs 1/S produced a straight line converging on the zero (Figure 10D), suggesting competitive and reversible inhibition of DWP16001. Similar results were shown in case of dapagliflozin and ipragliflozin (Figure 10B,C,E,F). The results collectively suggested that the inhibition of SGLT2 by DWP16001, dapagliflozin, and ipragliflozin is reversible and competitive.

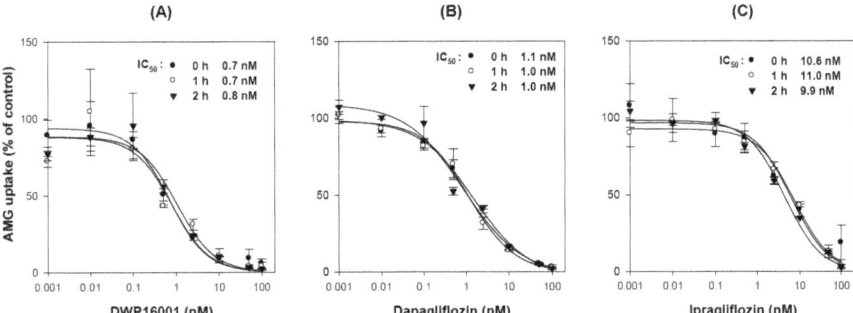

Figure 9. Inhibitory effect of (**A**) DWP16001, (**B**) dapagliflozin, and (**C**) ipragliflozin on the SGLT2-mediated uptake of 10 μM [^{14}C]methyl-a-D-glucopyranoside (AMG) was measured with preincubation time for 1 and 2 h or without preincubation of DWP16001, dapagliflozin, and ipragliflozin, respectively, in a concentration range of 0.001–100 nM. Each data point represents the mean±standard deviation of three independent experiments.

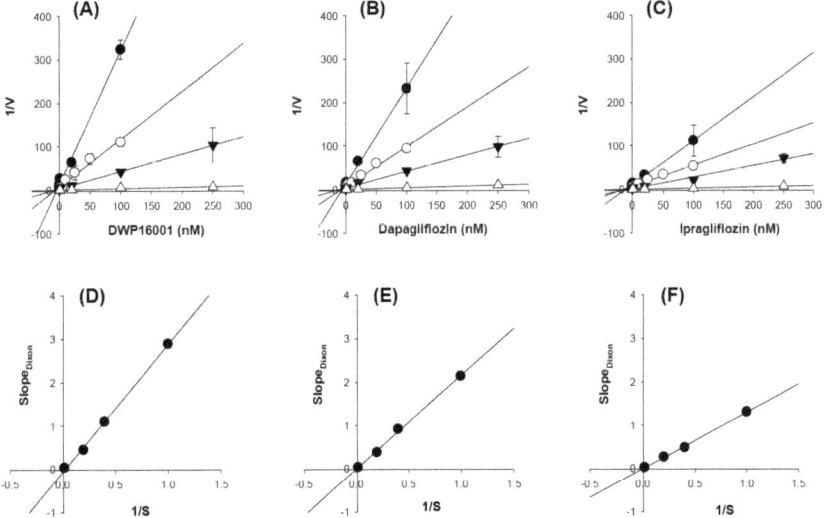

Figure 10. Dixon plot for the inhibitory effect of (**A**) DWP16001, (**B**) dapagliflozin, and (**C**) ipragliflozin on the uptake of [^{14}C]methyl-a-D-glucopyranoside (AMG) in CHO-SGLT2 cells. Each symbol represents the concentration of [^{14}C]AMG: ●, 1 μM; ○, 2.5 μM; ▼, 5 μM; △, 50 μM. Replot of the slopes of Dixon plot (slopes vs 1/[S]) was shown for (**D**) DWP16001, (**E**) dapagliflozin, and (**F**) ipragliflozin. V indicates the SGLT2-mediated uptake rate of [^{14}C]AMG and S indicates the concentration of [^{14}C]AMG. The data are the means±standard deviations of triplicate measurements.

3.4.3. Retained Inhibition Potential of DWP16001 Compared to Dapagliflozin and Ipragliflozin

The recovery of SGLT2 activities depending on the washout period after 24 h exposure of DWP16001, ipragliflozin, and dapagliflozin in CHO-SGLT2 cells was investigated. As shown in Figure 11, the activity of reduced SGLT2 by treatment with DWP16001, dapagliflozin, and ipragliflozin for 24 h in CHO-SGLT2 cells revealed differences in the recovery of SGLT2 depending on the time of drug removal from the medium, as well as SGLT2 inhibitors. In the case of DWP16001, the activity tended to gradually recover as the washout time increased. When treated at a high concentration (200 nM), the activity did not recover even 8 h after the drug was removed from the medium (Figure 11A). However, when dapagliflozin and ipragliflozin were used, SGLT2 activity was recovered to the control level 4 h after the removal of dapagliflozin and ipragliflozin (Figure 11B,C). The results indicate that the dissociation of DWP16001 to SGLT2 is slower and more incomplete than that of dapagliflozin and ipragliflozin and that the binding affinity to SGLT2 is stronger than that of dapagliflozin and ipragliflozin.

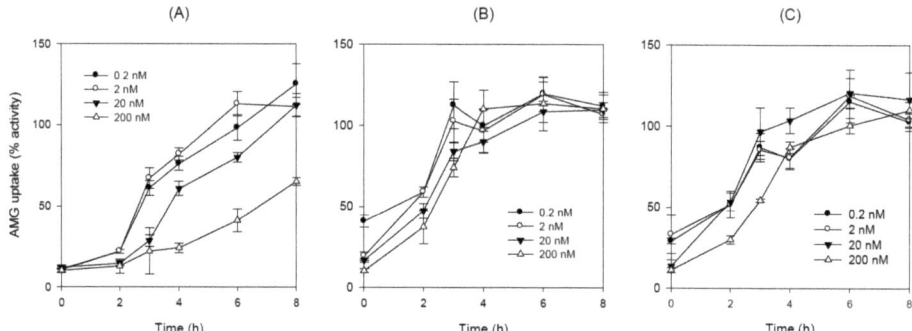

Figure 11. Recovery of SGLT2 transport function with different washout time following 24 h of incubation with (**A**) DWP16001, (**B**) dapagliflozin, and (**C**) ipragliflozin (0.2–200 nM) was measured through the uptake of [^{14}C]methyl-a-D-glucopyranoside (AMG) in CHO-SGLT2 cells. Each data point represents the mean±standard deviation of three independent experiments.

4. Discussion

DWP16001 is a candidate SGLT2 inhibitor that is currently under development. As a first step, the pharmacokinetic properties and in vitro SGLT2 inhibition were compared with currently used SGLT2 inhibitors. Dapagliflozin and ipragliflozin were selected based on their high kidney distributions and long elimination half-lives ($t_{1/2}$) in the kidney [5], which are thought to be important for the efficacy and duration of action of SGLT2 inhibitors. DWP16001 showed higher kidney distributions compared with dapagliflozin and ipragliflozin. DWP16001 also had longer $t_{1/2}$ in the kidney than dapagliflozin and ipragliflozin, as well as a comparable plasma profile with ipragliflozin (Table 1). Moreover, the kidney concentration of DWP16001 was maintained over 72 h following oral administration of 1 mg/kg DWP16001 (Figure 4). Taken together, these pharmacokinetic results show that the duration of action of DWP16001 is greater than that of dapagliflozin and ipragliflozin and that the oral therapeutic dose of DWP16001 could be reduced compared with both dapagliflozin and ipragliflozin.

To investigate the underlying mechanisms of highest kidney distribution and maintained concentration of DWP16001 in the kidney, we measured the kidney tissue binding and involvement of OAT1 and OAT3 transporters of the three SGLT2 inhibitors. All three SGLT2 inhibitors showed high protein binding, but the kidney tissue binding performances of these three SGLT2 inhibitors were not different from their plasma protein binding capabilities (Table 2). However, DWP16001 was a substrate for both OAT1 and OAT3, which are dominantly expressed in the kidney, whereas dapagliflozin and ipragliflozin were not (Figures 5 and 6). Although this could not solely explain the high kidney distribution, OAT1- and OAT3-mediated transport process may contribute to the high kidney distribution.

Next, we compared the in vitro SGLT2 inhibition and selectivity of SGLT2 inhibition over SGLT1. All three SGLT2 inhibitors inhibited SGLT2 and SGLT1 activity in a concentration-dependent manner and IC$_{50}$ values of dapagliflozin and ipragliflozin were in the range of previous reports (1.0–1.3 nM for dapagliflozin; 6.75–8.07 nM for ipragliflozin) [21,22]. IC$_{50}$ values of DWP16001 to SGLT2 and SGLT1 were lower than those of dapagliflozin and ipragliflozin, suggesting a greater affinity to SGLT2 inhibition for DWP16001 with a higher selectivity over SGLT1 than dapagliflozin and ipragliflozin. The mode of inhibition of DWP16001 was not different from the other SGLT2 inhibitors. They all showed reversible and competitive inhibition (Figure 10), which is consistent with other SGLT2 inhibitors [23,24]. However, the affinity to SGLT2 inhibition seemed to be different among the three SGLT2 inhibitors (Table 3). In addition, the recovery of SGLT2 transport activity following the pretreatment of DWP16001, dapagliflozin, and ipragliflozin for 24 h was retained at a higher concentration (200 nM) of DWP16001 compared with dapagliflozin and ipragliflozin. These results suggested that DWP16001 had the highest SGLT2 inhibition potential and that this inhibition potential retained for a longer time compared with dapagliflozin and ipragliflozin. Combined with the higher kidney distribution of DWP16001, retained SGLT2 inhibition with a high concentration of DWP16001 could also potentiate the efficacy of DWP16001 compared with dapagliflozin and ipragliflozin.

The comparative pharmacokinetics and in vitro SGLT2 inhibition findings suggest that DWP16001 might be a superior alternative to dapagliflozin and ipragliflozin; however, we should note that comparisons of the in vivo pharmacologic properties of these agents using therapeutic doses in animals and humans need to be further undertaken.

Author Contributions: Conceptualization, M.-K.C., H.-Y.J and I.-S.S.; Investigation, M.-K.C., S.J.N., H.-Y.J., M.J.P., J.-S.C. and I.-S.S.; Writing-Original Draft Preparation, M.-K.C.; Supervision, I.-S.S.; Writing-Review & Editing, I.-S.S. All authors have read and agreed to the published version of the manuscript.

Funding: This research received no external funding.

Conflicts of Interest: The authors declare no conflict of interest.

References

1. Choi, M.-K.; Jin, Q.-R.; Ahn, S.-H.; Bae, M.A.; Song, I.-S. Sitagliptin attenuates metformin-mediated AMPK phosphorylation through inhibition of organic cation transporters. *Xenobiotica* **2010**, *40*, 817–825. [CrossRef]
2. Chao, E.C.; Henry, R.R. SGLT2 inhibition—A novel strategy for diabetes treatment. *Nat. Rev. Drug Discov.* **2010**, *9*, 551–559. [CrossRef]
3. Ferrannini, E.; Solini, A. SGLT2 inhibition in diabetes mellitus: Rationale and clinical prospects. *Nat. Rev. Endocrinol.* **2012**, *8*, 495–502. [CrossRef]
4. Van Baar, M.J.B.; Van Ruiten, C.C.; Muskiet, M.H.A.; Van Bloemendaal, L.; Ijzerman, R.G.; Van Raalte, D.H. SGLT2 inhibitors in combination therapy: From mechanisms to clinical considerations in type 2 diabetes management. *Diabetes Care* **2018**, *41*, 1543–1556. [CrossRef]
5. Tahara, A.; Takasu, T.; Yokono, M.; Imamura, M.; Kurosaki, E. Characterization and comparison of sodium-glucose cotransporter 2 inhibitors: Part 2. Antidiabetic effects in type 2 diabetic mice. *J. Pharmacol. Sci.* **2016**, *131*, 198–208. [CrossRef]
6. Schuhmacher, J.; Buhner, K.; Witt-Laido, A. Determination of the free fraction and relative free fraction of drugs strongly bound to plasma proteins. *J. Pharm. Sci.* **2000**, *89*, 1008–1021. [CrossRef]
7. Jeon, J.H.; Lee, S.; Lee, W.; Jin, S.; Kwon, M.; Shin, C.H.; Choi, M.K.; Song, I.S. Herb-drug interaction of red ginseng extract and ginsenoside Rc with valsartan in rats. *Molecules* **2020**, *25*, 622. [CrossRef] [PubMed]
8. Mathialagan, S.; Piotrowski, M.A.; Tess, D.A.; Feng, B.; Litchfield, J.; Varma, M.V.; Litchfiled, J. Quantitative prediction of human renal clearance and drug-drug interactions of organic anion transporter substrates using in vitro transport data: A relative activity factor approach. *Drug Metab. Dispos.* **2017**, *45*, 409–417. [CrossRef] [PubMed]
9. Song, I.S.; Jeong, H.U.; Choi, M.K.; Kwon, M.; Shin, Y.; Kim, J.H.; Lee, H.S. Interactions between cyazofamid and human drug transporters. *J. Biochem. Mol. Toxic.* **2020**, e22459. [CrossRef]
10. Choi, M.K.; Kwon, M.; Ahn, J.H.; Kim, N.J.; Bae, M.A.; Song, I.S. Transport characteristics and transporter-based drug-drug interactions of TM-25659, a novel TAZ modulator. *Biopharm. Drug Dispos.* **2014**, *35*, 183–194. [CrossRef]
11. Grempler, R.; Thomas, L.; Eckhardt, M.; Himmelsbach, F.; Sauer, A.; Sharp, D.E.; Bakker, R.A.; Mark, M.; Klein, T.; Eickelmann, P. Empagliflozin, a novel selective sodium glucose cotransporter-2 (SGLT-2) inhibitor: Characterisation and comparison with other SGLT-2 inhibitors. *Diabetes Obes. Metab.* **2012**, *14*, 83–90. [CrossRef]

12. Jin, S.; Lee, S.; Jeon, J.H.; Kim, H.; Choi, M.K.; Song, I.S. Enhanced intestinal permeability and plasma concentration of metformin in rats by the repeated administration of red ginseng extract. *Pharmaceutics* **2019**, *11*, e189. [CrossRef] [PubMed]
13. Choi, M.K.; Jin, Q.R.; Choi, Y.L.; Ahn, S.H.; Bae, M.A.; Song, I.S. Inhibitory effects of ketoconazole and rifampin on OAT1 and OATP1B1 transport activities: Considerations on drug-drug interactions. *Biopharm. Drug Dispos.* **2011**, *32*, 175–184. [CrossRef] [PubMed]
14. Kim, S.; Choi, W.G.; Kwon, M.; Lee, S.; Cho, Y.Y.; Lee, J.Y.; Kang, H.C.; Song, I.S.; Lee, H.S. In vitro inhibitory effects of APINACA on human major Cytochrome P450, UDP-Glucuronosyltransferase enzymes, and drug transporters. *Molecules* **2019**, *24*, e3000. [CrossRef] [PubMed]
15. Harvey, A.L.; Edrada-Ebel, R.; Quinn, R.J. The re-emergence of natural products for drug discovery in the genomics era. *Nat. Rev. Drug Discov.* **2015**, *14*, 111–129. [CrossRef] [PubMed]
16. Vallon, V.; Eraly, S.A.; Rao, S.R.; Gerasimova, M.; Rose, M.; Nagle, M.; Anzai, N.; Smith, T.; Sharma, K.; Nigam, S.K.; et al. A role for the organic anion transporter OAT3 in renal creatinine secretion in mice. *Am. J. Physiol. Renal Physiol.* **2012**, *302*, F1293–F1299. [CrossRef] [PubMed]
17. Jeong, H.U.; Kwon, M.; Lee, Y.; Yoo, J.S.; Shin, D.H.; Song, I.S.; Lee, H.S. Organic anion transporter 3-and organic anion transporting polypeptides 1B1-and 1B3-mediated transport of catalposide. *Drug Des. Dev. Ther.* **2015**, *9*, 643–653.
18. Yamamoto, K.; Uchida, S.; Kitano, K.; Fukuhara, N.; Okumura-Kitajima, L.; Gunji, E.; Kozakai, A.; Tomoike, H.; Kojima, N.; Asami, J.; et al. TS-071 is a novel, potent and selective renal sodium-glucose cotransporter 2 (SGLT2) inhibitor with anti-hyperglycaemic activity. *Br. J. Pharmacol.* **2011**, *164*, 181–191. [CrossRef]
19. Meneilly, G.S.; Demuth, H.U.; McIntosh, C.H.S.; Pederson, R.A. Effect of ageing and diabetes on glucose-dependent insulinotropic polypeptide and dipeptidyl peptidase IV responses to oral glucose. *Diabetic Med.* **2000**, *17*, 346–350. [CrossRef]
20. Lorey, S.; Stockel-Maschek, A.; Faust, J.; Brandt, W.; Stiebitz, B.; Gorrell, M.D.; Kahne, T.; Mrestani-Klaus, C.; Wrenger, S.; Reinhold, D.; et al. Different modes of dipeptidyl peptidase IV (CD26) inhibition by oligopeptides derived from the N-terminus of HIV-1 Tat indicate at least two inhibitor binding sites. *Eur. J. Biochem.* **2003**, *270*, 2147–2156. [CrossRef]
21. Ohkura, T. Ipragliflozin: A novel sodium-glucose cotransporter 2 inhibitor developed in Japan. *World J. Diabetes* **2015**, *6*, 136–144. [CrossRef] [PubMed]
22. Obermeier, M.; Yao, M.; Khanna, A.; Koplowitz, B.; Zhu, M.; Li, K.; Komoroski, B.; Kasichayanula, S.; Discenza, L.; Washburn, W.; et al. In vitro characterization and pharmacokinetics of dapagliflozin (BMS-512148), a potent sodium-glucose cotransporter type II Inhibitor, in animals and humans. *Drug Metab. Dispos.* **2010**, *38*, 405–414. [CrossRef] [PubMed]
23. Demaris, K.M.; White, J.R. Dapagliflozin, an SGLT2 inhibitor for the treatment of type 2 diabetes. *Drugs Today* **2013**, *49*, 289–301. [CrossRef] [PubMed]
24. Takasu, T.; Yokono, M.; Tahara, A.; Takakura, S. In vitro pharmacological profile of ipragliflozin, a sodium glucose co-transporter 2 Inhibitor. *Biol. Pharm. Bull.* **2019**, *42*, 507–511. [CrossRef]

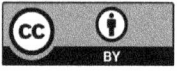

© 2020 by the authors. Licensee MDPI, Basel, Switzerland. This article is an open access article distributed under the terms and conditions of the Creative Commons Attribution (CC BY) license (http://creativecommons.org/licenses/by/4.0/).

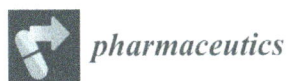

Article

Identification of Catalposide Metabolites in Human Liver and Intestinal Preparations and Characterization of the Relevant Sulfotransferase, UDP-glucuronosyltransferase, and Carboxylesterase Enzymes

Deok-Kyu Hwang [1,†], Ju-Hyun Kim [2,†], Yongho Shin [1], Won-Gu Choi [1], Sunjoo Kim [1], Yong-Yeon Cho [1], Joo Young Lee [1], Han Chang Kang [1] and Hye Suk Lee [1,*]

[1] BK21 PLUS Team for Creative Leader Program for Pharmacomics-based Future Pharmacy, College of Pharmacy, The Catholic University of Korea, Bucheon 14662, Korea
[2] College of Pharmacy, Yeungnam University, Gyeongsan 38541, Korea
* Correspondence: sianalee@catholic.ac.kr; Tel.: +82-2-2164-4061; Fax: +82-32-342-2013
† These authors contributed equally to this work.

Received: 24 June 2019; Accepted: 19 July 2019; Published: 22 July 2019

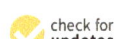

Abstract: Catalposide, an active component of *Veronica* species such as *Catalpa ovata* and *Pseudolysimachion lingifolium*, exhibits anti-inflammatory, antinociceptive, anti-oxidant, hepatoprotective, and cytostatic activities. We characterized the in vitro metabolic pathways of catalposide to predict its pharmacokinetics. Catalposide was metabolized to catalposide sulfate (M1), 4-hydroxybenzoic acid (M2), 4-hydroxybenzoic acid glucuronide (M3), and catalposide glucuronide (M4) by human hepatocytes, liver S9 fractions, and intestinal microsomes. M1 formation from catalposide was catalyzed by sulfotransferases (SULTs) 1C4, SULT1A1*1, SULT1A1*2, and SULT1E1. Catalposide glucuronidation to M4 was catalyzed by gastrointestine-specific UDP-glucuronosyltransferases (UGTs) 1A8 and UGT1A10; M4 was not detected after incubation of catalposide with human liver preparations. Hydrolysis of catalposide to M2 was catalyzed by carboxylesterases (CESs) 1 and 2, and M2 was further metabolized to M3 by UGT1A6 and UGT1A9 enzymes. Catalposide was also metabolized in extrahepatic tissues; genetic polymorphisms of the carboxylesterase (CES), UDP-glucuronosyltransferase (UGT), and sulfotransferase (SULT) enzymes responsible for catalposide metabolism may cause inter-individual variability in terms of catalposide pharmacokinetics.

Keywords: catalposide; in vitro human metabolism; UDP-glucuronosyltransferase; sulfotransferase; carboxylesterase

---

1. Introduction

Catalposide is an active iridoid glycoside of *Veronica* species including *Catalpa ovata* and *Pseudolysimachion lingifolium* [1–3]. Catalposide exhibits various biological effects including anti-inflammatory [4–9], anti-oxidant [10], antinociceptive [8], cytostatic [11], hypolipidemic via peroxisome proliferator-activated receptor-α activation [12], and hepatoprotective activities [13].

Catalposide had a short half-life (19.3 ± 9.5 min), and exhibited high systemic clearance (96.7 ± 44.1 mL/min/kg), and low urinary excretion (9.9 ± 4.1% of the dose) after intravenous administration of 10 mg/kg to male Sprague-Dawley rats [14]. This indicated that catalposide might be extensively metabolized in rats. However, catalposide remained stable after 1 h incubation with rat liver microsomes in the presence of NADPH [14]. Thus, catalposide may be catabolized via non-cytochrome P450 (CYP)-mediated mechanism. Catalposide was the substrate of OAT3, OATP1B1, and OATP1B3 transporters and weakly inhibited their transport activities with IC_{50} values of 83, 200, and 235 µM, respectively, suggesting that OAT3, OATP1B1, and OATP1B3 may regulate the pharmacokinetics and drug interactions of catalposide [15].

Pharmacokinetics and metabolism of potential active constituents in herbal drugs is helpful for the determination of dosage regimens and interpretation of pharmacological effects under clinical conditions [16]. It is important to establish the comparative metabolism and drug-metabolizing enzymes of active constituents for a full characterization of its pharmacokinetics, pharmacodynamics, and toxicity. The characterization of drug-metabolizing enzymes such as CYPs, carboxylesterases (CESs), UDP-glucuronosyltransferases (UGTs), and sulfotransferases (SULTs) responsible for the metabolism of a drug may reveal inter-individual variability in drug metabolism and the potential drug interactions [17–19]. However, catalposide metabolism has not been studied in humans and animals. We identified catalposide metabolites and drug-metabolizing enzymes involved to predict its pharmacokinetics and possible drug interactions.

We identified catalposide metabolites formed from in vitro incubations of catalposide with human hepatocytes, intestinal microsomes, and liver S9 fractions using liquid chromatography-high resolution mass spectrometry (LC-HRMS) and characterized the CES, UGT, and SULT enzymes involved in catalposide metabolism using human cDNA-expressed CES, UGT, and SULT supersomes, respectively.

2. Materials and Methods

2.1. Materials and Reagents

Catalposide (purity, 98%) was obtained from Aobious Inc. (Gloucester, MA, USA). Alamethicin, 3-phosphoadenosine-5-phosphosulfate (PAPS), and uridine 5′-diphosphoglucuronic acid (UDPGA) were from Sigma-Aldrich Co. (St. Louis, MO, USA). 4-hydroxybenzoic acid and 4-hydroxybenzoic acid glucuronide were purchased from Toronto Research Chemicals (North York, ON, Canada). Pooled human intestinal microsomes; pooled human liver S9 fractions; human cDNA-expressed UGTs 1A1/3/4/6/7/8/9/10 and 2B4/7/15/17 supersomes; human cDNA-expressed CESs 1b, 1c, and 2 supersomes; cryopreserved human hepatocytes; and hepatocyte purification kits were obtained from Corning Life Sciences (Woburn, MA, USA). Human cDNA-expressed SULT 1A1*1, 1A1*2, 1A2, 1A3, 1B1, 1C2, 1C4, 1E1, and 2A1 supersomes were purchased from Cypex Ltd. (Dundee, UK). Methanol (HPLC grade) was from Burdick & Jackson Inc. (SK Chemicals, Ulsan, Korea), and all other chemicals were of the highest quality available. Calibration mixtures for Exactive MS [ProteoMass LTQ/FT-hybrid ESI positive mode Cal Mix (MSCAL5) and negative mode Cal Mix (MSCAL6)] were obtained from Supelco (Bellefonte, PA, USA).

2.2. In Vitro Metabolism of Catalposide in Cryopreserved Human Hepatocytes

Cryopreserved human hepatocytes were recovered with the aid of a hepatocyte purification kit, and viable cells were resuspended in William's E buffer at a final concentration of 1.28×10^6 cells/mL [20]. Human hepatocyte suspensions (62.5 µL, 8.00×10^4 cells) and 62.5 µL of 400 µM catalposide in William's E buffer were added to the wells of a 96-well plate and the mixture was incubated for 120 min at 37 °C in a CO_2 incubator. Methanol (250 µL) was added to each well and the mixture was centrifuged at $3000\times g$ for 10 min. Aliquots of the supernatants (250 µL) were evaporated to dryness using a vacuum evaporator (Genevac Ltd., Ipswich, UK). Each residue was dissolved in 100 µL of 5% methanol and an aliquot (5 µL) was injected into the LC-HRMS system.

2.3. In Vitro Metabolism of Catalposide in Human Liver S9 Fractions and Intestinal Microsomes

Each reaction mixture contained 50 mM potassium phosphate buffer (pH 7.4), 10 mM magnesium chloride, human liver S9 fractions or human intestinal microsomes (100 µg protein), 2 mM UDPGA or

200 µM PAPS, 200 µM catalposide or a possible metabolite, and 1000 µM 4-hydroxybenzoic acid in a volume of 200 µL. Samples lacking UDPGA and PAPS served as controls. The mixtures were incubated at 37 °C for 60 min and the reactions were then quenched by adding 500 µL of methanol. The tubes were centrifuged and the supernatants evaporated to dryness using a vacuum concentrator. The residues were dissolved in 100 µL of 5% methanol and 5 µL aliquots were injected into the LC-HRMS system.

2.4. Characterization of Human SULTs Involved in Catalposide Sulfation

To screen for SULT enzymes involved in catalposide sulfation, each 100 µL of reaction mixture contained 20 µM PAPS; 10 mM dithiothreitol; 5 mM magnesium chloride; 50 mM phosphate buffer (pH 7.4); 150 µM catalposide; and the human liver S9 fraction (40 µg protein) or human cDNA-expressed SULT 1A1*1, 1A1*2, 1A2, 1A3, 2A1, 1B1, 1C2, 1C4, or 1E1 supersomes [1A1*1 (0.25), 1A1*2 (0.5), 1A2 (0.25), 1A3 (0.2), 2A1 (1.25), 1B1 (0.5), 1C2 (2.5), 1C4 (0.1), 1E1 (0.2 µg protein)]. Incubation proceeded at 37 °C for 5 min. The reactions were stopped by adding 100 µL of methanol containing 30 ng/mL 4-methylumbelliferone (an internal standard). After vortex-mixing and centrifugation, 50 µL of each supernatant was diluted with 50 µL deionized water. The mixture was transferred to an injection vial, and an aliquot (5 µL) was injected into the LC-HRMS system.

To explore the kinetics of the metabolism of catalposide to catalposide sulfate, various concentrations of catalposide (10 to 2000 µM) were incubated in duplicate with pooled human liver S9 fractions (40 µg protein) or human cDNA-expressed SULT1A1*1 (0.5 µg protein), SULT1A1*2 (0.5 µg protein), SULT1C4 (0.1 µg protein), or SULT1E1 (0.2 µg protein) in the presence of 20 µM PAPS, 10 mM dithiothreitol, and 5 mM magnesium chloride at 37 °C for 5 min to obtain K_m and V_{max} values.

2.5. Characterization of Human UGTs Involved in Catalposide and 4-Hydroxybenzoic Acid Glucuronidation

To identify the UGT enzymes responsible for formation of catalposide glucuronide (M4) from catalposide and 4-hydroxybenzoic acid glucuronide (M3) from 4-hydroxybenzoic acid (M2), 100 µL reaction mixtures containing human intestinal microsomes (40 µg protein), or human cDNA-expressed UGTs 1A1, 1A3, 1A4, 1A6, 1A7, 1A8, 1A9, 1A10, 2B4, 2B7, 2B15, or 2B17 (10 µg protein); 2 mM UDPGA; 0.025 mg/mL alamethicin; and 400 µM catalposide or 500 µM 4-hydroxybenzoic acid in 50 mM Tris buffer (pH 7.4) were incubated at 37 °C for 60 min. The reactions were stopped by addition of 100 µL methanol containing 30 ng/mL 4-methylumbelliferone (an internal standard). After vortex-mixing and centrifugation, 50 µL of each supernatant was diluted with an equal volume of water and a 5 µL aliquot was injected into the LC-HRMS system.

To explore the kinetics of the metabolism of catalposide to catalposide glucuronide, various concentrations of catalposide (10, 25, 100, 400, 800, 1200, 1600, and 2000 µM) were incubated in duplicate with 2 mM UDPGA, 0.025 mg/mL alamethicin, pooled human intestinal microsomes (40 µg protein), or human cDNA-expressed UGT1A8 or UGT1A10 supersomes (20 µg protein), to obtain K_m and V_{max} values.

2.6. Characterization of Carboxylesterases Involved in the Formation of 4-Hydroxybenzoic Acid from Catalposide

To identify the CES enzymes involved in hydrolysis of catalposide to 4-hydroxybenzoic acid, 100 µL reaction mixtures containing human liver S9 fractions; human intestinal microsomes; or human CES1b, CES1c, or CES2 enzymes (50 µg protein), and catalposide (200 or 400 µM) in 50 mM phosphate buffer (pH 7.4) were incubated at 37 °C for 30 min. Reactions were stopped by addition of 100 µL 4-methylumbelliferone (internal standard, 10 ng/mL) in methanol. After vortex-mixing and centrifugation, 50 µL of each supernatant was diluted with 50 µL of deionized water. Each mixture was transferred to an injection vial, and a 5 µL aliquot was injected into the LC-HRMS system.

2.7. LC-HRMS Analysis of Catalposide and Metabolites

To separate and identify catalposide and its metabolites, we used a Q-Exactive Orbitrap mass spectrometer coupled to an Accela UPLC system (Thermo Scientific, Waltham, MA, USA). Catalposide and its metabolites were optimally separated on a Halo C18 column via gradient elution using 5% (v/v) methanol in 1 mM ammonium formate (pH 3.1) (mobile phase A) and methanol (mobile phase B) at a flow rate of 0.5 mL/min: 5% mobile phase B for 2 min, 5–20% mobile phase B over 11.5 min, 20–90% mobile phase B over 0.5 min, 90% mobile phase B for 3 min, 90–5% mobile phase B over 0.5 min, and 5% mobile phase B for 2.5 min. The column and the autosampler were maintained at 40 and 6 °C, respectively. Accurate mass measurements of catalposide and its metabolites were derived via electrospray ionization in the negative mode using the following electrospray source settings: ion transfer capillary temperature, 330 °C; needle spray voltage, −3000 V; capillary voltage, −47.5 V; nitrogen sheath gas, 50 arbitrary units; auxiliary gas, 15 arbitrary units. The resolution and automatic gain control were scaled to 70,000 and 1,000,000, respectively. MS data were obtained using external calibration over the scan range *m/z* 100–700 and processed using Xcalibur software version 2.2 (Thermo Scientific). The Q-Exactive Orbitrap MS was calibrated using MSCAL5 and MSCAL6 for the positive and negative ion modes, respectively. Nitrogen gas was employed for higher-energy collision dissociation (HCD) at an energy of 25 eV to obtain product ion spectra of catalposide and its metabolites. Structures were determined using Mass Frontier software (version 6.0; HighChem Ltd., Bratislava, Slovakia). We used the extracted ion monitoring mode for quantification: *m/z* 481.1349 for catalposide, *m/z* 657.1674 for catalposide glucuronide, *m/z* 561.0921 for catalposide sulfate, *m/z* 137.0239 for 4-hydroxybenzoic acid, *m/z* 313.0569 for 4-hydroxybenzoic acid glucuronide, and *m/z* 175.0410 for 4-methylumbelliferone (the internal standard). The peak areas of all components were integrated using Xcalibur software. The calibration curve was linear over the catalposide concentration range 0.5–200 pmol. The concentrations of catalposide glucuronide and catalposide sulfate were calculated using the calibration curve for catalposide because we had no authentic standards.

2.8. Data Analysis

All results are the average of two determinations obtained using pooled human intestinal microsomes, pooled human liver S9 fractions, UGTs, and SULTs. The apparent kinetic parameters (K_m, V_{max}, n, and K_i) for formation of catalposide glucuronide or catalposide sulfate by human intestinal microsomes, liver S9 fractions, UGTs, or SULTs were determined by fitting the Hill equation model [$V = V_{max}S^n/(K_m^n + S^n)$], the substrate inhibition model [$V = V_{max}/(1 + K_m/S + S/K_i)$], or the single enzyme model [$V = V_{max}S/(K_m + S)$] to the unweighted formation rates of catalposide glucuronide and catalposide sulfate, respectively, over a range of catalposide concentrations using Enzyme Kinetics software (version 1.1 SPSS Science Inc., Chicago, IL, USA). In the above equations, V is the velocity of the reaction at substrate concentration [S], V_{max} is the maximum velocity, n is the Hill constant, K_m is the substrate concentration at which the reaction velocity is 50% of V_{max}, and K_i is the dissociation constant of the substrate binding to the inhibitory region within the enzyme active site.

3. Results

3.1. In Vitro Metabolic Profiles of Catalposide Incubated with Human Hepatocytes and Intestinal Microsomes

LC-HRMS analysis of extracts after incubation of catalposide with human hepatocytes revealed three metabolites (M1–M3) and residual catalposide (Figure 1A). LC-HRMS analysis of reaction mixtures after incubation of catalposide with human intestinal microsomes in the presence of UDPGA yielded M2, M3, and a new metabolite M4 (Figure 1B).

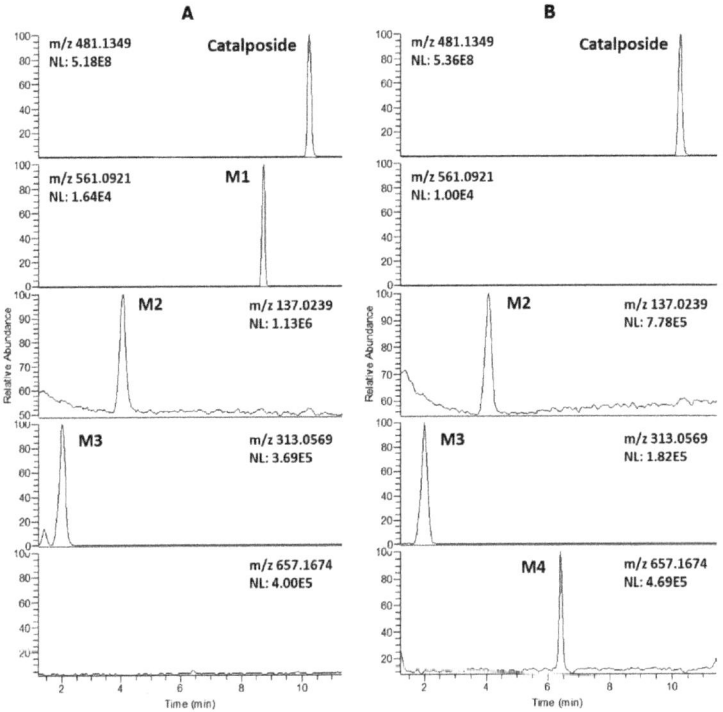

Figure 1. Extracted ion chromatograms of catalposide and its possible metabolites after incubation of 200 μM catalposide with (**A**) human hepatocytes for 2 h at 37 °C in a CO_2 incubator and (**B**) human intestinal microsomes in the presence of UDPGA at 37 °C for 1 h (mass accuracy: 5 ppm). The extracted ion chromatograms were reconstructed based on the [M−H]⁻ ions: m/z 481.1349 for catalposide, m/z 561.0921 for M1 (catalposide sulfate), m/z 137.0239 for M2 (4-hydroxybenzoic acid), m/z 313.0569 for M3 (4-hydroxybenzoic acid glucuronide), and m/z 657.1674 for M4 (catalposide glucuronide).

The formulae, deprotonated molecular ions ([M−H]⁻), mass errors, and retention times of catalposide and its four metabolites, M1–M4, are shown in Table 1. The four metabolite peaks were identified using the accurate mass values and the characteristic product ions of the product scan spectra (Table 1, Figure 2). The mass errors between the theoretical and observed m/z values for each metabolite were less than 5 ppm, indicating good correlations between the calculated theoretical masses and the experimentally observed masses obtained after full-scan MS analysis.

Table 1. Molecular formulae, deprotonated molecular ions ([M−H]⁻), mass errors, retention times (t_R), and product ions of catalposide and its metabolites were identified after incubation of catalposide with human hepatocytes and intestinal microsomes.

Metabolite	Formula	Exact Mass [M−H]⁻ (m/z)	Error (ppm)	t_R (min)	Product Ions (m/z)
Catalposide	$C_{22}H_{26}O_{12}$	481.1349	−0.6	10.26	319.0822, 205.0497, 137.0239
M1	$C_{22}H_{26}SO_{15}$	561.0921	0.2	8.74	481.1349, 319.0822, 205.0499, 137.0239
M2	$C_7H_6O_3$	137.0239	−3.6	4.07	93.0339
M3	$C_{13}H_{14}O_9$	313.0569	1.3	2.02	193.0345, 175.0240, 137.0239, 113.0239, 85.0283
M4	$C_{28}H_{34}O_{18}$	657.1674	0.3	6.41	481.1353, 319.0823, 205.0499, 175.0240, 137.0239, 113.0238, 85.0283

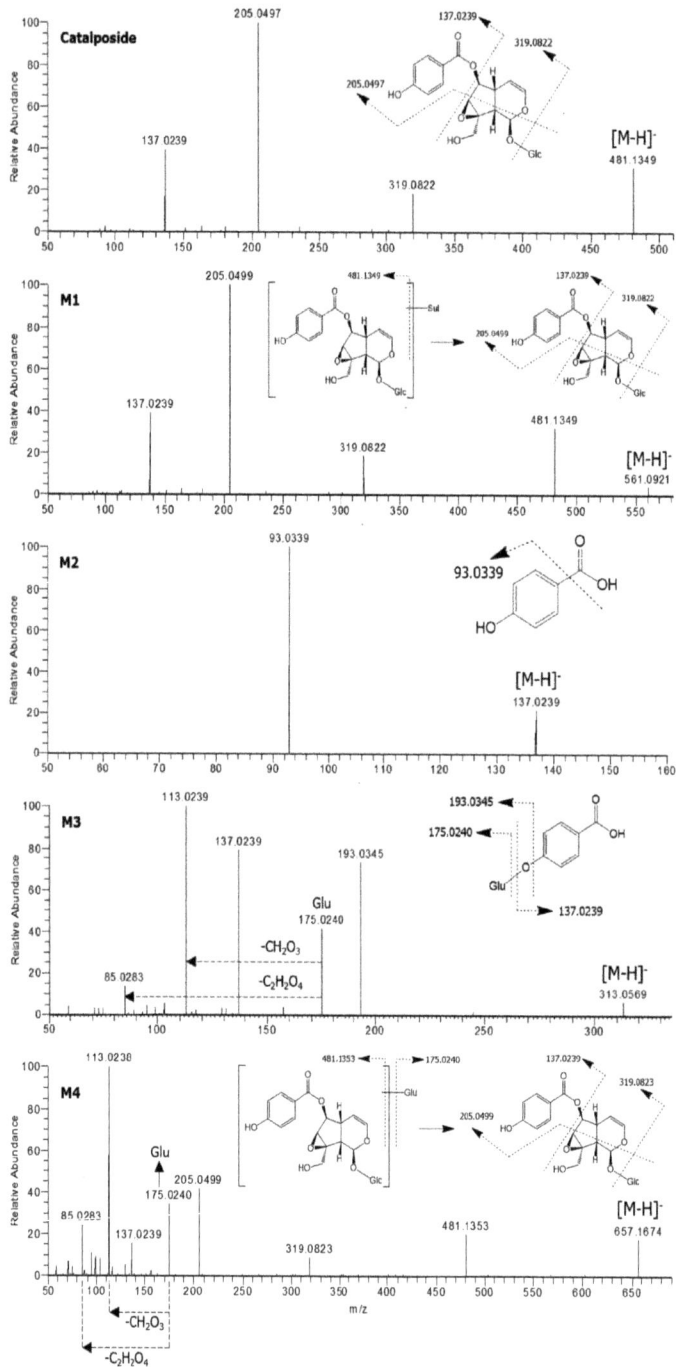

Figure 2. Product scan spectra of catalposide and its four metabolites, M1–M4 obtained via liquid chromatography-high resolution mass spectrometry (LC-HRMS) analysis of reaction mixtures obtained after incubation of catalposide with human intestinal microsomes in the presence of uridine 5′-diphosphoglucuronic acid (UDPGA) or human hepatocytes. Glc: glucose; Glu: glucuronosyl.

The product scan spectra of catalposide exhibiting the [M−H]⁻ ion at m/z 481.1349 generated characteristic product ions at m/z 319.0822 (reflecting loss of glucose from the [M−H]⁻ ion), m/z 205.0497 (loss of $C_5H_6O_3$ caused by the breakdown of the iridoid moiety of m/z 319.0822), and m/z 137.0239 (the 4-hydroxybenzoyl moiety) (Figure 2).

M1 exhibited an [M−H]⁻ ion at m/z 561.0921, that is, 80 amu higher than the [M−H]⁻ ion of catalposide, indicating that M1 was catalposide sulfate. The product scan spectra of M1 generated the characteristic product ions at m/z 481.1349 (loss of SO_3 from the [M−H]⁻ ion), m/z 319.0822 (loss of glucose from m/z 481.1349), m/z 205.0499, and m/z 137.0239 (Figure 2). M1 was also formed from catalposide after incubation with human liver S9 fractions in the presence of PAPS. Thus, M1 was identified as catalposide sulfate.

M2 exhibited an [M−H]⁻ ion at m/z 137.0239 and generated a characteristic product ion at m/z 93.0339 (reflecting loss of a carboxyl group from the [M−H]⁻ ion)(Figure 2). M2 was identified as 4-hydroxybenzoic acid by comparison with the mass, retention time, and product ion of the authentic standard.

M3 exhibited an [M−H]⁻ ion at m/z 313.0569, that is, 176 amu higher than the [M−H]⁻ ion of M2 (4-hydroxybenzoic acid), reflecting glucuronidation of M2. In the product scan spectrum of M3, characteristic product ions were observed at m/z 137.0239 (reflecting loss of the glucuronosyl moiety from the [M−H]⁻ ion), m/z 175.0240 (the glucuronosyl moiety), and m/z 113.0239 (loss of CO_2 and H_2O from m/z 175.0240) (Figure 2). Incubation of 4-hydroxybenzoic acid (M2) with human liver S9 fractions or intestinal microsomes in the presence of UDPGA yielded M3, which was identified as 4-hydroxybenzoic acid glucuronide by comparison with the mass, retention time, and product ions of the authentic standard.

M4 exhibited an [M−H]⁻ ion at m/z 657.1674, that is, 176 amu higher than the [M−H]⁻ ion of catalposide, reflecting catalposide glucuronidation. M4 yielded characteristic product ions at m/z 481.1353 (reflecting loss of the glucuronosyl moiety from the [M−H]⁻ ion), m/z 319.0823 (loss of glucose from m/z 481.1353), m/z 205.0499, m/z 175.0240, m/z 113.0238, and m/z 85.0283 (Figure 2). Thus, M4 was identified as catalposide glucuronide.

The possible in vitro metabolic pathways of catalposide in humans are shown in Figure 3. Catalposide is metabolized to catalposide sulfate (M1), catalposide glucuronide (M4), and 4-hydroxybenzoic acid (M2); the latter is then further metabolized to 4-hydroxybenzoic acid glucuronide (M3).

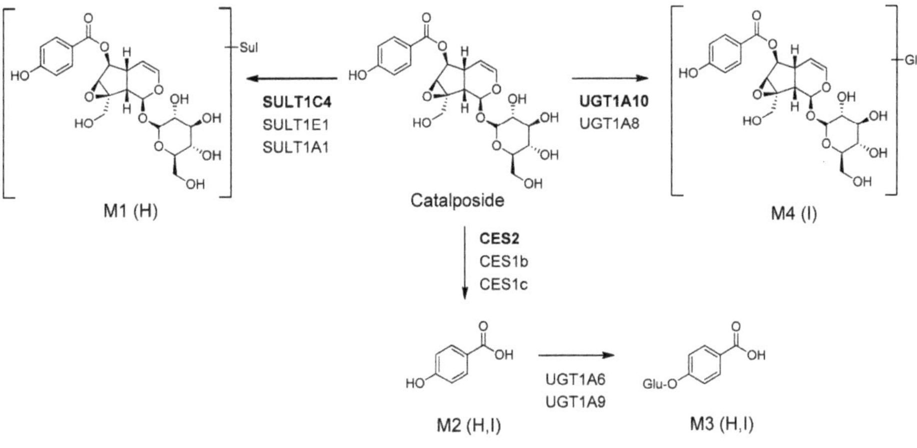

Figure 3. Possible in vitro metabolic pathways of catalposide incubated with human hepatocytes and intestinal microsomes. H: human hepatocytes; I: human intestinal microsomes; Sul: sulfate; Glu: glucuronic acid; CES: carboxylesterase; UGT: UDP-glucuronosyltransferase; SULT: sulfotransferase.

3.2. Characterization of Human SULT, UGT, and CES Enzymes Involved in Catalposide Metabolism

A screen using human cDNA-expressed SULTs 1A1*1, 1A1*2, 1A2, 1A3, 1B1, 1C2, 1C4, 1E1, and 2A1 to assess the formation of catalposide sulfate (M1) from catalposide identified possible roles for SULTs 1A1*1, 1A1*2, 1C4, and 1E1 (Figure 4).

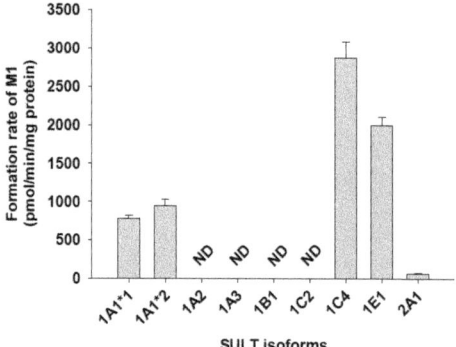

Figure 4. Rate of formation of catalposide sulfate (M1) from 150 μM catalposide by human cDNA-expressed SULT enzymes. All data are means ± SD (n = 3). ND: <32 pmol/min/mg protein.

The formation of catalposide sulfate from catalposide catalyzed by SULTs 1A1*1, 1A1*2, and 1E1 exhibited substrate inhibition kinetics, but the activities of SULT1C4 and pooled human liver S9 fractions fitted the Hill equation (Figure 5). The enzyme kinetic parameters for the formation of catalposide sulfate from catalposide are listed in Table 2. SULT1C4 exhibited a higher affinity for catalposide and more rapid sulfation than did SULT1A1*1, SULT1A1*2, and SULT1E1.

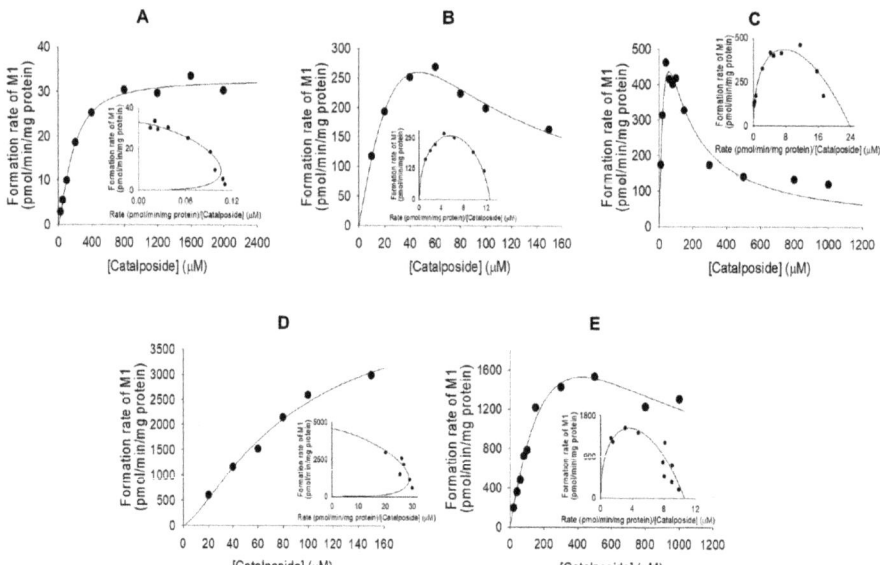

Figure 5. Michaelis–Menten plots of the sulfation of catalposide to catalposide sulfate (M1) by pooled human liver S9 fractions (**A**) and human cDNA-expressed SULT1A1*1 (**B**), SULT1A1*2 (**C**), SULT1C4 (**D**), and SULT1E1 (**E**). Insets: Eadie–Hofstee plots. Each data point represents the average of two determinations.

Table 2. Kinetic parameters for the formation of catalposide sulfate (M1) and catalposide glucuronide (M4) from catalposide in pooled human liver S9 fractions, intestinal microsomes, and human cDNA-expressed sulfotransferase (SULT) or UDP-glucuronosyltransferase (UGT) enzymes.

Enzyme	K_m (µM)	V_{max}	K_i (µM)	n	Cl_{int}
Sulfation of catalposide to M1					
SULT1A1*1	162.0	2046.8	13.7	-	12.6
SULT1A1*2	50.5	1203.2	65.5	-	23.8
SULT1C4	89.8	4576.2	-	1.4	51.0
SULT1E1	456.6	4840.0	391.4	-	10.6
Human liver S9 fractions	169.7	32.8	-	1.4	0.19
Glucuronidation of catalposide to M4					
UGT1A8	1230.1	48.7	-	0.9221	0.0396
UGT1A10	641.7	218.1	-	2.3	0.3399
Human intestinal microsomes	1341.3	106.2	-	-	0.0792

V_{max}: pmol/min/mg protein; Cl_{int}: µL/min/mg protein; n: Hill coefficient.

A screen using human cDNA-expressed UGTs 1A1, 1A3, 1A4, 1A6, 1A7, 1A8, 1A9, 1A10, 2B4, 2B7, 2B15, and 2B17 supersomes for the metabolism of 4-hydroxybenzoic acid (M2) to 4-hydroxybenzoic acid glucuronide (M3) identified possible roles of UGT1A6 and UGT1A9 (Figure 6A). The results show that 4-hydroxybenzoic acid glucuronide (M3) was produced on incubation of catalposide with human hepatocytes, liver S9 fractions, and intestinal microsomes.

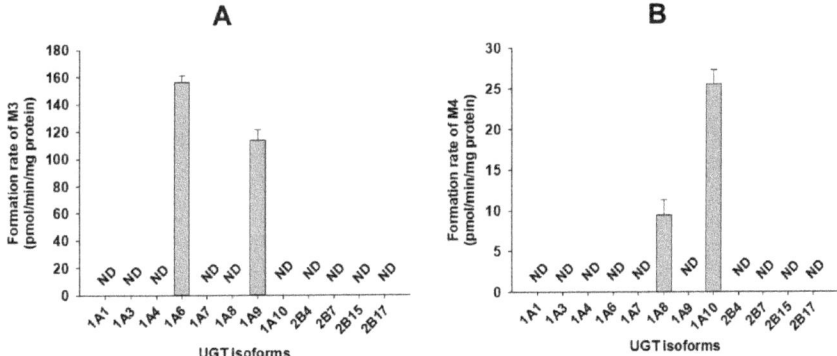

Figure 6. Rates of formation of (A) 4-hydroxybenzoic acid glucuronide (M3) from 500 µM 4-hydroxybenzoic acid (M2) and (B) catalposide glucuronide (M4) from 400 µM catalposide by human cDNA-expressed UGT enzymes. All data are means ± SD (n = 3). ND: <27 pmol/min/mg protein for M3, <0.83 pmol/min/mg protein for M4.

A screen using twelve human cDNA-expressed UGT supersomes, to assess the metabolism of catalposide to catalposide glucuronide (M4), identified possible roles of gastrointestinal tract-specific UGT1A8 and UGT1A10 (Figure 6B). The results show that catalposide glucuronide (M4) was produced after incubation of catalposide with pooled human intestinal microsomes, but not human liver S9 fractions.

Formation of catalposide glucuronide (M4) from catalposide by pooled human intestinal microsomes followed single enzyme kinetics; formation via UGT1A8 and UGT1A10 exhibited Hill equation kinetics (Figure 7, Table 2).

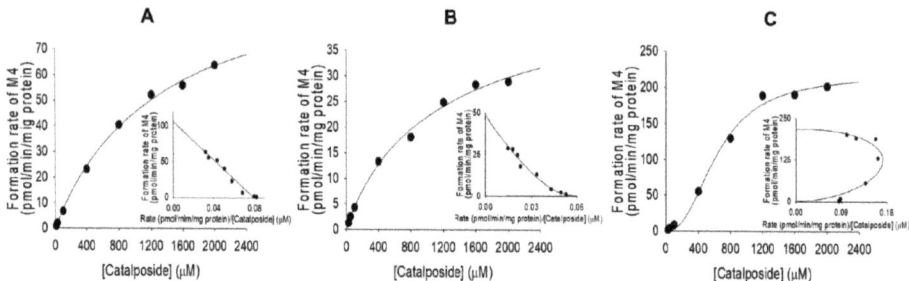

Figure 7. Michaelis–Menten plots for glucuronidation of catalposide to catalposide glucuronide (M4) by pooled human intestinal microsomes (**A**) and human cDNA-expressed UGT1A8 (**B**) and UGT1A10 (**C**). Insets: Eadie–Hofstee plots. Each data point represents the average of two determinations.

4-Hydroxybenzoic acid (M2) was formed from catalposide by pooled human liver S9 fractions; intestinal microsomes; and the CES1b, CES1c, and CES2 enzymes (Figure 8). The rate of formation of 4-hydroxybenzoic acid (M2) after incubation of catalposide with pooled human intestinal microsomes was higher than that after incubation with pooled human liver S9 fractions (Figure 8).

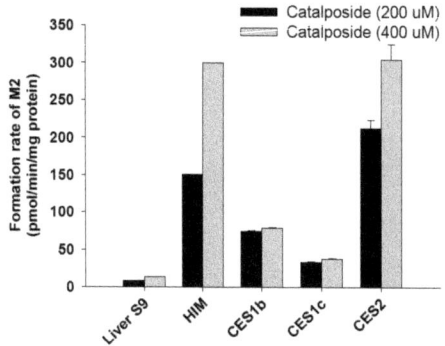

Figure 8. Rates of formation of 4-hydroxybenzoic acid (M2) from 200 μM and 400 μM catalposide in human liver S9 fractions (Liver S9); human intestinal microsomes (HIM); and human cDNA-expressed CES1b, CES1c, and CES2 enzymes. All data are means ± SD (n = 3).

4. Discussion

Catalposide was metabolized to catalposide sulfate (M1), catalposide glucuronide (M4), 4-hydroxybenzoic acid (M2), and M2 glucuronide (M3) by human hepatocytes or intestinal microsomes (Figure 3). On the basis of the kinetics of catalposide sulfate (M1) formation from catalposide catalyzed by human cDNA-expressed SULTs 1A1*1, 1A1*2, 1C4, and 1E1 (Figure 4, Table 2), we suggest that SULT1A1, SULT1C4, and SULT1E1 may play major roles in this metabolism. SULT1C4 exhibited higher activity (Cl_{int}, 51.0 μL/min/mg protein) in terms of catalposide sulfation than did SULT1A1*1, SULT1A1*2, or SULT1E1 (Cl_{int}, 10.6~23.8 μL/min/mg protein) (Table 2). SULT1C4 is highly expressed in the fetal lung and kidney, and at lower levels in the fetal heart, adult kidney, ovary, brain, and spinal cord [21–23]. SULT1A1 is the major hepatic SULT (53% of total hepatic SULTs), but is also present in substantial quantities in the small intestine (19% of total SULTs) [23,24]. SULT1E1 is expressed at relatively low levels in the liver (6% of total SULTs) and small intestine (8% of total SULTs), but is the most abundant enzyme in the lung (40% of total SULTs) [23,24]. Catalposide was metabolized to M1 by cytosolic SULTs of both hepatic and extrahepatic tissues. There may be inter-individual variability in catalposide sulfation, given that SULT1A1, SULT1C4, and SULT1E1 polymorphisms are known in humans [25]. SULT1A1, SULT1C4, and SULT1E1 are induced or inhibited by various drugs and chemicals [26,27]; therefore, co-administration of drugs that inhibit or induce expression of these enzymes may affect catalposide sulfation and thus catalposide pharmacokinetics.

Metabolism of catalposide to catalposide glucuronide (M4) was mediated by human cDNA-expressed UGT1A8 and UGT1A10 enzymes, which are confined to the gastrointestinal tract [28–32] (Figure 7), indicating that catalposide glucuronidation was gastrointestinal tract-specific; glucuronidation was not detected after incubation of catalposide with human hepatocytes and liver S9 fractions. UGT1A10-catalyzed catalposide glucuronidation was more extensive (Cl_{int}, 0.3399 µL/min/mg protein) than UGT1A8-catalyzed glucuronidation (Cl_{int}, 0.0396 µL/min/mg protein) (Table 2). UGT1A10 is more abundant than UGT1A8 in the small intestine (17.3% vs. 0.8% of total UGT protein) and colon (27.4% vs. 1.5% of total UGT protein) [32]. Thus, UGT1A10 may play the major role in glucuronidation of catalposide and UGT1A8 only a minor role. The human UGT1A8 and UGT1A10 enzymes are inhibited by various drugs [30,32–35]. Therefore, co-administration of drugs that inhibit or induce UGT1A8 and UGT1A10 may affect catalposide glucuronidation.

CES2, the predominant CES of the intestine, was more active in terms of hydrolysis of catalposide to 4-hydroxybenzoic acid (M2) than were the hepato-predominant CES1b and CES1c enzymes [32,36]. Thus, the rate of formation of 4-hydroxybenzoic acid (M2) was higher when catalposide was incubated with pooled human intestinal microsomes than with pooled human liver S9 fractions.

UGT1A6 and UGT1A9 play major roles in the formation of 4-hydroxybenzoic acid glucuronide (M3) from 4-hydroxybenzoic acid (Figure 6A). Abbas et al. [37] found that UGT1A9 played the major role in metabolism of 4-hydroxybenzoic acid to 4-hydroxybenzoic acid glucuronide. UGT1A6 and UGT1A9 are major enzymes of both the liver and intestine; therefore, 4-hydroxybenzoic acid glucuronide (M3) was identified after incubation of catalposide with either human hepatocytes or intestinal microsomes.

5. Conclusions

Catalposide was metabolized to catalposide sulfate (M1), 4-hydroxybenzoic acid (M2), M2 glucuronide (M3), and catalposide glucuronide (M4) via sulfation, glucuronidation, and hydrolysis, on incubation with human hepatocytes, liver S9 fractions, or intestinal microsomes. SULT1A1, SULT1C4, and SULT1E1 formed catalposide sulfate (M1) from catalposide. Gastrointestine-specific UGT1A8 and UGT1A10 played major roles in formation of catalposide glucuronide (M4). CES2 and CES1 catalyzed hydrolysis of catalposide to 4-hydroxybenzoic acid (M2), which was further metabolized to M2 glucuronide (M3) by UGT1A6 and UGT1A9. These results suggest that SULT1A1, SULT1C4, SULT1E1, UGT1A8, UGT1A10, CES2, and CES1 enzymes may play important roles in the pharmacokinetics and drug–drug interaction of catalposide in humans. The pharmacokinetics of catalposide may be dramatically affected by the co-administration of inhibitors or inducers of UGTs, CESs, or SULTs.

Author Contributions: Conceptualization, D.-K.H. and H.S.L.; methodology, D.-K.H., W.-G.C., Y.S., and S.K.; software, D.-K.H. and J.-H.K.; investigation, D.-K.H., W.-G.C., Y.S., and S.K.; data curation, D.-K.H., Y.S., J.-H.K., and H.S.L.; writing—original draft preparation, D.-K.H., J.-H.K., and Y.S.; writing—review and editing, Y.-Y.C., J.Y.L., H.C.K., and H.S.L.; supervision, H.S.L.; project administration, H.S.L.; funding acquisition, H.C.K. and H.S.L.

Funding: This work was supported by the National Research Foundation of Korea (NRF) grant funded by the Korea government (MSIT) (NRF-2015M3A9E1028325, NRF-2017M3A9F5028608, and NRF-2017R1A4A1015036).

Conflicts of Interest: The authors declare no conflict of interest.

References

1. Harput, U.S.; Saracoglu, I.; Inoue, M.; Ogihara, Y. Phenylethanoid and Iridoid Glycosides from Veronica persica. *Chem. Pharm. Bull.* **2002**, *50*, 869–871. [CrossRef] [PubMed]
2. Harput, U.S.; Saracoglu, I.; Nagatsu, A.; Ogihara, Y. Iridoid Glucosides from Veronica hederifolia. *Chem. Pharm. Bull.* **2002**, *50*, 1106–1108. [CrossRef] [PubMed]
3. Harput, U.; Varel, M.; Nagatsu, A.; Saracoglu, I. Acylated iridoid glucosides from Veronica anagallis-aquatica. *Phytochemistry* **2004**, *65*, 2135–2139. [CrossRef] [PubMed]

4. Oh, H.; Pae, H.O.; Oh, G.S.; Lee, S.Y.; Chai, K.Y.; Song, C.E.; Kwon, T.O.; Chung, H.T.; Lee, H.S. Inhibition of Inducible Nitric Oxide Synthesis by Catalposide from Catalpa ovata. *Planta Med.* **2002**, *68*, 685–689. [CrossRef] [PubMed]
5. An, S.; Pae, H.; Oh, G.; Choi, B.; Jeong, S.; Jang, S.; Oh, H.; Kwon, T.; Song, C.E.; Chung, H. Inhibition of TNF-α, IL-1β, and IL-6 productions and NF-κB activation in lipopolysaccharide-activated RAW 264.7 macrophages by catalposide, an iridoid glycoside isolated from Catalpa ovata G. Don (Bignoniaceae). *Int. Immunopharmacol.* **2002**, *2*, 1173–1181. [CrossRef]
6. Moon, M.K.; Choi, B.M.; Oh, G.S.; Pae, H.O.; Kim, J.D.; Oh, H.; Oh, C.S.; Kim, D.H.; Rho, Y.D.; Shin, M.K.; et al. Catalposide protects Neuro 2A cells from hydrogen peroxide-induced cytotoxicity via the expression of heme oxygenase-1. *Toxicol. Lett.* **2003**, *145*, 46–54. [CrossRef]
7. Kim, S.W.; Choi, S.C.; Choi, E.Y.; Kim, K.S.; Oh, J.M.; Lee, H.J.; Oh, H.M.; Kim, S.; Oh, B.S.; Kimm, K.C.; et al. Catalposide, a Compound Isolated from Catalpa Ovata, Attenuates Induction of Intestinal Epithelial Proinflammatory Gene Expression and Reduces the Severity of Trinitrobenzene Sulfonic Acid-Induced Colitis in Mice. *Inflamm. Bowel Dis.* **2004**, *10*, 564–572. [CrossRef]
8. Kupeli, E.; Harput, U.S.; Varel, M.; Yesilada, E.; Saracoglu, I. Bioassay-guided isolation of iridoid glucosides with antinociceptive and anti-inflammatory activities from *Veronica anagallis-aquatica* L. *J. Ethnopharmacol.* **2005**, *102*, 170–176. [CrossRef]
9. Lu, Q.; Sun, Y.; Shu, Y.; Tan, S.; Yin, L.; Guo, Y.; Tang, L. HSCCC Separation of the Two Iridoid Glycosides and Three Phenolic Compounds from Veronica ciliata and Their in Vitro Antioxidant and Anti-Hepatocarcinoma Activities. *Molecules* **2016**, *21*, 1234. [CrossRef]
10. Kwak, J.H.; Kim, H.J.; Lee, K.H.; Kang, S.C.; Zee, O.P. Antioxidative iridoid glycosides and phenolic compounds from Veronica peregrina. *Arch. Pharmacal Res.* **2009**, *32*, 207–213. [CrossRef]
11. Saracoglu, I.; Harput, U.S. In vitro cytotoxic activity and structure activity relationships of iridoid glucosides derived from Veronica species. *Phytother. Res.* **2012**, *26*, 148–152. [CrossRef] [PubMed]
12. Lee, J.H.; Jun, H.J.; Hoang, M.H.; Jia, Y.; Han, X.H.; Lee, D.H.; Lee, H.J.; Hwang, B.Y.; Lee, S.J. Catalposide is a natural agonistic ligand of peroxisome proliferator-activated receptor-α. *Biochem. Biophys. Res. Commun.* **2012**, *422*, 568–572. [CrossRef] [PubMed]
13. Tan, S.; Lu, Q.; Shu, Y.; Sun, Y.; Chen, F.; Tang, L. Iridoid Glycosides Fraction Isolated from Veronica ciliata Fisch. Protects against Acetaminophen-Induced Liver Injury in Mice. *Evid. Based Complement. Alternat. Med.* **2017**, *2017*. [CrossRef] [PubMed]
14. Ji, H.Y.; Lee, H.W.; Kim, H.H.; Lee, H.I.; Chung, H.T.; Lee, H.S. Determination of Catalposide in Rat Plasma by Liquid Chromatography-Mass Spectrometry. *Anal. Lett.* **2003**, *36*, 2999–3009. [CrossRef]
15. Jeong, H.U.; Kwon, M.; Lee, Y.; Yoo, J.S.; Shin, D.H.; Song, I.S.; Lee, H.S. Organic anion transporter 3- and organic anion transporting polypeptides 1B1- and 1B3-mediated transport of catalposide. *Drug Des. Dev. Ther.* **2015**, *9*, 643–653.
16. Choi, W.G.; Kim, J.H.; Kim, D.K.; Lee, Y.; Yoo, J.S.; Shin, D.H.; Lee, H.S. Simultaneous Determination of Chlorogenic Acid Isomers and Metabolites in Rat Plasma Using LC-MS/MS and Its Application to A Pharmacokinetic Study Following Oral Administration of Stauntonia Hexaphylla Leaf Extract (YRA-1909) to Rats. *Pharmaceutics* **2018**, *10*, 143. [CrossRef] [PubMed]
17. Cerny, M.A. Prevalence of Non-Cytochrome P450-Mediated Metabolism in Food and Drug Administration-Approved Oral and Intravenous Drugs: 2006–2015. *Drug Metab. Dispos.* **2016**, *44*, 1246–1252. [CrossRef] [PubMed]
18. Foti, R.S.; Dalvie, D.K. Cytochrome P450 and non-Cytochrome P450 Oxidative Metabolism: Contributions to the Pharmacokinetics, Safety and Efficacy of Xenobiotics. *Drug Metab. Dispos.* **2016**, *44*, 1229–1245. [CrossRef] [PubMed]
19. Kim, J.H.; Hwang, D.K.; Moon, J.Y.; Lee, Y.; Yoo, J.S.; Shin, D.H.; Lee, H.S. Multiple UDP-Glucuronosyltransferase and Sulfotransferase Enzymes are Responsible for the Metabolism of Verproside in Human Liver Preparations. *Molecules* **2017**, *22*, 670. [CrossRef] [PubMed]
20. Jeong, H.U.; Kim, J.H.; Kong, T.Y.; Choi, W.G.; Lee, H.S. Comparative metabolism of honokiol in mouse, rat, dog, monkey, and human hepatocytes. *Arch. Pharmacal Res.* **2016**, *39*, 516–530. [CrossRef] [PubMed]
21. Suiko, M.; Kurogi, K.; Hashiguchi, T.; Sakakibara, Y.; Liu, M.C. Updated perspectives on the cytosolic sulfotransferases (SULTs) and SULT-mediated sulfation. *Biosci. Biotech. Biochem.* **2017**, *81*, 63–72. [CrossRef] [PubMed]

22. Guidry, A.L.; Tibbs, Z.E.; Runge-Morris, M.; Falany, C.N. Expression, Purification, and Characterization of Human Cytosolic Sulfotransferase (Sult) 1c4. *Horm. Mol. Boil. Clin. Investig.* **2017**, *29*, 27–36. [CrossRef] [PubMed]
23. Coughtrie, M.W. Function and organization of the human cytosolic sulfotransferase (SULT) family. *Chem. Interact.* **2016**, *259*, 2–7. [CrossRef] [PubMed]
24. Riches, Z.; Stanley, E.L.; Bloomer, J.C.; Coughtrie, M.W.H. Quantitative Evaluation of the Expression and Activity of Five Major Sulfotransferases (SULTs) in Human Tissues: The SULT "Pie". *Drug Metab. Dispos.* **2009**, *37*, 2255–2261. [CrossRef] [PubMed]
25. Marto, N.; Morello, J.; Monteiro, E.C.; Pereira, S.A.; Morello, J.B. Implications of Sulfotransferase Activity in Interindividual Variability in Drug Response: Clinical Perspective on Current Knowledge. *Drug Metab. Rev.* **2017**, *49*, 357–371. [CrossRef] [PubMed]
26. James, M.O.; Ambadapadi, S. Interactions of cytosolic sulfotransferases with xenobiotics. *Drug Metab. Rev.* **2013**, *45*, 401–414. [CrossRef] [PubMed]
27. Zhou, T.; Chen, Y.; Huang, C.; Chen, G. Caffeine Induction of Sulfotransferases in Rat Liver and Intestine. *J. Appl. Toxicol.* **2012**, *32*, 804–809. [CrossRef] [PubMed]
28. Lv, X.; Zhang, J.B.; Hou, J.; Dou, T.Y.; Ge, G.B.; Hu, W.Z.; Yang, L. Chemical probes fpr human UDP-glucuronosyltransferases: A comprehensive review. *Biotechnol. J.* **2019**, *14*. [CrossRef] [PubMed]
29. Wang, H.; Cao, G.; Wang, G.; Hao, H. Regulation of Mammalian UDP-Glucuronosyltransferases. *Curr. Drug Metab.* **2018**, *19*, 490–501. [CrossRef]
30. Meech, R.; Hu, D.G.; McKinnon, R.A.; Mubarokah, S.N.; Haines, A.Z.; Nair, P.C.; Rowland, A.; MacKenzie, P.I. The UDP-Glycosyltransferase (UGT) Superfamily: New Members, New Functions, and Novel Paradigms. *Physiol. Rev.* **2019**, *99*, 1153–1222. [CrossRef]
31. Fallon, J.K.; Neubert, H.; Goosen, T.C.; Smith, P.C. Targeted Precise Quantification of 12 Human Recombinant Uridine-Diphosphate Glucuronosyl Transferase 1A and 2B Isoforms Using Nano-Ultra-High-Performance Liquid Chromatography/Tandem Mass Spectrometry with Selected Reaction Monitoring. *Drug Metab. Dispos.* **2013**, *41*, 2076–2080. [CrossRef] [PubMed]
32. Argikar, U.A.; Potter, P.M.; Hutzler, J.M.; Marathe, P.H. Challenges and opportunities with Non-CYP enzymes aldehyde oxidase, carboxylesterase, and UDP-Glucuronosyltransferase: Focus on reaction phenotyping and prediction of human clearance. *AAPS J.* **2016**, *18*, 1391–1405. [CrossRef] [PubMed]
33. Kiang, T.K.; Ensom, M.H.; Chang, T.K. UDP-glucuronosyltransferases and clinical drug-drug interactions. *Pharmacol. Ther.* **2005**, *106*, 97–132. [CrossRef]
34. Miners, J.O.; Mackenzie, P.I.; Knights, K.M. The prediction of drug-glucuronidation parameters in humans: UDP-glucuronosyltransferase enzyme-selective substrate and inhibitor probes for reaction phenotyping and in vitro-in vivo extrapolation of drug clearance and drug-drug interaction potential. *Drug Metab. Rev.* **2010**, *42*, 196–208. [CrossRef]
35. Parkinson, A.; Kazmi, F.; Buckley, D.B.; Yerino, P.; Ogilvie, B.W.; Paris, B.L. System-Dependent Outcomes during the Evaluation of Drug Candidates as Inhibitors of Cytochrome P450 (CYP) and Uridine Diphosphate Glucuronosyltransferase (UGT) Enzymes: Human Hepatocytes versus Liver Microsomes versus Recombinant Enzymes. *Drug Metab. Pharmacok.* **2010**, *25*, 16–27. [CrossRef]
36. Chen, F.; Zhang, B.; Parker, R.B.; Laizure, S.C. Clinical implications of genetic variation in carboxylesterase drug metabolism. *Expert Opin. Drug Metab. Toxicol.* **2018**, *14*, 131–142. [CrossRef]
37. Abbas, S.; Greige-Gerges, H.; Karam, N.; Piet, M.H.; Netter, P.; Magdalou, J. Metabolism of Parabens (4-Hydroxybenzoic Acid Esters) by Hepatic Esterases and UDP-Glucuronosyltransferases in Man. *Drug Metab. Pharmacok.* **2010**, *25*, 568–577. [CrossRef]

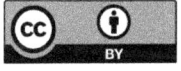

© 2019 by the authors. Licensee MDPI, Basel, Switzerland. This article is an open access article distributed under the terms and conditions of the Creative Commons Attribution (CC BY) license (http://creativecommons.org/licenses/by/4.0/).

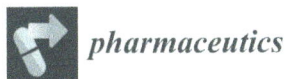

Article

Mertansine Inhibits mRNA Expression and Enzyme Activities of Cytochrome P450s and Uridine 5′-Diphospho-Glucuronosyltransferases in Human Hepatocytes and Liver Microsomes

Won-Gu Choi, Ria Park, Dong Kyun Kim, Yongho Shin, Yong-Yeon Cho and Hye Suk Lee *

Drug Metabolism and Bioanalysis Laboratory, College of Pharmacy, The Catholic University of Korea, Bucheon 14662, Korea; cwg0222@catholic.ac.kr (W.-G.C.); hyacinthy7@catholic.ac.kr (R.P.); kdk3124@catholic.ac.kr (D.K.K.); driger6103@catholic.ac.kr (Y.S.); yongyeon@catholic.ac.kr (Y.-Y.C.)
* Correspondence: sianalee@catholic.ac.kr

Received: 18 February 2020; Accepted: 1 March 2020; Published: 2 March 2020

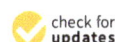

Abstract: Mertansine, a tubulin inhibitor, is used as the cytotoxic component of antibody–drug conjugates (ADCs) for cancer therapy. The effects of mertansine on uridine 5′-diphospho-glucuronosyltransferase (UGT) activities in human liver microsomes and its effects on the mRNA expression of cytochrome P450s (CYPs) and UGTs in human hepatocytes were evaluated to assess the potential for drug–drug interactions (DDIs). Mertansine potently inhibited UGT1A1-catalyzed SN-38 glucuronidation, UGT1A3-catalyzed chenodeoxycholic acid 24-acyl-β-glucuronidation, and UGT1A4-catalyzed trifluoperazine N-β-D-glucuronidation, with K_i values of 13.5 µM, 4.3 µM, and 21.2 µM, respectively, but no inhibition of UGT1A6, UGT1A9, and UGT2B7 enzyme activities was observed in human liver microsomes. A 48 h treatment of mertansine (1.25–2500 nM) in human hepatocytes resulted in the dose-dependent suppression of mRNA levels of CYP1A2, CYP2B6, CYP3A4, CYP2C8, CYP2C9, CYP2C19, UGT1A1, and UGT1A9, with IC_{50} values of 93.7 ± 109.1, 36.8 ± 18.3, 160.6 ± 167.4, 32.1 ± 14.9, 578.4 ± 452.0, 539.5 ± 233.4, 856.7 ± 781.9, and 54.1 ± 29.1 nM, respectively, and decreased the activities of CYP1A2-mediated phenacetin O-deethylase, CYP2B6-mediated bupropion hydroxylase, and CYP3A4-mediated midazolam 1′-hydroxylase. These in vitro DDI potentials of mertansine with CYP1A2, CYP2B6, CYP2C8/9/19, CYP3A4, UGT1A1, and UGT1A9 substrates suggest that it is necessary to carefully characterize the DDI potentials of ADC candidates with mertansine as a payload in the clinic.

Keywords: mertansine; human hepatocytes; cytochrome P450; UDP-glucuronosyltransferases; drug–drug interaction

1. Introduction

Maytansine was first isolated in 1972 from the plant *Maytenus* ovatus [1] and showed potent cytotoxic effects in cell-based systems and efficacy in animal tumor models by binding to tubulin and blocking microtubule assembly [1–5]. However, maytansine failed as an anticancer drug in human clinical trials because of its unacceptable systemic toxicity [5–7]. Many maytansinoids, chemical derivatives of maytansine, showed higher cytotoxicity—by 100–1000 times—than other tubulin inhibitors, vincristine and vinblastine, in cancer cell lines in vitro [7,8]. The structure–antitumor activity relationship revealed that the ester side chain of maytansine plays an important role in the anti-tumor activity as well as tubulin binding [8]. Maytansinoids with potent cytotoxicity are clinically used and studied as the cytotoxic component of antibody–drug conjugates (ADCs) or aptamer-drug conjugates to reduce side effects and increase treatment effectiveness [7–15]. Mertansine

(Figure 1, called DM1), a thiol-containing maytansinoid, is attached to a monoclonal antibody through a reaction of the thiol group with a linker to create an ADC. Several ADCs containing mertansine have been developed, including bivatuzumab mertansine, cantuzumab mertansine, lorvotuzummab mertansine, and trastuzumab emtansine (T-DM1, Kadcyla®) [6–15]. T–DM1 is an ADC drug approved in early 2013 for the treatment of human epidermal growth factor receptor 2 (HER2)-positive metastatic breast cancer that combines the biological activity of HER2 antibody (Herceptin or trastuzumab) with the targeted delivery of a potent antimicrotubule agent mertansine to HER2-expressing breast cancer cells [16–20]. A meta-analysis of a total of five randomized clinical trials involving 3720 patients with HER2-positive metastatic breast cancer revealed that T-DM1 significantly prolonged the progression-free survival and overall survival with tolerated toxicity compared to other anti-HER2 therapies [20]. However, patients who received T-DM1 treatment exhibited a significantly higher risk ratio of hepatotoxicity and thrombocytopenia [20].

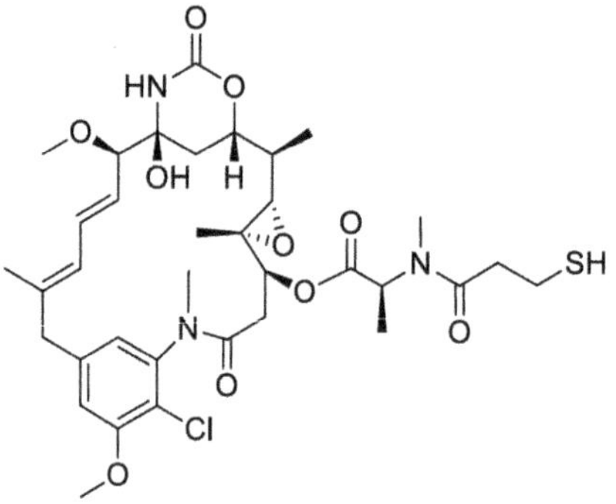

Figure 1. The chemical structure of mertansine.

Cytochrome P450s (CYPs) and uridine-5′-diphospho-glucuronosyltransferases (UGTs) are critical drug-metabolizing enzymes and are often involved in drug–drug interactions (DDIs) [21–27]. The in vitro inhibitory and induction potentials of drugs on CYPs and UGTs in human liver microsomes and hepatocytes have been evaluated to help identify clinical DDIs [26].

After an intravenous injection of [^{3}H]-mertansine at 0.2 mg/kg in rats, the radioactivity of mertansine was rapidly cleared from the blood and extensively distributed to highly perfused organs such as liver, kidney, spleen, lungs, heart, adrenal, and the gastrointestinal tract with high tissue-to-blood radioactivity ratios (ca. 1~11) for 24 h, declining to minimal levels by 120 h [28]. The majority of dosed mertansine radioactivity was recovered in feces over 120 h, with biliary excretion as the major route (~46% of dosed radioactivity over 72 h), but 5% of dosed radioactivity was recovered in urine over 120 h [28,29]. Mertansine was extensively metabolized to 11 metabolites via S-oxidation, hydrolysis, S-methylation, and glutathione conjugation [28,30,31]. It competitively inhibited CYP2C8-mediated paclitaxel 6α-hydroxylation and CYP2D6-mediated dextromethorphan O-demethylation with K_i values of 11 and 14 µM, respectively, in human liver microsomes; mertansine also inactivated midazolam 1′-hydroxylation in recombinant human CYP3A4 with a K_i of 3.4 µM and a k_{inact} of 0.058 min^{-1}, but it exhibited no induction potential up to 1 µM [31,32].

Other tubulin inhibitors, such as colchicine and monomethyl auristatin E (MMAE), have been reported to downregulate CYP mRNA expression through the disruption of the microtubulin cellular skeletal structure that is necessary for the proper functioning of nuclear receptor signaling cascades [33–35]. However, to our knowledge, no studies have investigated the inhibitory potential of mertansine on UGTs, the second major group of enzymes responsible for drug metabolism [27], in human liver microsomes and the suppression potential of mertansine on mRNA expression or activities of major CYPs and UGTs in human hepatocytes.

The purpose of this study was to investigate the in vitro inhibitory potentials of mertansine on human UGT activities including UGT1A1, UGT1A3, UGT1A4, UGT1A6, UGT1A9, and UGT2B7 in ultrapooled human liver microsomes and to evaluate the effect of mertansine on the mRNA levels of human CYP1A2, CYP2B6, CYP3A4, CYP2C8, CYP2C9, CYP2C19, UGT1A1, UGT1A4, and UGT1A9 in human hepatocytes to assess the potential for mertansine-induced drug interactions.

2. Materials and Methods

2.1. Materials

Mertansine (96.9% purity) was obtained from BrightGene Biomedical Technology (Jiangsu, China). Acetaminophen, N-acetylserotonin, alamethicin, chenodeoxycholic acid, 6-(4-chlorophenyl)imidazo[2,1-b](1,3)thiazole-5-carbaldehyde-O-(3,4-dichlorobenzyl)oxime (CITCO), dimethyl sulfoxide (DMSO), L-glutamine, meloxicam, mycophenolic acid, naloxone, naloxone 3-β-D-glucuronide, omeprazole, phenacetin, rifampin, trifluoperazine, Trizma HCl, Trizma Base, uridine 5′-diphosphoglucuronic acid (UDPGA), and William's Medium E were obtained from Sigma-Aldrich (St. Louis, MO, USA). $^{13}C_2, ^{15}N$-acetaminophen, d_9-1′-hydroxybufuralol, 1′-hydroxymidazolam, bupropion, hydroxy-bupropion, trypan blue, matrigel, ultrapooled human liver microsomes (150 donors, mixed gender), Biocoat™ Hepatocyte Culture Medium, Biocoat™ Collagen 96-well and 48-well plates, and cryopreserved plateable human hepatocytes (lots 319, 53-year-old male donor; 321, 58-year-old female donor; and 361, 48-year-old female donor) were purchased from Corning Life Sciences (Woburn, MA, USA). N-acetylserotonin β-D-glucuronide, chenodeoxycholic acid 24-acyl-β-glucuronide, diclofenac, ketoconazole, mycophenolic acid β-D-glucuronide, propofol β-D-glucuronide, SN-38 glucuronide, and trifluoperazine N-β-D-glucuronide were obtained from Toronto Research Chemicals (Toronto, ON, Canada). SN-38 was obtained from Santa Cruz Biotechnology (Dallas, TX, USA). TaqMan® RNA-to-C_T™ 1-Step Kit, TaqMan® Gene Expression Assays, and gene-specific probes and primers for real-time reverse transcription polymerase chain reaction (RT-PCR) were obtained from Applied Biosystems (Foster City, CA, USA). Midazolam was purchased from Cayman Chemical (Ann Arbor, MI, USA). Cryopreserved hepatocyte recovery medium, cryopreserved hepatocyte plating medium, and fetal bovine serum (FBS) were purchased from Invitrogen (Carlsbad, CA, USA). CellTiter 96® AQueous One Solution Cell Proliferation Assay (MTS) kit was obtained from Promega (Madison, WI, USA). Acetonitrile, methanol, and water (LC-MS grade) were obtained from Fisher Scientific Co. (Fair Lawn, NJ, USA). RNeasy Micro Kit was purchased from QIAZEN (Germantown, MD, USA). All other reagents used were the highest quality available.

2.2. Inhibitory Potential of Mertansine on Human Major UGTs in Human Liver Microsomes

The inhibitory potential of mertansine on UGT1A1, UGT1A3, UGT1A4, UGT1A6, UGT1A9, and UGT2B7 activities was evaluated using liquid chromatography–tandem mass spectrometry (LC-MS/MS) with a cocktail of UGT substrates and ultrapooled human liver microsomes [36]. Each incubation mixture was prepared to a final volume of 100 µL as follows: ultrapooled human liver microsomes (0.2 mg/mL), 5 mM UDPGA, 10 mM magnesium chloride, alamethicin (25 µg/mL), 50 mM Tris buffer (pH 7.4), various concentrations of mertansine in methanol (final concentrations of 0.01–50 µM), and the cocktail sets of UGT enzyme-specific substrates. Two cocktail sets were used: set A contained 0.5 µM SN-38 for UGT1A1, 2 µM chenodeoxycholic acid for UGT1A3, and 0.5 µM trifluoperazine for UGT1A4; and set B contained 1 µM N-acetylserotonin for UGT1A6, 0.2 µM mycophenolic acid for UGT1A9, and 1 µM naloxone for UGT2B7. The reactions were initiated by adding UDPGA and incubated in a shaking water bath for 60 min at 37 °C. Reactions were terminated by adding 50 µL of ice-cold acetonitrile containing internal standards (IS, propofol glucuronide for set A and meloxicam for set B). Incubation mixtures were centrifuged at 13,000 g for 8 min at 4 °C. Next, 50 µL of each supernatant of sets A and B was mixed, and aliquots (5 µL) were analyzed using LC-MS/MS. All assays were performed in triplicate and average values were used in the analysis.

The LC-MS/MS system was comprised of an Agilent 6495 triple quadrupole mass spectrometer coupled with an Agilent 1290 Infinity system (Agilent Technologies, Wilmington, DE, USA). The column and autosampler temperatures were set to 40 °C and 4 °C, respectively. Six glucuronide metabolites and two ISs were simultaneously separated using an Atlantis dC$_{18}$ system (3 µm, 2.1 mm i.d. ×100 mm, Waters Technologies, Milford, MA, USA) with a gradient elution of 5% acetonitrile in 0.1% formic acid (MP A) and 95% acetonitrile in 0.1% formic acid (MP B) at a flow rate of 0.3 mL/min. Separation was achieved using the following sequence: 10% MP B for 1 min, 10% to 60% MP B for 1 min, 60% to 95% MP B for 1 min, 95% MP B for 2 min, 95% to 10% MP B for 0.1 min, and 10% MP B for 2.9 min. The electrospray ionization (ESI) source settings in both positive and negative ion modes were as follows: gas temperature, 200 °C; gas flow, 14 L/min; nebulizer, 40 psi; sheath gas temperature, 380 °C; sheath gas flow, 11 L/min; capillary voltage, 4500 V; and nozzle voltage, 500 V. Each metabolite was quantified via selected reaction monitoring in the negative ion mode (chenodeoxycholic acid 24-acyl-β-glucuronide, *m/z* 567.1 to 391.2; mycophenolic acid β-D-glucuronide, *m/z* 495.0 to 319.0; propofol glucuronide (IS), *m/z* 353.0 to 177.0) and in the positive ion mode (SN-38 glucuronide, *m/z* 568.9 to 392.9; trifluoperazine N-β-D-glucuronide, *m/z* 583.9 to 407.9; N-acetylserotonin β-D-glucuronide, *m/z* 394.0 to 219.0; naloxone 3-β-D-glucuronide, *m/z* 503.9 to 309.9; meloxicam (IS), *m/z* 351.9 to 115.0). Data were processed using MassHunter software (Version B.07.00, Agilent Technologies, Wilmington, DE, USA).

2.3. Kinetic Analysis for the Inhibition of UGT1A1, UGT1A3, and UGT1A4 by Mertansine

Kinetic analysis was conducted to determine the K_i values and inhibition mode of mertansine for UGT1A1, UGT1A3, and UGT1A4 enzymes. Human liver microsomes (0.1 mg/mL) were incubated with various concentrations of SN-38 (0.2–2 µM) for UGT1A1, chenodeoxycholic acid (0.5–5 µM) for UGT1A3 or trifluoperazine (0.2–2 µM) for UGT1A4, 5 mM UDPGA, 25 µg/mL alamethicin, 10 mM MgCl$_2$, and various concentrations of mertansine (2.5, 5, 10, 20 µM for UGT1A1; 1, 2, 5, 10, 20 µM for UGT1A3; and 2.5, 5, 10, 20, 40 µM for UGT1A4) in 50 mM Tris buffer (pH 7.4) to a total incubation volume of 100 µL. Reactions were initiated by addition of UDPGA at 37 °C and stopped after 30 min by placing the incubation tubes on ice and adding 100 µL of internal standard (500 ng/mL meloxicam for SN-38 glucuronide and trifluoperazine N-β-D-glucuronide or propofol glucuronide for chenodeoxycholic acid 24-acyl-β-glucuronide) in ice-cold acetonitrile. The incubation mixtures were then centrifuged at 13,000 g for 4 min, and 50 µL of the supernatant was diluted with 50 µL of water. Aliquots (5 µL) were then analyzed using LC-MS/MS.

2.4. Induction of Mertansine on Human Major CYPs and UGTs in Human Hepatocytes

Plateable cryopreserved human hepatocytes (lots 319, 321, and 361) were thawed in cryopreserved hepatocyte recovery medium according to the manufacturer's protocol.

2.4.1. Cytotoxicity of Mertansine in Human Hepatocytes

To estimate the cytotoxicity of mertansine, viable hepatocytes (lot 319) cells were seeded in a collagen type 1 precoated 96-well plate in 100 µL of hepatocyte plating medium (6×10^4 cells/well) and incubated for 4 h at 37 °C in 5% CO$_2$. Next, the plating medium was removed, and a matrigel medium containing 0.25 mg/mL of Matrigel™ matrix was applied to each cell prior to incubation for 24 h at 37 °C in 5% CO$_2$. The hepatocytes were incubated with 0.0125, 0.0625, 0.125, 0.250, 0.625, 1.25, 2.5, and 6.25 µM mertansine in triplicate for 48 h at 37 °C in 5% CO$_2$. The medium was exchanged with fresh medium containing mertansine every 24 h. Then, 20 µL of MTS solution was added to each well and the plate was incubated for 1 h at 37 °C in 5% CO$_2$. The absorbance of the reaction mixture was measured at 492 nm.

2.4.2. Treatment of Mertansine in Human Hepatocytes

To evaluate the induction effect of mertansine on drug-metabolizing enzymes, three different cryopreserved human hepatocytes (lots 319, 321, and 361) were thawed in cryopreserved hepatocyte recovery medium, and viable cells were seeded in collagen type 1 precoated 48-well plates in 250 µL of hepatocyte plating medium (6×10^5 cells/well) and incubated for 4 h at 37 °C in 5% CO_2. Next, the plating medium was removed and replaced with matrigel medium containing 0.25 mg/mL of Matrigel™ matrix prior to incubation at 37 °C for 24 h. The hepatocytes were incubated with 1.25, 12.5, 125, 625, 1250, and 2500 nM mertansine, vehicle (0.1% DMSO in hepatocyte culture media), and prototypical inducers including 50 µM omeprazole, 10 nM CITCO, and 10 µM rifampicin in triplicate. Samples were incubated for 48 h at 37 °C in 5% CO_2, and the medium was exchanged with 250 µL of fresh medium containing drugs or the vehicle every 24 h.

2.4.3. CYP1A2, CYP2B6, and CYP3A4 Activity Measurement

The effects of mertansine on CYP1A2, CYP2B6, and CYP3A4 activities were evaluated. Plates were prepared with a vehicle, omeprazole, CITCO, rifampin, and mertansine, and incubated for 48 h. Next, 150 µL of a CYP cocktail solution containing 40 µM phenacetin (CYP1A2 substrate), 20 µM bupropion (CYP2B6 substrate), and 20 µM midazolam (CYP3A4 substrate) in William's E buffer was added to each well and incubated for 30 min, and then 100 µL aliquots of the incubate from each well were stored at −80 °C until LC-MS/MS analysis. $^{13}C_2, ^{15}N$-acetaminophen (0.1 µg/mL, IS for acetaminophen), and d_9-1'-hydroxybufuralol (0.01 µg/mL, IS for hydroxybupropion and 1'-hydroxymidazolam) in methanol were added to 50 µL of the medium obtained from each well. Mixtures were vortexed for 2 min and then centrifuged at 13,000 g for 4 min at 4 °C. The supernatant (40 µL) was diluted with 60 µL of deionized water and then mixed for 2 min by vortexing. An aliquot (5 µL) was analyzed using LC-MS/MS [37], and CYP1A2, CYP2B6, and CYP3A4 enzyme activities were expressed as formation rates (pmol/million cells/min).

2.4.4. RNA Purification and RT-PCR Analysis

At the end point of the experiment, total RNA was immediately isolated using an RNeasy Micro Kit, and RNA concentration and purity were determined using an absorbance test at 260 nm/280 nm using a NanoVue Plus spectrophotometer (GE Healthcare Bio-Sciences Corp., Piscataway, NJ, USA). Samples were stored at −80 °C until RT-PCR analysis.

RT-PCR analysis was performed using an RT-PCR detection system (Bio-Rad, Hercules, CA, USA) with a TaqMan® RNA-to-CT™ 1-Step Kit and TaqMan® Gene Expression Assay Kits (CYP1A2, Hs01070369_m1; CYP2B6, Hs03044634_m1; CYP3A4, Hs00430021_m1; CYP2C8, Hs00426387_m1; CYP2C9, Hs00426397_m1; CYP2C19, Hs00559368_m1; UGT1A1, Hs02511055_s1; UGT1A4, Hs01655285_s1; UGT1A9, Hs02516855_sH) according to the manufacturer's protocol. Total RNA (15 ng) in each reaction sample was used for RT-PCR: 25 min for reverse transcription at 48 °C, 15 min for enzyme activation at 95 °C, 44 cycles of denaturation (each 15 s) at 95 °C, and 1 min annealing/extension at 60 °C. The relative threshold cycle (ΔC_t) values of all samples, including CYP1A2, CYP2B6, CYP3A4, CYP2C8, CYP2C9, CYP2C19, UGT1A1, UGT1A4, and UGT1A9, were normalized to the ΔC_t value of glyceraldehyde 3-phosphate dehydrogenase (GAPDH). The relative mRNA abundance was then calculated with the normalized relative C_t value ($\Delta\Delta C_t$) of each sample using the formula: $2^{-(\Delta\Delta C_t)}$.

2.5. Data Analysis

The percentage changes in enzymatic activities were calculated as (CYP activity with test compound treatment/CYP activity with vehicle control treatment) × 100. The IC_{50} (the concentration of the inhibitor needed for half-maximal inhibition) values were calculated using SigmaPlot ver. 12.5 (Systat Software, Inc.; San Jose, CA, USA). K_i (the inhibition constant) and the inhibition mode of UGT1A1, UGT1A3, and UGT1A4 activities were determined using Enzyme Kinetics ver. 1.1 (Systat Software, Inc.).

3. Results

3.1. Inhibition of UGT Enzyme Activities by Mertansine in Human Liver Microsomes

Mertansine inhibited UGT1A1-catalyzed SN-38 glucuronidation, UGT1A3-catalyzed chenodeoxycholic acid 24-acyl-β-glucuronidation, and UGT1A4-catalyzed trifluoperazine N-β-D-glucuronidation with IC_{50} values of 16.2 μM, 6.4 μM, and 23.3 μM, respectively, but negligibly inhibited UGT1A6-catalyzed N-acetylserotonin β-D-glucuronidation, UGT1A9-catalyzed mycophenolic acid β-D-glucuronidation, and UGT2B7-catalyzed naloxone 3-β-D-glucuronidation in human liver microsomes at 50 μM (Figure 2, Table 1).

Mertansine noncompetitively inhibited UGT1A1-catalyzed SN-38 glucuronidation with a K_i value of 13.5 μM, and competitively inhibited UGT1A3-catalyzed chenodeoxycholic acid 24-acyl-glucuronidation and UGT1A4-catalyzed trifluoperazine N-β-D-glucuronidation, with K_i values of 4.3 and 21.2 μM, respectively (Figure 3, Table 1).

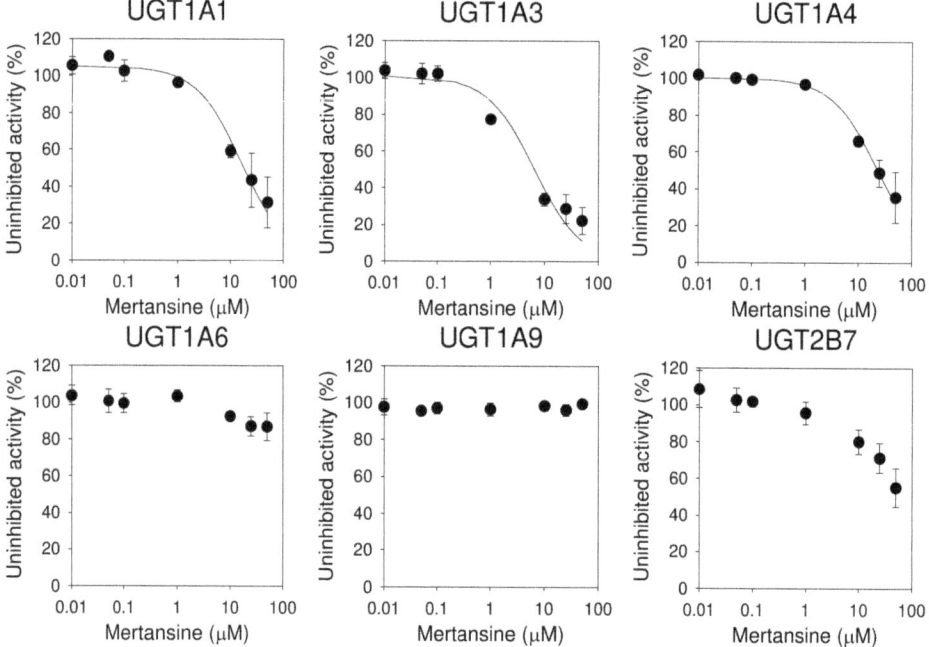

Figure 2. Inhibitory effects of mertansine on six uridine 5′-diphospho-glucuronosyltransferase (UGT) enzyme activities in ultrapooled human liver microsomes. The cocktail UGT substrate concentrations contained 0.5 μM SN-38 for UGT1A1, 2 μM chenodeoxycholic acid for UGT1A3, 0.5 μM trifluoperazine for UGT1A4, 1 μM N-acetylserotonin for UGT1A6, 0.2 μM mycophenolic acid for UGT1A9, and 1 μM naloxone for UGT2B7. Data are expressed as means ± SD (n = 3).

Table 1. Inhibitory potentials of mertansine on six UGT enzyme activities in ultrapooled human liver microsomes.

UGTs	Enzyme Activities	IC$_{50}$ (μM)	K_i (μM)	Inhibition Mode
1A1	SN-38 glucuronidation	16.2	13.5	Noncompetitive
1A3	Chenodeoxycholic acid 24-acyl-β-glucuronidation	6.4	4.3	Competitive
1A4	Trifluoperazine N-β-D-glucuronidation	23.3	21.2	Competitive
1A6	N-acetylserotonin β-D-glucuronidation	No inhibition	-	-
1A9	Mycophenolic acid β-D-glucuronidation	No inhibition	-	-
2B7	Naloxone 3-β-D-glucuronidation	No inhibition	-	-

-: not assayed.

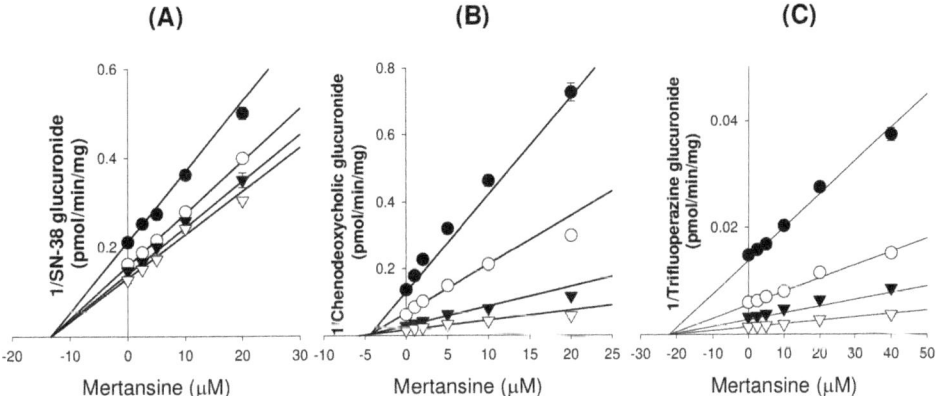

Figure 3. Dixon plots for the inhibitory effects of mertansine on (**A**) UGT1A1-catalyzed SN-38 glucuronidation, (**B**) UGT1A3-catalyzed chenodeoxycholic acid 24-acyl glucuronidation, and (**C**) UGT1A4-catalyzed trifluoperazine N-β-D-glucuronidation in ultrapooled human liver microsomes. Several substrate concentrations were evaluated: (**A**) SN-38; 0.2 μM (●); 0.5 μM (○); 1 μM (▼); 2 μM (▽); (**B**) chenodeoxycholic acid; 0.5 μM (●); 1 μM (○); 2 μM (▼); 5 μM (▽); and (**C**) trifluoperazine; 0.2 μM (●); 0.5 μM (○); 1 μM (▼); 2 μM (▽). Data are expressed as means ± SD (n = 3).

3.2. Effects of Mertansine on CYP and UGT mRNA Levels in Human Hepatocytes

In the MTS colorimetric assay, mertansine did not cause toxicity in human hepatocytes (lot 319), as the viability of hepatocytes following 48 h mertansine treatment (1.25–6250 nM) was over 96.2%.

The functionality of the hepatocyte was confirmed by the increase of mRNA levels and enzyme activities of CYPs following 48 h treatment with prototypical inducers using RT-PCR and LC-MS/MS, respectively, compared to the vehicle (Table 2). Fifty micromoles of omeprazole, a representative aromatic hydrocarbon receptor inducer (AHR), increased the CYP1A2 mRNA levels by enhancing the AHR binding to the promoter region of CYP1A2 [38] and CYP1A2-mediated phenacetin O-deethylase activity by 58.7–299.3 and 11.7–61.8 fold, respectively (Table 2). 10 μM rifampin, a potent pregnane X receptor (PXR) inducer, increased mRNA levels of CYP3A4 by enhancing the PXR binding to the promoter region of CYP3A4 [39] and CYP3A4-mediated midazolam 1'-hydroxylase by 74.0–146.7 and 3.6–9.8 fold, respectively (Table 2). Additionally, 10 nM CITCO increased CYP2B6 mRNA levels and CYP2B6-mediated bupropion hydroxylase activity by 5.6–8.7 and 3.8–15.7 fold, respectively (Table 2), which was mediated by the transcriptional activation by the enhancement of constitutive androstane receptor binding to the promoter region of CYP2B6 [40]. 10 μM rifampin increased mRNA levels of CYP2C8, CYP2C9, CYP2C19, UGT1A1, UGT1A4, and UGT1A9 by 3.7–4.8, 2.9–5.3, 2.0–2.2, 2.5–3.0,

3.9–4.5, and 2.0–2.2 fold, respectively, and 50 µM omeprazole increased the mRNA levels of UGT1A1 and UGT1A4 by 3.9–7.0 and 3.3–4.1 fold, respectively, in three human hepatocytes (Table 2).

Table 2. Effects of prototypical inducers such as omeprazole, 6-(4-chlorophenyl)imidazo[2,1-b] (1,3)thiazole-5-carbaldehyde-O-(3,4-dichlorobenzyl)oxime (CITCO), and rifampicin on the mRNA expression of cytochrome p450s (CYPs) and UGTs and the enzyme activities of CYP1A2, CYP2B6, and CYP3A4 after 48 h treatment in three human hepatocytes (lots 319, 321, and 361). Data are expressed as means ± SD ($n = 3$).

Enzymes	mRNA (Fold Change)			Enzyme Activities (pmol/10^6 Cells/min)		
	Lot 319	Lot 321	Lot 361	Lot 319	Lot 321	Lot 361
Omeprazole 50 µM						
Vehicle control	1.0	1.0	1.0	1.6 ± 0.40 [a]	3.10 ± 0.26 [a]	1.3 ± 0.16 [a]
CYP1A2	132.4 ± 0.22	58.7 ± 4.7	299.3 ± 49.0	18.5 ± 3.3 [a]	89.45 ± 4.52 [a]	81.0 ± 0.53 [a]
UGT1A1	6.97 ± 0.94	4.05 ± 0.53	3.9 ± 0.24	-	-	-
UGT1A4	3.31 ± 0.35	4.13 ± 0.66	3.7 ± 0.62	-	-	-
CITCO 10 nM						
Vehicle control	1.0	1.0	1.0	0.68 ± 0.23 [b]	0.72 ± 0.10 [b]	3.43 ± 0.48 [b]
CYP2B6	7.4 ± 1.9	5.6 ± 1.6	8.7 ± 0.32	9.2 ± 0.28 [b]	11.3 ± 0.49 [b]	12.9 ± 0.51 [b]
Rifampin 10 µM						
Vehicle control	1.00	1.00	1.00	16.6 ± 3.78 [c]	4.3 ± 0.09 [c]	7.1 ± 0.67 [c]
CYP3A4	74.0 ± 10.3	146.7 ± 24.9	129.8 ± 0.5	74.9 ± 3.36 [c]	42.0 ± 9.8 [c]	25.6 ± 1.0 [c]
CYP2C8	3.7 ± 0.57	4.8 ± 0.84	4.0 ± 0.16	-	-	-
CYP2C9	5.3 ± 0.02	2.9 ± 0.11	3.7 ± 0.36	-	-	-
CYP2C19	2.2 ± 0.09	2.0 ± 0.18	2.1 ± 0.25	-	-	-
UGT1A1	2.9 ± 0.13	3.0 ± 0.11	2.5 ± 0.37	-	-	-
UGT1A4	4.0 ± 0.22	4.5 ± 0.59	4.5 ± 0.87	-	-	-
UGT1A9	2.0 ± 0.23	2.2 ± 0.31	2.1 ± 0.23	-	-	-

-: not assayed; vehicle control: 0.1% DMSO treatment; [a]: CYP1A2-catalyzed phenacetin O-deethylase activity; [b]: CYP2B6-catalyzed bupropion 1'-hydroxylase activity; [c]: CYP3A4-catalyzed midazolam 1'-hydroxylase activity.

Mertansine led to the dose-dependent suppression of mRNA expression of CYP1A2 (from 1.2 to 0.22 fold), CYP2B6 (from 1.2 to 0.18 fold), and CYP3A4 (from 1.1 to 0.29 fold) in three human hepatocytes (Figure 4A). Mertansine decreased the activities of CYP1A2-mediated phenacetin O-deethylase by 27.8–79.0%, CYP2B6-mediated bupropion hydroxylase by 23.9–93.1%, and CYP3A4-mediated midazolam 1'-hydroxylase by 30.8–62.7%, compared to the enzyme activities treated with the vehicle in three human hepatocytes (Figure 4B).

Mertansine dose-dependently suppressed the mRNA levels of CYP2C8 (from 1.2 to 0.09 fold), CYP2C9 (from 1.2 to 0.32 fold), CYP2C19 (from 1.3 to 0.23 fold), UGT1A1 (from 1.1 to 0.37 fold), UGT1A4 (from 1.1 to 0.45 fold), and UGT1A9 (from 1.2 to 0.09 fold), in three human hepatocytes (Figure 5). Table 3 lists the IC_{50} values for mertansine on the suppression of mRNA expression of CYPs and UGTs in three human hepatocytes.

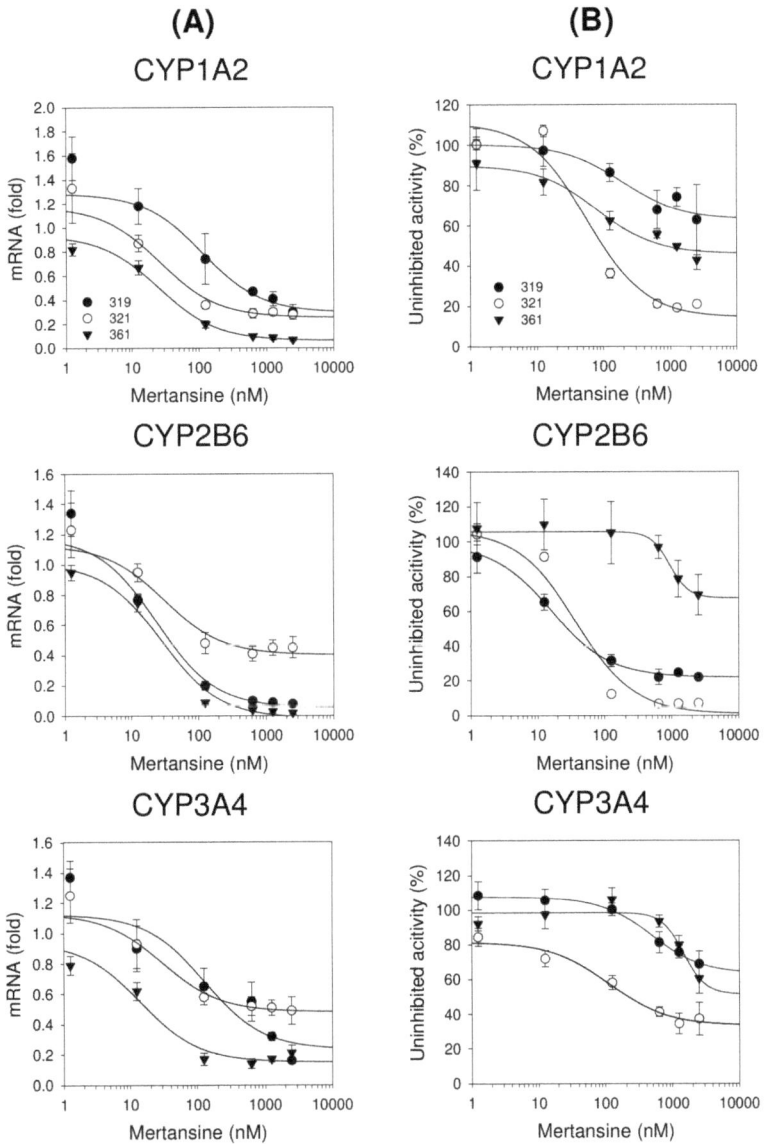

Figure 4. Effects of mertansine on (**A**) the mRNA levels of CYP1A2, CYP2B6, and CYP3A4; and (**B**) the activities of CYP1A2-catalyzed phenacetin O-deethylase, CYP2B6-catalyzed bupropion hydroxylase, and CYP3A4-catalyzed midazolam hydroxylase compared to the vehicle (0.1% DMSO) after 48 h mertansine treatment (1.25–2500 nM) in three human hepatocytes: lots 319 (●), 321 (○), and 361 (▼). Data are expressed as means ± SD (n = 3).

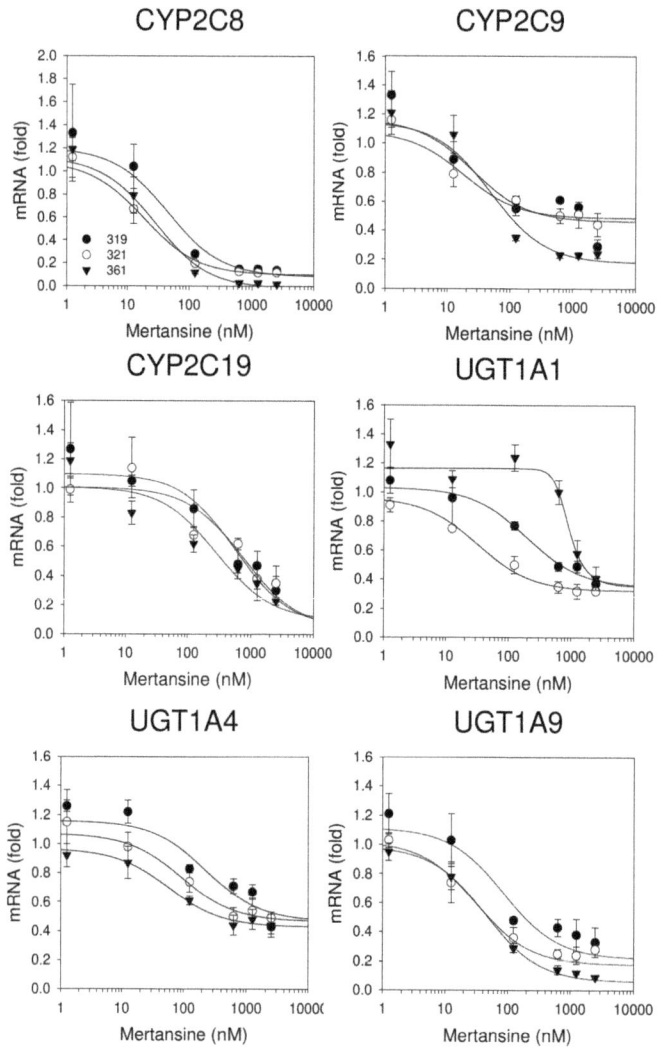

Figure 5. Effects of mertansine on mRNA levels of CYP2C8, CYP2C9, CYP2C19, UGT1A1, UGT1A4, and UGT1A9 after 48 h treatment in three human hepatocytes: lots 319 (●), 321 (○), and 361 (▼). Data are expressed as means ± SD (n = 3).

Table 3. IC$_{50}$ values for mertansine on the suppression of mRNA expression of CYPs and UGTs after 48 h mertansine treatment (1.25–2500 nM) in three human hepatocytes (lots 319, 321, and 361).

Enzymes	IC$_{50}$ (nM)			
	Lot 319	Lot 321	Lot 361	Mean ± SD
CYP1A2	219.7	34.3	27.3	93.7 ± 109.1
CYP2B6	25.0	57.8	27.6	36.8 ± 18.3
CYP3A4	344.5	120.5	16.8	160.6 ± 167.4
CYP2C8	48.7	20.0	27.5	32.1 ± 14.9
CYP2C9	788.2	887.5	59.6	578.4 ± 452.0
CYP2C19	573.5	754.1	291.0	539.5 ± 233.4
UGT1A1	784.5	113.4	1672.1	856.7 ± 781.9
UGT1A4	>2500	>2500	>2500	>2500
UGT1A9	86.9	31.4	44.1	54.1 ± 29.1

4. Discussion

In this study, the effects of mertansine on the inhibition of UGT activities in human liver microsomes and its effects on mRNA expression of CYPs and UGTs in human hepatocytes were evaluated to assess the potential for mertansine-induced drug interactions.

Mertansine was a noncompetitive inhibitor of UGT1A1-catalyzed SN-38 glucuronidation with a K_i value of 13.5 µM, and a competitive inhibitor of UGT1A3-catalyzed 24-acyl-β-glucuronidation and UGT1A4-catalyzed trifluoperazine N-β-D-glucuronidation with K_i values of 4.3 and 21.2 µM, respectively, in human liver microsomes (Figure 3). These findings suggest the potential for DDIs between mertansine and UGT1A1, UGT1A3, or UGT1A4 substrates when used concomitantly. However, the maximum plasma concentrations of mertansine were 7.2 ± 2.7 nM, with the highest level of 30 nM after the intravenous infusion of 3.6 mg/kg T-DM1 every 3 weeks in HER2-positve breast cancer patients [16–19]. Therefore, the ratio of maximal unbound plasma concentrations of mertansine to K_i values (0.00004–0.0002) was much lower than the ratio indicating the likelihood of drug interaction (0.1), suggesting that mertansine-induced drug interactions via the inhibition of UGT activity are unlikely during T-DM1 therapies.

In addition, although mertansine is a competitive inhibitor of CYP2C8 and CYP2D6 activities with K_i values of 11 and 14 µM, respectively, and it also irreversibly inhibits CYP3A4 activity with K_i of 3.4 µM and k_{inact} of 0.058 min^{-1}, mertansine would not cause serious CYP-mediated DDI during the T-DM1 therapies considering the plasma concentrations [32].

The mRNA levels and enzyme activities of CYP1A2, CYP2B6, and CYP3A4 were induced to levels comparable to typical inducers, such as omeprazole, CITCO, and rifampin, following 48 h treatment in three human hepatocytes (Table 2), indicating that the induction system used herein was reliable. The induction effects of mertansine on CYPs and UGTs were assessed using therapeutic to clinically non-achievable high concentrations (1.25–2500 nM) in three human hepatocytes. Mertansine dose-dependently suppressed the mRNA expression of CYP1A2, CYP2B6, and CYP3A4 with IC$_{50}$ values of 93.7 ± 109.1, 36.8 ± 18.3, and 160.6 ± 167.4 nM, respectively, in thee human hepatocytes (Figure 4A, Table 3). Additionally, mertansine decreased the activities of CYP1A2-mediated phenacetin O-deethylase, CYP2B6-mediated bupropion hydroxylase, and CYP3A4-mediated midazolam 1'-hydroxylase by mean values of 48.3%, 63.5%, and 39.7%, respectively, at the highest concentration (2500 nM) in three human hepatocytes (Figure 4B). Mertansine dose-dependently suppressed the mRNA expression of CYP2C8, CYP2C9, CYP2C19, UGT1A1, and UGT1A9 mRNA levels with IC$_{50}$ values of 32.1 ± 14.9, 578.4 ± 452.0, 539.5 ± 233.4, 856.7 ± 781.9, and 54.1 ± 29.1 nM, respectively, with a little suppression of UGT1A4 mRNA levels (IC$_{50}$ value > 2500 nM) (Figure 5, Table 3). These suppressions were not likely to be due to cytotoxic effects because the viability of hepatocytes was not affected by mertansine treatment (1.25–6250 nM). The suppression of CYP mRNA by mertansine was similar to those of other tubulin inhibitors, such as MMAE and colchicine [33–35]. In previous studies, 100 and 1000 nM MMAE treatment suppressed CYP1A2, CYP2B6, and CYP3A4 mRNA expression by 61–90%

and 95–97%, respectively, and decreased CYP activities by 40–71% and 45–81%, respectively, in three human hepatocytes [32]. These findings support the idea that the suppression of CYP and UGT mRNA levels by mertansine may result from the disruption of cytoskeletal structures formed by microtubule networks, which are important for the functioning of the nuclear receptor signaling cascade [33–35,41]. These in vitro results suggest the clinical evaluation of the DDI potential of mertansine with CYP1A2, CYP2B6, CYP3A4, CYP2C8/9/19, UGT1A1, and UGT1A9 substrates.

Several ADCs with mertansine as a payload have been under clinical trials since the approval of T-DM1 [7,10–14]. Liver is the major organ for the distribution and metabolism of antibody maytansinoid conjugates and its catabolites, and the hepatic concentrations of mertansine or ravtansine therefore depend on the catabolism of ADC within the liver [7,18,29,42]. The extensive tissue distribution of mertansine after the administration of mertansine itself in rats led to higher hepatic levels of mertansine compared to plasma levels [28]. Although the maximal plasma concentration of the catabolite mertansine is low ($\leq 7.2 \pm 2.7$ nM) in T-DM1 treated cancer patients [16–19], a clinical evaluation of DDIs regarding the reduced mRNA levels by repeated treatment of T-DM1 and the CYP1A2, CYP2B6, CYP2C8/9/19, CYP3A4, UGT1A1, and UGT1A9 substrates may be necessary on the basis of these in vitro findings.

5. Conclusions

Mertansine inhibited UGT1A1, UGT1A3, and UGT1A4 enzyme activities in human liver microsomes and dose-dependently suppressed the mRNA levels of CYP1A2, CYP2B6, CYP3A4, CYP2C8, CYP2C9, CYP2C19, UGT1A1, UGT1A4, and UGT1A9 after 48 h treatment of 1.25–2500 nM mertansine in three human hepatocytes. Additionally, mertansine treatment resulted in the decrease of CYP1A2, CYP2B6, and CYP3A4 enzyme activities. These in vitro DDI potentials of mertansine with substrate drugs for major CYPs and UGTs enzymes indicate that the evaluation of the DDI potentials of ADC candidates with mertansine as a payload is necessary.

Author Contributions: Conceptualization, W.-G.C. and H.S.L.; methodology, W.-G.C., R.P., D.K.K., Y.S., and Y.-Y.C.; software, W.-G.C., R.P. and H.S.L.; investigation, W.-G.C., R.P., D.K.K., and Y.S.; data curation, W.-G.C. and H.S.L.; writing—original draft preparation, W.-G.C. and D.K.K.; writing—review and editing, Y.-Y.C. and H.S.L.; supervision, H.S.L.; project administration, H.S.L.; funding acquisition, H.S.L. All authors have read and agreed to the published version of the manuscript.

Funding: This work was supported by the Korea Health Technology R&D Project through the Korea Health Industry Development Institute (KHIDI), funded by the Ministry of Health & Welfare, Republic of Korea (HI12C1852) and the National Research Foundation of Korea (NRF) grant funded by the Korea government (MSIT) (NRF-2015M3A9E1028325).

Conflicts of Interest: The authors declare no conflicts of interest. The funders had no role in the design of the study; in the collection, analyses, or interpretation of data; in the writing of the manuscript; or in the decision to publish the results.

References

1. Kupchan, S.M.; Komoda, Y.; Court, W.A.; Thomas, G.J.; Smith, R.M.; Karim, A.; Gilmore, C.J.; Haltiwanger, R.C.; Bryan, R.F. Tumor inhibitors. LXXIII. Maytansine, a novel antileukemic ansa macrolide from Maytenus ovatus. *J. Am. Chem. Soc.* **1972**, *94*, 1354–1356. [CrossRef]
2. Huang, A.B.; Lin, C.M.; Hamel, F. Maytansine inhibits nucleotide binding at the exchangeable site of tubulin. *Biochem. Biophys. Res. Commun.* **1985**, *128*, 1239–1246. [CrossRef]
3. Hamel, E. Natural products which interact with tubulin in the vinca domain: Maytansine, rhizoxin, phomopsin A, dolastatins 10 and 15 and halichondrin B. *Pharm. Ther.* **1992**, *55*, 31–51. [CrossRef]
4. Sawada, T.; Kato, Y.; Kobayashi, H.; Hashimoto, Y.; Watanabe, T.; Sugiyama, Y.; Iwasaki, S. A fluorescent probe and a photoaffinity labeling reagent to study the binding site of maytansine and rhizoxin on tubulin. *Bioconjugate Chem.* **1993**, *4*, 284–289. [CrossRef] [PubMed]

5. Widdison, W.C.; Wilhelm, S.D.; Cavanagh, E.E.; Whiteman, K.R.; Leece, B.A.; Kovtun, Y.; Goldmacher, V.S.; Xie, H.; Steeves, R.M.; Lutz, R.J.; et al. Semisynthetic maytansine analogues for the targeted treatment of cancer. *J. Med. Chem.* **2006**, *49*, 4392–4408. [CrossRef] [PubMed]
6. Lopus, M.; Oroudjev, E.; Wilson, L.; Wilhelm, S.; Widdison, W.; Chari, R.; Jordan, M.A. Maytansine and cellular metabolites of antibody-maytansinoid conjugates strongly suppress microtubule dynamics by binding to microtubules. *Mol. Cancer Ther.* **2010**, *9*, 2689–2699. [CrossRef]
7. Taplin, S.; Vashisht, K.; Walles, M.; Calise, D.; Kluwe, W.; Bouchard, P.; Johnson, R. Hepatotoxicity with antibody maytansinoid conjugates: A review of preclinical and clinical findings. *J. Appl. Toxicol.* **2018**, *38*, 600–615. [CrossRef] [PubMed]
8. Cassady, J.M.; Chan, K.K.; Floss, H.G.; Leistner, E. Recent developments in the maytansinoid antitumor agents. *Chem. Pharm. Bull.* **2004**, *52*, 1–26. [CrossRef]
9. Sun, X.; Widdison, W.; Mayo, M.; Wilhelm, S.; Leece, B.; Chari, R.; Singh, R.; Erickson, H. Design of antibody-maytansinoid conjugates allows for efficient detoxification via liver metabolism. *Bioconj. Chem.* **2011**, *22*, 728–735. [CrossRef]
10. Chen, H.; Lin, Z.; Arnst, K.E.; Miller, D.D.; Li, W. Tubulin inhibitor-based antibody-drug conjugates for cancer therapy. *Molecules* **2017**, *22*, 1281. [CrossRef]
11. Dan, N.; Setua, S.; Kashyap, V.K.; Khan, S.; Jaggi, M.; Yallapu, M.M.; Chauhan, S.C. Antibody-drug conjugates for cancer therapy: Chemistry to clinical implications. *Pharmaceuticals* **2018**, *11*, 32. [CrossRef]
12. Lambert, J.M.; Morris, C.Q. Antibody-drug conjugates (ADCs) for personalized treatment of solid tumors: A review. *Adv. Ther.* **2017**, *34*, 1015–1035. [CrossRef] [PubMed]
13. Marcucci, F.; Casterta, C.A.; Romeo, E.; Rumio, C. Antibody-drug conjugates (ADC) against cancer stem-like cells (CSC): Is there still room for optimism? *Front. Oncol.* **2019**, *9*, 167. [CrossRef]
14. Wolska-Washer, A.; Robak, T. Safety and tolerability of antibody-drug conjugates in cancer. *Drug Saf.* **2019**, *42*, 295–314. [CrossRef] [PubMed]
15. Collins, D.M.; Bossenmaier, B.; Kollmorgen, G.; Niederfellner, G. Acquired resistance to antibody-drug conjugates. *Cancers* **2019**, *11*, 394. [CrossRef] [PubMed]
16. Krop, I.E.; Beeram, M.; Modi, S.; Jones, S.F.; Holden, S.N.; Yu, W.; Girish, S.; Tibbitts, J.; Yi, J.H.; Sliwkowski, M.X.; et al. Phase I study of trastuzumab-DM1, an HER2 antibody-drug conjugate, given every 3 weeks to patients with HER2-positive metastatic breast cancer. *J. Clin. Oncol.* **2010**, *28*, 2698–2704. [CrossRef] [PubMed]
17. Burris, H.A., 3rd; Rugo, H.S.; Vukelja, S.J.; Vogel, C.L.; Borson, R.A.; Limentani, S.; Tan-Chiu, E.; Krop, I.E.; Michaelson, R.A.; Girish, S.; et al. Phase II study of the antibody drug conjugate trastuzumab-DM1 for the treatment of human epidermal growth factor receptor 2 (HER2)-positive breast cancer after prior HER2-directed therapy. *J. Clin. Oncol.* **2011**, *29*, 398–405. [CrossRef]
18. Yamamoto, H.; Ando, M.; Aogi, K.; Iwata, H.; Tamura, K.; Yonemori, K.; Shimizu, C.; Hara, F.; Takabatake, D.; Hattori, M.; et al. Phase I and pharmacokinetic study of trastuzumab emtansine in Japanese patients with HER2-positive metastatic breast cancer. *Jpn. J. Clin. Oncol.* **2015**, *45*, 12–18. [CrossRef]
19. Girish, S.; Gupta, M.; Wang, B.; Lu, D.; Krop, I.E.; Vogel, C.L.; Burris, H.A., 3rd; LoRusso, P.M.; Yi, J.H.; Saad, O.; et al. Clinical pharmacology of trastuzumab emtansine (T-DM1): An antibody-drug conjugate in development for the treatment of HER2-positive cancer. *Cancer Chemother. Pharmacol.* **2012**, *69*, 1229–1240. [CrossRef]
20. Yan, H.; Yu, K.; Zhang, K.; Liu, L.; Li, Y. Efficacy and safety of trastuzumab emtansine (T-DM1) in the treatment of HER2-positive metastatic breast cancer (MBC): A meta-analysis of randomized controlled trial. *Oncotarget* **2017**, *8*, 102458–102467. [CrossRef]
21. Zanger, U.M.; Schwab, M. Cytochrome P450 enzymes in drug metabolism: Regulation of gene expression, enzyme activities, and impact of genetic variation. *Pharmacol. Ther.* **2013**, *138*, 103–141. [CrossRef] [PubMed]
22. Sychev, D.A.; Ashraf, G.M.; Svistunov, A.A.; Maksimov, M.L.; Tarasov, V.V.; Chubarev, V.N.; Otdelenov, V.A.; Denisenko, N.P.; Barreto, G.E.; Aliev, G. The cytochrome P450 isoenzyme and some new opportunities for the prediction of negative drug interaction in vivo. *Drug Des. Dev.* **2018**, *12*, 1147–1156. [CrossRef] [PubMed]
23. Manikandan, P.; Nagini, S. Cytochrome P450 structure, function and clinical significance: A review. *Curr. Drug Targets* **2018**, *19*, 38–54. [CrossRef] [PubMed]

24. Fowler, S.; Morcos, P.N.; Cleary, Y.; Martin-Facklam, M.; Parrott, N.; Gertz, M.; Yu, L. Progress in prediction and interpretation of clinically relevant metabolic drug–drug interactions: A minireview illustrating recent developments and current opportunities. *Curr. Pharmacol. Rep.* **2017**, *3*, 36–49. [CrossRef]
25. Hu, D.G.; Hulin, J.U.; Nair, P.C.; Haines, A.Z.; McKinnon, R.A.; Mackenzie, P.I.; Meech, R. The UGTome: The expanding diversity of UDP glycosyltransferases and its impact on small molecule metabolism. *Pharmacol. Ther.* **2019**, *204*, 107414. [CrossRef]
26. Hariparsad, N.; Ramsden, D.; Palamanda, J.; Dekeyser, J.G.; Fahmi, O.A.; Kenny, J.R.; Einolf, H.; Mohutsky, M.; Pardon, M.; Amy Siu, Y.; et al. Considerations from the IQ induction working group in response to drug-drug interaction guidance from regulatory agencies: Focus on downregulation, CYP2C induction, and CYP2B6 positive control. *Drug Metab. Dispos.* **2017**, *45*, 1049–1059. [CrossRef]
27. Cerny, M.A. Prevalence of non-cytochrome P450-mediated metabolism in food and drug administration-approved oral and intravenous drugs: 2006–2015. *Drug Metab. Dispos.* **2016**, *44*, 1246–1252. [CrossRef]
28. Shen, B.Q.; Bumbaca, D.; Yue, Q.; Saad, O.; Tibbitts, J.; Khojasteh, S.C.; Girish, S. Non-clinical disposition and metabolism of DM1, a component of trastuzumab emtansine (T-DM1), in Sprague Dawley rats. *Drug Metab. Lett.* **2015**, *9*, 119–131. [CrossRef]
29. Shen, B.Q.; Bumbaca, D.; Saad, O.; Yue, Q.; Pastuskovas, C.V.; Khojasteh, S.C.; Tibbitts, J.; Kaur, S.; Wang, B.; Chu, Y.W.; et al. Catabolic fate and pharmacokinetic characterization of trastuzumab emtansine (T-DM1): An emphasis on preclinical and clinical catabolism. *Curr. Drug Metab.* **2012**, *13*, 901–910. [CrossRef]
30. Erickson, H.K.; Lambert, J.M. ADME of antibody-maytansinoid conjugates. *AAPS J.* **2012**, *14*, 799–805. [CrossRef]
31. Han, T.H.; Zhao, B. Absorption, metabolism, and excretion considerations for the development of antibody-drug conjugates. *Drug Metab. Dispos.* **2014**, *42*, 1914–1920. [CrossRef] [PubMed]
32. Davis, J.A.; Rock, D.A.; Wienkers, L.C.; Pearson, J.T. In vitro characterization of the drug-drug interaction potential of catabolites of antibody-maytansinoid conjugates. *Drug Metab. Dispos.* **2012**, *40*, 1927–1934. [CrossRef] [PubMed]
33. Wolenski, F.S.; Xia, C.Q.; Ma, B.; Han, T.H.; Shyu, W.C.; Balani, S.K. CYP suppression in human hepatocytes by monomethyl auristatin E, the payload in brentuximab vedotin (Adcetris®), is associated with microtubule disruption. *Eur. J. Drug Metab. Pharmacok.* **2018**, *43*, 347–354. [CrossRef] [PubMed]
34. Dvorak, Z.; Modriansky, M.; Pichard-Garcia, L.; Balaguer, P.; Vilarem, M.J.; Ulrichová, J.; Maurel, P.; Pascussi, J.M. Colchicine down-regulates Cytochrome P450 2B6, 2C8, 2C9, and 3A4 in human hepatocytes by affecting their glucocorticoid receptor-mediated regulation. *Mol. Pharm.* **2003**, *64*, 160–169. [CrossRef] [PubMed]
35. Dvorak, Z.; Ulrichova, J.; Modriansky, M. Role of microtubules network in CYP gene expression. *Curr. Drug Metab.* **2005**, *6*, 545–552. [CrossRef] [PubMed]
36. Kwon, S.S.; Kim, J.H.; Jeong, H.U.; Cho, Y.Y.; Oh, S.R.; Lee, H.S. Inhibitory effects of aschantin on cytochrome P450 and uridine 5′-diphospho-glucuronosyltransferase enzyme activities in human liver microsomes. *Molecules* **2016**, *21*, 554. [CrossRef]
37. Cho, Y.Y.; Jeong, H.U.; Kim, J.H.; Lee, H.S. Effect of honokiol on the induction of drug metabolizing enzymes in human hepatocytes. *Drug Des. Devel. Ther.* **2014**, *8*, 2137–2145.
38. Yoshinari, K.; Ueda, R.; Kusano, K.; Yoshimura, T.; Nagata, K.; Yamazoe, Y. Omeprazole transactivates human CYP1A1 and CYP1A2 expression through the common regulatory region containing multiple xenobiotic-responsive elements. *Biochem. Pharm.* **2008**, *76*, 139–145. [CrossRef]
39. Luo, G.; Cunningham, M.; Kim, S.; Burn, T.; Lin, J.; Sinz, M.; Hamilton, G.; Rizzo, C.; Jolley, S.; Gilbert, D.; et al. CYP3A4 induction by drugs: Correlation between a pregnane X receptor reporter gene assay and CYP3A4 expression in human hepatocytes. *Drug Metab. Dispos.* **2002**, *30*, 795–804. [CrossRef]
40. Wang, H.; Faucette, S.; Moore, R.; Sueyoshi, T.; Negishi, M.; LeCluyse, E. Human constitutive androstane receptor mediates induction of CYP2B6 gene expression by phenytoin. *J. Biol. Chem.* **2004**, *279*, 29295–29301. [CrossRef]

41. Lu, Y.; Chen, J.; Xiao, M.; Li, W.; Miller, D.D. An overview of tubulin inhibitors that interact with the colchicine binding site. *Pharm. Res.* **2012**, *29*, 2943–2971. [CrossRef] [PubMed]
42. Walles, M.; Rudolph, B.; Wolf, T.; Bourgailh, J.; Suetterlin, M.; Moenius, T.; Peraus, G.; Heudi, O.; Elbast, W.; Lanshoeft, C.; et al. New insights in tissue distribution, metabolism, and excretion of [3H]-labeled antibody maytansinoid conjugates in female tumor-bearing nude rats. *Drug Metab. Dispos.* **2016**, *44*, 897–910. [CrossRef] [PubMed]

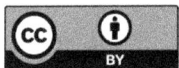

© 2020 by the authors. Licensee MDPI, Basel, Switzerland. This article is an open access article distributed under the terms and conditions of the Creative Commons Attribution (CC BY) license (http://creativecommons.org/licenses/by/4.0/).

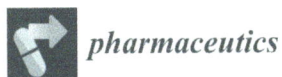

Article

Pharmacokinetic Interaction between Metformin and Verapamil in Rats: Inhibition of the OCT2-Mediated Renal Excretion of Metformin by Verapamil

Seung Yon Han and Young Hee Choi *

College of Pharmacy and Integrated Research Institute for Drug Development, Dongguk University_Seoul, 32 Dongguk-lo, Ilsandong-gu, Goyang-si 10326, Korea; hsyglory@gmail.com
* Correspondence: choiyh@dongguk.edu

Received: 2 May 2020; Accepted: 19 May 2020; Published: 21 May 2020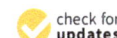

Abstract: The incidence of hypertension in diabetic patients has been increasing and contributing to the high mortality of diabetic patients. Recently, verapamil use was found to lower fasting blood glucose levels in diabetic patients, which led to a new indication of verapamil as combination treatment with anti-diabetic agents such as metformin. As pharmacokinetic (PK) interaction can affect drug efficacy and safety in drug combination, their PK-based interaction is recommended to be evaluated in preclinical levels as well as clinical levels. In case of metformin and verapamil, organic cation transporter (OCT) 1 and 2 primarily mediate metformin distribution to the liver and its elimination into urine, whereas cytochrome P450 is responsible for the hepatic metabolism of verapamil. Verapamil is also known as a potential OCT2 inhibitor. Thus, PK interaction between metformin (30 mg/kg) and verapamil (20 mg/kg) were investigated after their simultaneous administration to rats. In our results, verapamil inhibited the OCT2-mediated renal excretion of metformin, subsequently leading to increase of the systemic exposure of metformin. In contrast, metformin did not influence the pharmacokinetic pattern of verapamil. Although the further clinical investigation is required, our finding suggests a possibility of OCT2-mediated interaction of metformin and verapamil.

Keywords: metformin; verapamil; drug interaction; organic cation transporter 2; renal excretion

1. Introduction

The incidences of diabetic mellitus and hypertension are rapidly growing worldwide, and hypertension is an important cardiovascular risk factor in patients with type 2 diabetes mellitus (T2DM) [1–3]. The dramatically increased (two- to four-fold) risk of cardiovascular diseases in T2DM patients is their leading cause of mortality [4–6]. Insulin resistance and compensatory hyperinsulinemia are also frequent findings in hypertensive patients [7,8]. Since blood pressure-lowering treatment is important to reduce the risk of developing cardiovascular complications in T2DM patients, a combination of anti-diabetic and anti-hypertension drugs is needed and increasingly used [9].

Metformin, an oral biguanide antihyperglycemic agent, increases hepatic and skeletal muscle insulin sensitivity and decreases hepatic glucose production without causing hypoglycemia [10–12]. Metformin also reduces cardiovascular disease complications such as high blood pressure in patients with type 2 diabetic mellitus (T2DM) [3,13,14]. Metformin pharmacokinetics (PK) and pharmacodynamics (PD) rely on the organic cation transporter (OCT) 1 in the sinusoidal membrane of hepatocytes to transport metformin into the liver, its pharmacological target site. The metformin concentration in the liver determines the metformin's effect on inhibiting glucose production [15–17]. OCT2 in the basolateral membrane of the renal proximal tubules mediates the renal excretion of metformin as ~70% of the metformin dose [16,18]. Reduced renal excretion of metformin via renal

OCT2 inhibition causes an increase of systemic exposure (i.e., plasma concentration of metformin), which can result in lactic acidosis [19]. Previous reports that metformin suppresses P-glycoprotein (P-gp) and pregnane X receptor (PXR)-regulated transactivation of the cytochrome P450 (CYP) 3A4 gene [20,21] suggest that the potential for a PK-based drug-drug interaction (DDI) occurrence between metformin and verapamil.

Verapamil, as a calcium channel blocker, is recently emerged as a combination drug in DM patients with hypertension, because verapamil lowers fasting blood glucose levels and enhances insulin secretion in T2DM patients [22,23]. In particular, it is an important issue to regulate insulin secretion as a compensatory mechanism of hyperinsulinemia in hypertensive patients [7,8]. Verapamil has been popularly used for treatment of hypertension and supraventricular tachyarrhythmias [22–27]. Orally administered verapamil is rapidly and well-absorbed, and then it is eliminated via extensive cytochrome P450 (CYP)-mediated hepatic metabolism [25–29]. An N-methylated metabolite, norverapamil, has been shown to have a vasodilator effect in vitro [13]. Verapamil also has an inhibitory effect on P-gp and OCT2 in in vitro and clinical studies [16,30,31]. Although it was reported that verapamil reduced the maximum blood glucose concentration and area under the blood glucose concentration-time curve in healthy adults orally administered with metformin and verapamil together [32], there was no direct measurement of metformin concentration in liver, which may be a substantial evidence on its glucose tolerance activity. Moreover, there has been no report to explain whether transporter and/or metabolic enzyme-mediated PK changes of metformin and verapamil in their combination. In the meantime, new findings regarding positive effect of verapamil for the treatment of hypertension in DM patients have been introduced [22,23], there is a need to investigate how the plasma and tissue concentrations of metformin and verapamil change in DDI events, especially at preclinical levels [33,34]. Since changes in plasma and tissue concentrations of these drugs in combination are associated with their efficacy and toxicity [35,36], the PK interactions of metformin and verapamil were evaluated in rats based on their plasma and tissue concentration changes.

2. Materials and Methods

2.1. Chemicals

Metformin hydrochloride was donated from Daelim Pharmaceutical Company (Seoul, Korea). Verapamil hydrochloride, norverapamil, ipriflavone (internal standard (IS) for the high-performance liquid chromatography (HPLC) analysis of metformin) and propranolol (IS for the HPLC analysis of verapamil and norverapamil), the reduced form of β-nicotinamide adenine dinucleotide phosphate, tris(hydroxymethyl)-aminomethane (Tris) buffer and ethylenediamine tetraacetic acid were purchased from Sigma–Aldrich Corporation (St. Louis, MO, USA). HEK-293 cells overexpressing OCT1 (SLC22A1) and OCT2 (SLC22A2) were purchased from Corning Life Sciences (Corning, NY, USA). Other chemicals were of reagent or HPLC grade.

2.2. Animals

The protocol for the animal studieswas approved by the Animal Care and Use Committee of the College of Pharmacy, Dongguk University-Seoul, Korea (approval no. IACUC-2013-006, 15 December 2013). Male Sprague–Dawley rats (5–7 weeks old, weighing 190–260 g) were purchased from Taconic Farms Inc. (Samtako Bio Korea, O-San, Korea). The rats were housed and handled similarly based on the reported methods [17,33,34].

2.3. Pharmacokinetic Studies of Metformin, Verapamil and Both Drugs in Rats

Early in the morning, the carotid artery (for blood sampling in the intravenous and oral studies) and the jugular vein (for intravenous drug administration only in the intravenous study) of the rats were cannulated, similar to previously reported methods [17,33,34]. The rats were not restrained during the experimental period.

For the intravenous study, 30 mg (2 mL)/kg of metformin (as metformin hydrochloride dissolved in 0.9% NaCl-injectable solution; $n = 6$), 20 mg (2 mL)/kg of verapamil (as verapamil hydrochloride dissolved in 0.9% NaCl-injectable solution; $n = 6$) and both drugs together ($n = 6$) were administered to the rats. Blood samples (approximately 0.12 or 0.22 mL for each drug alone or both drugs together, respectively) were collected via the carotid artery at 0, 1, 5, 15, 30, 60, 90, 120, 180, 240, 300 or 360 min after the start of the drug administration. After each blood sampling, 0.3 mL of 0.9% NaCl-injectable solution containing heparin (20 U/mL) was immediately flushed into each cannula to prevent blood clotting. The blood samples were immediately centrifuged and a 50 μL (or two 50 μL for both drugs) of plasma sample was stored at −80 °C (Revco ULT 1490 D-N-S; Western Mednics, Asheville, NC, USA). The 24-h urine sample ($Ae_{0-24\,h}$) and the gastrointestinal tract (including its contents and feces) sample at 24 h ($GI_{24\,h}$) were prepared following previously reported methods [17,33,34], and the samples were also stored at −80 °C.

For the oral study, after overnight fasting with free access to water, the same doses of metformin ($n = 5$), verapamil ($n = 5$) and both drugs together ($n = 5$) were orally administered (total oral volume of 6 mL/kg) to the rats using a gastric gavage tube. Blood samples were collected via the carotid artery at 0, 5, 15, 30, 60, 90, 120, 180, 240, 360, 480 or 600 min after the drug administration. Other procedures were similar to those for the intravenous study.

2.4. Effect of Verapamil on Metformin Uptake in HEK-293 Cells Overexpressing OCT1 or OCT2

To investigate whether OCT1 and OCT2, as the main transporters affecting metformin pharmacokinetics, were changed by verapamil, the effect of verapamil on OCT1- or OCT2-mediated metformin uptake was investigated in HEK-293 cells overexpressing OCT1 or OCT2 following previously published procedures [33,34]. Briefly, a density of 4.0×10^5 cells/well of HEK-293 cells overexpressing either OCT1 or OCT2 were seeded into 24-well plates coated with poly-D-lysine (Corning Incorporated, Corning, NY, USA) and incubated with Dulbecco's Modified Eagle Medium supplemented with 10% fetal bovine serum for 24 h. After washing twice with pre-warmed Hank's Balanced Salt Solution with Ca^{2+} and Mg^{2+} (Hank's buffer) and pre-incubating the cells with Hank's buffer for 10 min, Hank's buffer was replaced to Hank's buffer containing 10 μM metformin with verapamil added as an inhibitor (0–100 μM). The concentrations of metformin and verapamil were chosen in the ranges of concentrations used in HEK-293 cells overexpressing OCT1 or OCT2 in the previous reports [33,34] and a protocol of in vitro screening method for human SLC uptake transporter inhibition (OCT1 and OCT2) by Cyprotex. Metformin uptake was initiated at this time and the cells were incubated at 37 °C for 10 min. At 10 min after starting metformin uptake, Hank's buffer was removed and the cells were immediately washing twice with ice-cold Hank's buffer to stop metformin uptake. The cells were lysed with distilled water and harvested by scraping them off in 200 μL distilled water followed by ultra-sonification at 4 °C for 10 s. After centrifuging the cells at $15,000 \times g$ for 10 min at 4 °C, the supernatant was determined by LC/MS/MS analysis of metformin [33,34]. The half-maximal inhibitory constant (IC_{50}) values of verapamil for the inhibition of OCT1 or OCT2-mediated metformin uptake are expressed as % of metformin uptake without verapamil (exposed to vehicle instead of verapamil) in HEK-293 cells overexpressing OCT1 or OCT2, arbitrarily set at 100% ($n = 2$ for each dose). From percentages of metformin uptake versus inhibitor concentrations, a sigmoid shaped curve was fitted to the data and IC_{50} was calculated by fitting Hill equation to the data using GraphPad Prism 5 (GraphPad Software Inc., San Diego, CA, USA).

2.5. Effect of Verapamil on Metformin Concentration in the Liver and Kidneys

To investigate whether verapamil changes the metformin concentration in the liver and kidneys, a tissue distribution study of metformin with and without verapamil was conducted following a previously reported method [17,33,34]. At 0.5, 1, 3 and 6 h after intravenous or oral administration of metformin with and without verapamil at the same doses as in the pharmacokinetic study, as much blood as possible was collected and each rat was then sacrificed by lethal blood loss. The liver and kidneys were excised, weighed and homogenized in a 4-fold volume of 0.9% NaCl-injectable solution ($n = 4$ for each organ). After centrifuging each homogenate at 15,000× g for 10 min at 4 °C, the supernatant was collected and stored at −80 °C.

2.6. Effect of Metformin on Verapamil Metabolism in Rat Hepatic and Intestinal Microsomes

To investigate the effect of metformin on verapamil metabolism, the measurement of kinetic constants, such as V_{max} (maximum velocity) and K_m (apparent Michaelis–Menten constant; the concentration at which the rate is one half of the V_{max}) for verapamil metabolism, with and without metformin, in hepatic and intestinal microsomes were conducted. Hepatic and intestinal microsomes were prepared by the previously reported method as followings [17,37,38]: freshly excised livers were cut in pieces, washed extensively with ice-cold solution (KCl 0.15 M) to remove remaining blood and were homogenized with Tris-HCl buffer (pH 7.5) containing 0.15 M KCl + 50 mM Tris, 1 mM EDTA in a Potter-Elvehjem glass homogenizer for 30 s. The homogenate was centrifuged for 10 min at 10,000× g and 4 °C and then followed by ultracentrifugation of the remaining supernatant for 1 h at 100,000× g and 4 °C. Microsomal pellets were then re-suspended in the same buffer with a hand homogenizer and re-centrifuged for 1 h at 100,000× g and 4 °C. The supernatant was discarded, and the microsomal pellets were carefully overlaid with 0.15 mol KCl buffer and stored at −80 °C. Intestinal microsomes were prepared using freshly excised proximal and middle sections of the small intestine. This part of intestine was excised, rinsed with ice-cold 0.01 M potassium phosphate buffer with 1.15% KCl (pH 7.4), filled with solution A (1.5 mM KCl + 96 mM NaCl + 27 mM sodium citrate + 8 mM KH_2PO_4 + 5.6 mM Na_2HPO_4 + 40 µg/mL PMSF). The intestine filled with solution A was incubated in a 37 °C water bath for 15 min. After discarding solution A, the intestine was filled with ice-cold solution B (phosphate-buffered saline + 1.5 mM EDTA + 0.5 mM dithiothreitol + 40 µg/mL PMSF), wound around a middle finger and tapped against the finger three times. The upper villus cells were released into solution B during this process, and the collected cells were pooled. The pooled solution was centrifuged at 10× g and 4 °C for 5 min. After discarding the supernatant, approximately 15 mL of ice-cold solution C (5 mM histidine + 0.25 M sucrose + 0.5 mM EDTA + 40 µg/mL PMSF) was added into each centrifuge tube, which was inverted twice. Following the discard of the supernatant, the cells were resuspended in fresh ice-cold solution C, homogenized with a Pyrex glass Potter-Elvehjem homogenize and centrifuged at 10,000× g and 4 °C for 20 min. The supernatant was then centrifuged at 100,000× g and 4 °C for 65 min. The pellet of intestinal microsome was resuspended in 0.2 mM EDTA/20% glycerol/80% 0.1 M phosphate buffer (pH 7.4), homogenized and stored at −80 °C. Protein contents in hepatic and intestinal microsomes were measured by the reported method [39].

In hepatic microsomes (equivalent to 1 mg protein), 2.5 µL of 0.9% NaCl-injectable solution containing 2.5, 5, 10, 20 or 50 µM verapamil (the substrate) as final concentrations, 2.5 µL of 0.9% NaCl-injectable solution containing 10 µM metformin (the inhibitor) as a final concentration and 50 µL of 1 mM of NADPH dissolved in 0.1 M phosphate buffer of pH 7.4 were added. The total volume, 0.5 mL, was adjusted by adding 0.1 M phosphate buffer (pH 7.4), and then the components were incubated at 37 °C using a thermomixer at 500 opm. In intestinal microsomes, verapamil (as the substrate) concentrations of 5, 10, 20, 50 or 200 µM were used and the other conditions were the same as in the hepatic microsome study. After incubation for 15 or 30 min of the hepatic and intestinal microsomes, respectively, 1 mL of diethylether containing 1 µg/mL of propranolol, as an IS, was added to terminate the reaction. The verapamil concentration in each sample was determined by HPLC analysis [29].

The K_m and V_{max} for the verapamil metabolism were calculated using a non-linear regression method [40]. The unweighted kinetic data from the hepatic and intestinal microsomes were fitted using a single-site Michaelis–Menten equation; $V = V_{max} \times [S]/(K_m + [S])$, in which [S] was the substrate concentration. The intrinsic clearance (CL_{int}) was calculated by dividing the V_{max} by the K_m.

2.7. Rat Plasma Protein Binding of Metformin and Verapamil Using Equilibrium Dialysis

Protein binding values of metformin and verapamil with and without each other were measured in the fresh plasma of control rats using equilibrium dialysis ($n = 4$ for each; [17]). A 1 mL aliquot of the plasma was dialyzed against 1 mL of isotonic Sørensen phosphate buffer (pH 7.4) containing 3% dextran (w/v) in a dialysis cell (Spectrum Medical Industries, Laguna Hills, CA, USA) using a Spectra/Por 4 membrane (mol. wt. cutoff 12–14 KDa; Spectrum Medical Industries, USA). After 24 h incubation, two 50 µL aliquots were collected from each compartment, and the samples were stored at −80 °C.

2.8. Analytical Methods for Metformin, Verapamil and Norverapamil

In the HPL-UV system, the metformin concentration in the sample was determined using the analytical method developed by Choi et al. [17]. The quantitation limits of metformin in rat plasma, urine and GI samples were 0.05, 0.1 and 0.1 µg/mL, respectively. The inter- and intra-day coefficients of variation were below 8.94%. Additionally, the metformin concentration in the sample from the metformin uptake study was determined by LC-MS/MS analysis [33,34]. The quantitation limits of metformin in rat plasma, urine and GI samples were 0.01, 0.02 and 0.02 µg/mL, respectively. The inter- and intra-day coefficients of variation were below 9.53%. Verapamil and norverapamil concentrations in the sample were also determined by the HPLC-UV analytical method of Hong et al. [29]. The quantitation limits of verapamil in rat plasma, urine and GI samples were 0.01, 0.05 and 0.05 µg/mL, respectively. The corresponding values of norverapamil in all biological samples was 0.02 µg/mL; the inter- and intra-day coefficients of variation were below 12.9%.

2.9. Pharmacokinetic Analysis

Standard methods [41] were used to calculate the following pharmacokinetic parameters using non-compartmental analysis (WinNonlin; Pharsight Corporation, Mountain View, CA, USA): the total area under the plasma concentration–time curve from time zero to infinity (AUC), terminal half-life, time-averaged total body, renal, and non-renal clearances (CL, CL_R and CL_{NR}, respectively), and apparent volume of distribution at a steady state (V_{ss}). The peak plasma concentration (C_{max}) and time to reach C_{max} (T_{max}) were directly read from the experimental data.

2.10. Statistical Analysis

A p-value < 0.05 was deemed to be statistically significant using a Student's t-test between the two means for the unpaired data. All results are expressed as mean ± standard deviation (S.D.) except the medians (ranges) for T_{max}.

3. Results

3.1. Effect of Verapamil on Metformin Pharmacokinetics

The mean arterial plasma concentration–time profiles and relevant pharmacokinetic parameters of metformin after its intravenous administration with and without verapamil are shown in Figure 1 and Table 1, respectively. After intravenous administration of metformin with verapamil, the AUC was significantly greater (by 66.7%); CL and CL_R were significantly slower (by 50.8 and 70.7%, respectively); and $Ae_{0-24\,h}$ was significantly smaller (by 43.0%) than those without verapamil.

After oral administration of metformin with verapamil, the AUC was significantly greater (by 73.5%), C_{max} was significantly higher (by 60.5%), CL_R was significantly slower (by 68.4%) and $Ae_{0-24\,h}$ was significantly smaller (by 46.0%) than those without verapamil.

Table 1. Mean (± S.D.) pharmacokinetic parameters of metformin after its intravenous and oral administration with and without verapamil to rats. Doses of metformin and verapamil were 30 and 20 mg/kg, respectively.

Parameter	Intravenous (n = 6 for Each)		Parameter	Oral (n = 5 for Each)	
	Without Verapamil	With Verapamil		Without Verapamil	With Verapamil
Body weight (g)	203 ± 8.80	209 ± 6.65	Body weight (g)	228 ± 19.2	217 ± 13.0
AUC (μg min/mL)	1590 ± 613	2650 ± 449 [a]	AUC (μg min/mL)	472 ± 40.2	819 ± 82.3 [b]
Terminal half-life (min)	92.4 ± 26.4	80.5 ± 34.6	Terminal half-life (min)	137 ± 44.4	101 ± 48.0
MRT (min)	21.4 ± 5.28	18.4 ± 7.69	C_{max} (μg/mL)	2.00 ± 0.328	3.21 ± 1.04 [c]
V_{SS} (mL/kg)	349 ± 128	286 ± 92.4	T_{max} (min)	60 (60–120)	60 (60–120)
CL (mL/min/kg)	24.2 ± 3.02	11.9 ± 2.00 [b]	CL_R (mL/min/kg)	45.6 ± 5.66	14.4 ± 5.45 [b]
CL_{NR} (mL/min/kg)	8.12 ± 3.03	7.13 ± 0.932	$Ae_{0-24\,h}$ (% of dose)	71.3 ± 5.86	38.5 ± 9.96 [b]
CL_R (mL/min/kg)	16.1 ± 3.18	4.72 ± 2.52 [b]	$GI_{24\,h}$ (% of dose)	3.57 ± 2.84	1.53 ± 1.57
$Ae_{0-24\,h}$ (% of dose)	66.5 ± 11.3	37.9 ± 14.9 [a]	F (%)	29.7	30.9
$GI_{24\,h}$ (% of dose)	0.471 ± 0.782	0.831 ± 0.787			

AUC, total area under the plasma concentration–time curve from time zero to infinity; MRT, mean residence time; V_{ss}, apparent volume of distribution at steady state; CL, time-averaged total body clearance; CL_{NR}, time-averaged non-renal clearance; CL_R, time-averaged renal clearance; $Ae_{0-24\,h}$, percentage of the dose excreted in the urine up to 24 h; $GI_{24\,h}$, percentage of the dose recovered from the gastrointestinal tract (including its contents and feces) at 24 h; C_{max}, peak plasma concentration of docetaxel; T_{max}, time to reach C_{max}; F, extent of absolute oral bioavailability. [a] Significantly different (p < 0.01) from with verapamil. [b] Significantly different (p < 0.001) from with verapamil. [c] Significantly different (p < 0.05) from with verapamil.

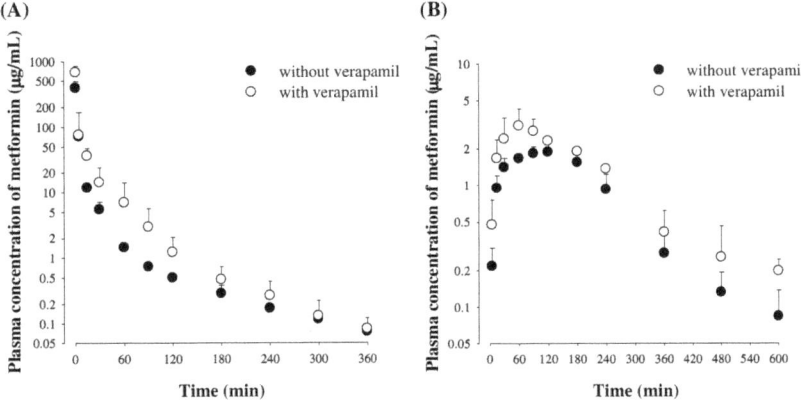

Figure 1. Mean (± S.D.) arterial plasma concentration–time profiles of metformin after intravenous (**A**; $n = 6$ for each) and oral (**B**; $n = 5$ for each) administration of metformin with (○) or without (●) verapamil to rats. Doses of metformin and verapamil were 30 and 20 mg/kg, respectively.

3.2. Effect of Verapamil on OCT1- or OCT2-Mediated Metformin Uptake in HEK-293 Cells Overexpressing OCT1 or OCT2

To examine the verapamil effect on OCT1 and OCT2 activities, the changes of metformin uptake with and without verapamil were compared in HEK-293 cells overexpressing OCT1 or OCT2. As shown in Figure 2, verapamil considerably inhibited metformin uptake in HEK-293 cells overexpressing either OCT1 or OCT2. The IC_{50} values of verapamil for inhibiting OCT1- and OCT2-mediated metformin uptake were 51.9 ± 1.09 and 19.3 ± 0.220 μM, respectively.

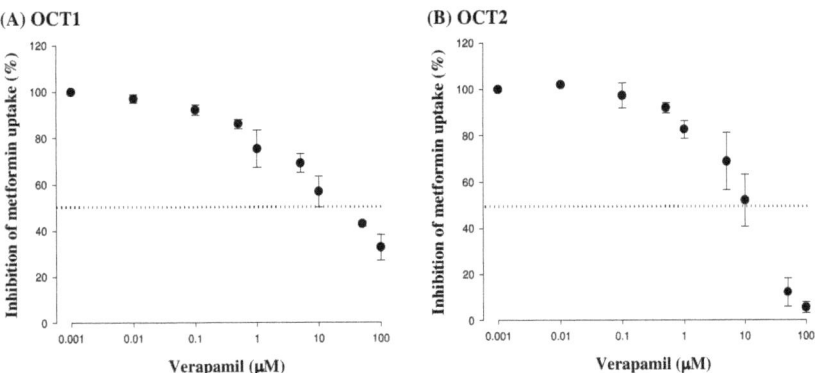

Figure 2. Mean (± S.D.) inhibitory effect of verapamil on metformin uptake in HEK293 cells overexpressing OCT1 (**A**, $n = 2$) or OCT2 (**B**, $n = 2$).

3.3. Effect of Verapamil on Metformin Concentrations in the Liver and Kidneys

After intravenous and oral administration of metformin with and without verapamil, metformin concentrations in the liver and kidneys are shown in Figure 3 and Table 2, respectively. After intravenous and oral administration of both drugs together, verapamil did not cause any change of the metformin concentration in the liver, but the metformin concentration in the kidneys was significantly decreased (by 38.6 and 48.7% at 1 and 3 h in the intravenous study and 42.9, 41.1 and 30.2% at 1, 3 and 6 h in the oral study, respectively) compared to metformin alone. Metformin concentrations in the plasma after intravenous and oral co-administration of metformin and verapamil were significantly lower than those after administration of metformin alone, showing similar patterns to the pharmacokinetic study.

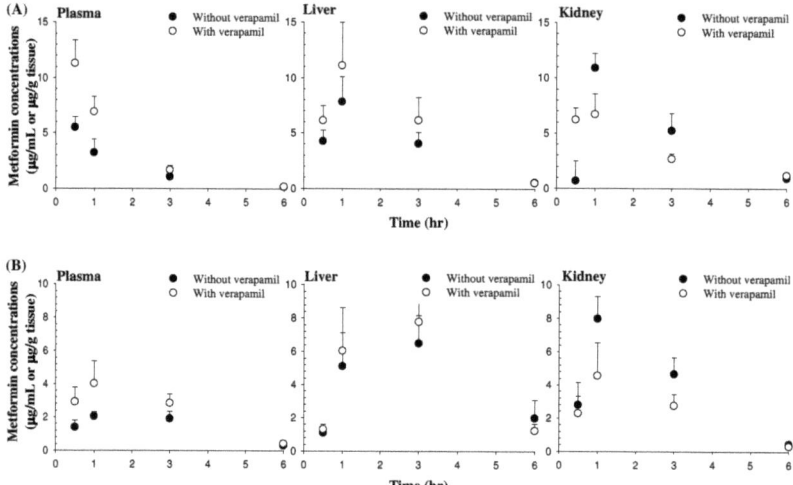

Figure 3. Mean (± S.D.) concentrations of metformin in the plasma, liver and kidneys after its intravenous (**A**, $n = 4$ for each) or oral (**B**, $n = 4$ for each) administration with (○) or without (●) verapamil. The dose of metformin and verapamil were 30 and 20 mg/kg, respectively.

Table 2. Mean (± S.D.) concentrations (μg/mL or μg/g tissue) of metformin in the plasma, liver and kidneys after intravenous or oral administration of metformin with and without verapamil.

Parameter	Intravenous ($n = 4$ for Each)		Oral ($n = 4$ for Each)	
	Without Verapamil	With Verapamil	Without Verapamil	With Verapamil
Plasma				
0.5	5.50 ± 0.988	11.3 ± 2.09 [a]	1.39 ± 0.415	2.91 ± 0.894 [b]
1	3.22 ± 1.22	6.94 ± 1.34 [a]	2.04 ± 0.281	4.03 ± 1.38 [b]
3	1.06 ± 0.214	1.68 ± 0.377 [b]	1.91 ± 0.455	2.84 ± 0.564 [b]
6	0.158 ± 0.0530	0.184 ± 0.0789	0.306 ± 0.0724	0.421 ± 0.0570 [b]
Liver				
0.5	4.25 ± 0.978	6.12 ± 1.39	1.09 ± 0.207	1.31 ± 0.300
1	7.84 ± 2.25	11.1 ± 3.84	5.11 ± 2.03	6.04 ± 2.60
3	4.04 ± 1.04	6.14 ± 2.10	6.49 ± 1.68	7.78 ± 1.11
6	0.553 ± 0.108	0.510 ± 0.222	1.99 ± 1.10	1.24 ± 0.407
Kidney				
0.5	0.706 ± 1.80	6.20 ± 1.12	2.78 ± 1.36	2.28 ± 1.01
1	10.9 ± 1.34	6.69 ± 1.87 [b]	7.97 ± 1.36	4.55 ± 1.98 [b]
3	5.22 ± 1.57	2.68 ± 0.471 [b]	4.65 ± 1.01	2.74 ± 0.675 [b]
6	0.935 ± 0.284	1.20 ± 0.342	0.443 ± 0.0640	0.309 ± 0.0767 [b]

[a] Significantly different ($p < 0.01$) from metformin. [b] Significantly different ($p < 0.05$) from metformin.

3.4. Effect of Metformin on Verapamil Pharmacokinetics

The mean arterial plasma concentration–time profiles and relevant pharmacokinetic parameters of verapamil and norverapamil after intravenous administration of verapamil with and without metformin are shown in Figure 4 and Table 3, respectively. After intravenous and oral administration of verapamil with metformin, all pharmacokinetic parameters of verapamil and norverapamil including the $AUC_{norverapamil}/AUC_{verapamil}$ ratio were comparable to those without metformin. The absorption of verapamil from the gastrointestinal tract and the formation of norverapamil were rapid based on the C_{max} of verapamil and norverapamil, respectively.

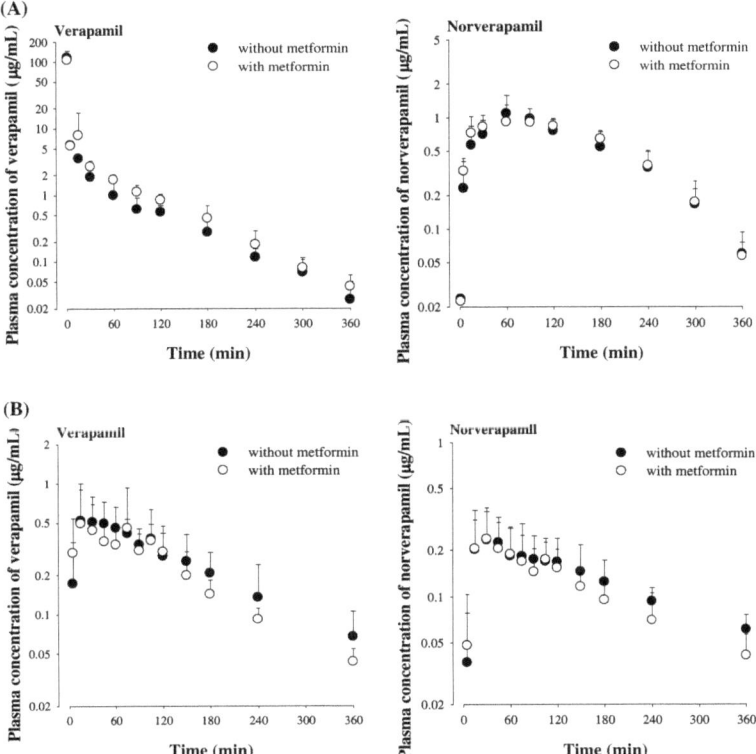

Figure 4. Mean (± S.D.) arterial plasma concentration–time profiles of verapamil and norverapamil after intravenous (**A**, $n = 6$ for each) or oral (**B**, $n = 5$ for each) administration of verapamil with (○) or without (●) metformin to rats. The doses of metformin and verapamil were 30 and 20 mg/kg, respectively.

Table 3. Mean (± S.D.) pharmacokinetic parameters of verapamil and norverapamil after intravenous or oral administration of verapamil without and with metformin to rats. The doses of metformin and verapamil were 30 and 20 mg/kg, respectively.

Parameter	Intravenous (n = 6 for Each)		Parameter	Oral (n = 5 for Each)	
	Without Metformin	With Metformin		Without Metformin	With Metformin
Verapamil			**Verapamil**		
Body weight (g)	205 ± 8.37	209 ± 6.65	Body weight (g)	214 ± 9.62	217 ± 13.0
AUC (μg·min/mL)	441 ± 69.5	527 ± 134	AUC (μg·min/mL)	103 ± 21.6	96.0 ± 30.6
Terminal half-life (min)	71.1 ± 19.0	79.1 ± 24.7	Terminal half-life (min)	128 ± 59.1	121 ± 57.5
MRT (min)	40.9 ± 7.75	42.4 ± 20.4	C_{max} (μg/mL)	0.678 ± 0.386	0.714 ± 0.452
V_{ss} (mL/kg)	1600 ± 861	1860 ± 535	T_{max} (min)	45 (15–105)	30 (15–75)
CL (mL/min/kg)	46.3 ± 7.14	40.0 ± 9.45	CL_R (mL/min/kg)	0.671 ± 0.748	0.489 ± 0.256
CL_{NR} (mL/min/kg)	46.1 ± 7.08	39.8 ± 9.40	Ae_{0-24h} (% of dose)	0.308 ± 0.215	0.231 ± 0.102
CL_R (mL/min/kg)	0.147 ± 0.121	0.108 ± 0.0726	GI_{24h} (% of dose)	0.291 ± 0.339	0.200 ± 0.135
Ae_{0-24h} (% of dose)	0.306 ± 0.219	0.258 ± 0.125	F (%)	23.4	18.2
GI_{24h} (% of dose)	0.148 ± 0.201	0.117 ± 0.0759			
Norverapamil			**Norverapamil**		
AUC (μg·min/mL)	188 ± 34.7	199 ± 38.7	AUC (μg·min/mL)	68.3 ± 38.6	53.9 ± 24.8
Terminal half-life (min)	50.8 ± 10.2	63.3 ± 15.2	Terminal half-life (min)	168 ± 73.2	117 ± 44.5
C_{max} (μg/mL)	1.24 ± 0.386	1.09 ± 0.308	C_{max} (μg/mL)	0.267 ± 0.141	0.273 ± 0.123
T_{max} (min)	60 (30–120)	60 (30–90)	T_{max} (min)	45 (15–120)	45 (15–105)
CL_R (mL/min/kg)	0.109 ± 0.102	0.0626 ± 0.0535	CL_R (mL/min/kg)	0.336 ± 0.107	0.562 ± 0.445
Ae_{0-24h} (% of dose)	0.0872 ± 0.0691	0.0585 ± 0.0453	Ae_{0-24h} (% of dose)	0.104 ± 0.0567	0.113 ± 0.0522
GI_{24h} (% of dose)	0.146 ± 0.0841	0.126 ± 0.0927	GI_{24h} (% of dose)	0.0870 ± 0.0665	0.0782 ± 0.0514
$AUC_{norverapamil}/AUC_{verapamil}$	43.0 ± 7.68	38.5 ± 11.6	$AUC_{norverapamil}/AUC_{verapamil}$	87.3 ± 26.7	89.7 ± 27.0

AUC, total area under the plasma concentration–time curve from time zero to infinity; MRT, mean residence time; V_{ss}, apparent volume of distribution at steady state; CL, time-averaged total body clearance; CL_{NR}, time-averaged non-renal clearance; CL_R, time-averaged renal clearance; Ae_{0-24h}, percentage of the dose excreted in the urine up to 24 h; GI_{24h}, percentage of the dose recovered from the gastrointestinal tract (including its contents and feces) at 24 h; C_{max}, peak plasma concentration of docetaxel; T_{max}, time to reach C_{max}; F, extent of absolute oral bioavailability.

3.5. Effect of Metformin on Verapamil Metabolism in Rat Hepatic and Intestinal Microsomes

The V_{max}, K_m and CL_{int} for the metabolism of verapamil with and without metformin in rat hepatic and intestinal microsomes are shown in Figure 5 and Table 4, respectively. There was no change of V_{max}, K_m or CL_{int} for verapamil metabolism in the presence of metformin, indicating that metformin did not affect verapamil metabolism in rat hepatic and intestinal microsomes under these conditions.

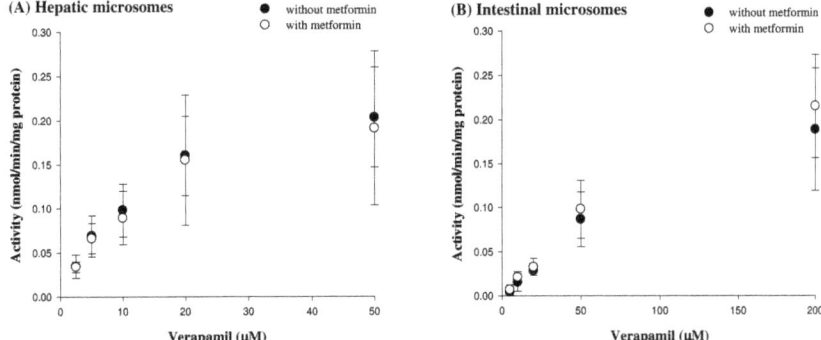

Figure 5. Nonlinear regression for mean values (± S.D.) of verapamil metabolism activity with (○) or without (●) metformin in rat hepatic (**A**, n = 5 for each) or intestinal (**B**, n = 4 for each) microsomes.

Table 4. Mean (± S.D.) K_m, V_{max} and CL_{int} for the metabolism of verapamil with and without metformin in hepatic and intestinal microsomes.

Parameter	Without Metformin	With Metformin
Hepatic	n = 5 for Each	
K_m (μM)	11.0 ± 3.11	13.8 ± 1.26
V_{max} (nmol/min/mg protein)	0.225 ± 0.0951	0.289 ± 0.151
CL_{int} (μL/min/mg protein)	0.0199 ± 0.00419	0.0205 ± 0.00911
Intestinal	n = 4 for Each	
K_m (μM)	148 ± 53.5	171 ± 11.4
V_{max} (nmol/min/mg protein)	0.332 ± 0.125	0.412 ± 0.0908
CL_{int} (μL/min/mg protein)	0.00181 ± 0.00150	0.00240 ± 0.000409

K_m, the concentration at which the rate is one-half of the V_{max}; V_{max}, maximum velocity; CL_{int}, intrinsic clearance.

3.6. Rat Plasma Protein Binding of Verapamil and Metformin Using Equilibrium Dialysis

The concentration of 5 g/mL of each drug was chosen based on previous reports [17,42]. Protein binding values of metformin with and without verapamil were 13.5% ± 5.39% and 11.6% ± 6.10%, respectively. The corresponding values for verapamil with and without metformin were 93.0% ± 38.9% and 85.1% ± 26.3%, respectively. Metformin and verapamil did not affect the rat plasma protein binding to each other.

4. Discussion

The ratio of AUC of a drug with an inhibitor (AUC_i)/ AUC of a drug without an inhibitor (AUC_0) of over 1.25 is classified as a relevant drug interaction by an inhibitor in U.S. FDA criteria [43]. In our study, the ratios of AUC_i/AUC of metformin with and without verapamil were 1.67 and 1.74 (i.e., relative bioavailability) after the intravenous and oral administration of both drugs (Table 1), indicating that verapamil might act as an inhibitor to cause a pharmacokinetic interaction with metformin.

In the intravenous study, the contribution of CL_R to CL, 66.5%, was a large portion of the metformin elimination pathway (Table 1), indicating that renal excretion is the main route of metformin elimination. The estimated CL_Rs of metformin considering the free fractions of metformin in the plasma ($CL_{R/fu}$s) were 4.08 and 14.2 mL/min/kg with and without verapamil, respectively. The $CL_{R/fu}$ of metformin without verapamil was faster than the reported glomerular filtration rate (GRF, represented by creatinine clearance), 5.24 mL/min/kg, in rats [44], indicating that active secretion of metformin as its renal excretion mechanism is changed by verapamil to glomerular filtration. Verapamil slowed the $CL_{R/fu}$ of metformin, 4.08 mL/min/kg, to the creatinine clearance level in rats, indicating that verapamil might cause metformin reabsorption in the renal tubules. The inhibited renal excretion pathway caused a dramatic increase in the systemic exposure (e.g., AUC) of metformin in this study similar as other references [18,45].

To investigate the inhibitory mechanism of verapamil on renal excretion of metformin, the IC_{50} of verapamil against metformin uptake in HEK-293 cells overexpressing OCT2 was conducted based on the known facts that metformin is an OCT2 substrate and verapamil inhibits OCT2 [15,16]. The inhibitory effect of verapamil on OCT2-mediated metformin uptake in HEK-293 cells overexpressing OCT2 (Figure 2) supported the reduced CL_R of metformin when co-administered with verapamil (Table 1). Verapamil significantly reduced the metformin concentration in the kidneys after intravenous and oral administration of metformin with verapamil (Table 2 and Figure 3), probably due to the inhibition of OCT2-mediated metformin uptake into the proximal renal tubules, as shown in the IC_{50} of verapamil in HEK-293 cells over-expressing OCT2 (Figure 2).

Considering that the metformin concentration in the liver is important to preserve the glucose-lowering effect of metformin [11,46,47], the metformin concentration in the liver was also measured after intravenous and oral administration of both drugs (Table 2 and Figure 3). However, the metformin concentration in the liver was not changed by verapamil, which might be due to verapamil not sufficiently inhibiting OCT1-mediated metformin uptake in the sinusoidal membrane of hepatocytes. Since OCT1 in the basolateral membrane uptakes metformin from the sinusoidal blood into hepatocytes, comparable metformin concentrations in the liver with and without verapamil could be supported by the relatively high IC_{50} of verapamil for inhibiting metformin uptake by HEK-293 cells over-expressing OCT1 (Figure 2). In other words, verapamil might have a stronger potential to inhibit OCT2 activity than OCT1 activity. Although verapamil inhibited OCT1 and OCT2-mediated metformin uptake in vitro (Figure 2), the inhibitory effect of verapamil on OCT1-mediated metformin uptake in hepatocytes might be almost negligible in in vivo studies (Table 2 and Figure 3). Therefore, verapamil is an OCT2 inhibitor in the renal proximal tubules, resulting in reduced renal excretion and increased systemic exposure of metformin.

On the other hand, the contribution of gastrointestinal (including biliary) excretion of unchanged metformin to its CL_{NR} was almost negligible; the GI_{24h} was less than 0.471% of the intravenous dose (Table 1). Similarly, it has been reported that metformin is mainly eliminated via renal excretion, but the biliary excretion of metformin as a parent form into feces was negligible [11,17]. In the aspect of metformin and verapamil interactions, the unchanged CL_{NR} and GI_{24h} of metformin by verapamil indicted that verapamil did not influence the non-renal elimination pathway (e.g., biliary excretion and metabolism) of metformin in rats.

After oral administration of metformin with and without verapamil, oral absorption of metformin was rapid and extensive regardless of co-administration of verapamil. For comparison, we estimated the mean 'true' unabsorbed fractions ('F_{unabs}') after oral metformin administration to rats with and without verapamil based on the following reported equation [48]:

$$0.0357 = 'F_{unabs}' + (0.00471 \times 0.297) \quad \text{without verapamil}$$
$$0.0153 = 'F_{unabs}' + (0.00831 \times 0.309) \quad \text{with verapamil} \tag{1}$$

where 0.0357 (0.0153), 0.00471 (0.00831) and 0.297 (0.309) are the oral GI_{24h}, intravenous GI_{24h} and F, respectively, of metformin without verapamil (with verapamil). The 'F_{unabs}' values thus estimated were 1.27% and 3.43% with and without verapamil, respectively, indicating that verapamil probably does not affect metformin absorption in the intestine (Table 1). Thus, the reduced AUC of metformin with verapamil could be due to the inhibition of renal excretion of metformin by verapamil, for the same reason as in the intravenous study.

In contrast, metformin did not change any pharmacokinetic profile of verapamil after intravenous and oral administration of metformin and verapamil together compared to verapamil alone. Metformin also did not affect the formation of norverapamil as an active metabolite of verapamil (Table 3). As hepatic metabolism via CYP3A is the main route of elimination of verapamil [28,49], and a suppressive effect of metformin on PXR-regulating CYP3A4 has been reported [21], the change of verapamil metabolism by metformin was evaluated with greater focus in this study. In parallel to the unchanged CL_{NR} of verapamil by metformin in the intravenous co-administration of metformin and verapamil (Table 3), metformin showed a negligible interaction with verapamil metabolism in in vitro hepatic and microsomal studies (Table 4). Considering that verapamil is a drug with a high (or intermediate) hepatic extraction ratio in rats [44], its hepatic clearance (metabolism) depends on the hepatic CL_{int} and free fraction (unbound to plasma proteins) of verapamil, and hepatic blood flow rate [50]. In our study, the unchanged CL_{NR}s of verapamil with and without metformin (Table 3) were supported by the comparable hepatic CL_{int}s and free unfound fractions of verapamil, and constant hepatic blood flow rate with and without metformin in rats. Metformin might not affect the hepatic blood flow rate based on studies in humans [51]. In other words, these findings indicated that metformin might inhibit the hepatic metabolism of verapamil including the formation of norverapamil (Table 3). Additionally, the unchanged K_ms and V_{max}s of verapamil with metformin compared to those without metformin in in vitro hepatic microsomal studies indicated that metformin did not affect the affinity between metabolic enzyme and verapamil and maximum rate of metabolism of verapamil.

Although the contribution of renal excretion of verapamil is minor in regards to its elimination, the renal excretion of verapamil with and without metformin was estimated as follows: the $CL_{R,fu}$s of verapamil with and without metformin adjusted by the free fraction of verapamil in the plasma were 0.00756 and 0.219 mL/min/kg, respectively. Both $CL_{R,fu}$s of verapamil were significantly slower than the reported GFR, indicating that glomerular filtration was a renal excretion mechanism of verapamil regardless of the presence of metformin and metformin did not inhibit its renal excretion in rats (Table 3).

After oral administration of both drugs, no effect of metformin on the pharmacokinetic profiles of verapamil and norverapamil was observed. The comparable AUCs of verapamil with and without metformin (Table 3) were likely due to the unchanged absorption of verapamil; the estimated 'F_{unabs}' values of verapamil were 0.00179 and 0.00256% for with and without metformin, respectively, from the equations [48]:

$$\begin{aligned} 0.00291 &= {'F_{unabs}'} + (0.00148 \times 0.234) \quad \text{without metformin} \\ 0.00200 &= {'F_{unabs}'} + (0.00117 \times 0.182) \quad \text{with metformin} \end{aligned} \quad (2)$$

where 0.00291 (0.00200), 0.00148 (0.00117) and 0.234 (0.182) are the oral GI_{24h}, intravenous GI_{24h} and F of verapamil, respectively, without metformin (with metformin). Thus, metformin might not affect verapamil absorption in the intestine (Table 3). Orally administered metformin might also not inhibit verapamil metabolism in the liver and intestine, as supported by the unchanged verapamil metabolism by metformin in the in vitro hepatic and intestinal microsome studies (Table 4).

Although Cho et al. [32] reported the inhibitory effect of verapamil on the glucose tolerance activity of metformin without any change of metformin's AUC in healthy adults, verapamil has recently emerged as a new indication for the treatment of hypertension in DM patients [22,23]. Extrapolating the rat dose to human equivalent dose based on the equation by FDA [52], there is a slight difference: the estimated human equivalent doses of metformin and verapamil in our study are 340 mg/70 kg and 227 mg/70 kg, respectively, and the corresponding doses in Cho et al. [32] were 1000 mg and 180 mg per patient (average body weight of patients was 70.5 kg). This inconsistency of doses can be one reason for the result in the different PK interaction pattern in metformin and verapamil combination. In addition, the relatively lower doses were used to emphasize the potential for the occurrence of metformin and verapamil interaction, which can provide a clue to cause OCT mediated drug interaction as underlying mechanism for the further investigations using various dosage regimens in preclinical as well as clinical studies.

5. Conclusions

After intravenous and oral administration of both drugs, the significantly greater AUC of metformin could be due to the inhibition of OCT2-mediated renal excretion of metformin by verapamil, leading to increased systemic exposure of metformin. Interestingly, there was no interaction effect on the metformin concentration in the liver in spite of the inhibitory effect of verapamil on OCT1-mediated metformin uptake in vitro. In contrast, metformin did not influence the pharmacokinetic profile of verapamil. These results can provide essential knowledge about the drug interaction potential between metformin and verapamil for their clinical applications.

Author Contributions: Conceptualization, methodology and writing—original draft preparation, S.Y.H. and Y.H.C.; investigation, S.Y.H.; writing—review and editing, S.Y.H. and Y.H.C.; resources and supervision, Y.H.C. All authors have read and agreed to the published version of the manuscript.

Funding: This research was supported by the National Research Foundation of Korea (NRF) grant funded by the Korea government (MSIT) (NRF-2016R1C1B2010849 and NRF-2018R1A5A2023127).

Conflicts of Interest: The authors declare no conflict of interest.

References

1. De Boer, I.H.; Bangalore, S.; Benetos, A.; Davis, A.M.; Michos, E.D.; Muntner, P.; Rossing, P.; Zoungas, S.; Bakris, G. Diabetes and hypertension: A position statement by the American Diabetes Association. *Diabetes Care* **2017**, *40*, 1273–1284. [CrossRef]
2. Ferrannini, E.; Cushman, W.C. Diabetes and hypertension: The bad companions. *Lancet* **2012**, *380*, 601–610. [CrossRef]
3. Junior, V.C.; Fuchs, F.D.; Schaan, B.D.; Moreira, L.B.; Fuchs, S.C.; Gus, M. Effect of metformin on blood pressure in patients with hypertension: A randomized clinical trial. *Endocrine* **2019**, *63*, 252–258. [CrossRef] [PubMed]
4. Beckmman, J.A.; Creager, M.A.; Libby, P. Diabetes and antherosclerosis: Epidemiology, pathophysiology, and management. *JAMA* **2002**, *287*, 2570–2581. [CrossRef] [PubMed]
5. Hayward, R.A.; Reaven, P.D.; Wiitala, W.L.; Bahn, G.D.; Reda, D.J.; Ge, L.; McCarren, M.; Duckworth, W.C.; Emanuele, N.V.; VADT Investigators. Follow-up of glycemic control and cardiovascular outcomes in type 2 diabetes. *N. Engl. J. Med.* **2015**, *372*, 2197–2206. [CrossRef] [PubMed]
6. Reaven, G.M.; Lithell, H.; Landsberg, L. Hypertension and associated metabolic abnormalities-the role of insulin resistance and the sympathoadrenale. *N. Engl. J. Med.* **1996**, *334*, 374–381. [CrossRef]
7. Sun, D.; Zhou, T.; Heianza, Y.; Li, X.; Fan, M.; Fonseca, V.A.; Qi, L. Type 2 Diabetes and Hypertension: A Study on Bidirectional Causality. *Circ. Res.* **2019**, *124*, 930–937. [CrossRef]
8. He, J.; Whelton, P.K. Epidemiology and prevention of hypertension. *Med. Clin. N. Am.* **1997**, *81*, 1077–1097. [CrossRef]
9. Sharma, S.K.; Ruggeneti, P.; Remuzzi, G. Managing hypertension in diabetic patients-focus on trandolapril/verapamil combination. *Vasc. Health Risk Manag.* **2007**, *3*, 453–465.
10. Dunn, D.J.; Peters, D.H. Metformin. A review of is pharmacological properties and therapeutic use in non-insulin-dependent diabetes mellitus. *Drugs* **1995**, *49*, 721–749. [CrossRef]
11. Gong, L.; Goswami, S.; Giacomini, K.M.; Altman, R.B.; Klein, T.E. Metformin pathway: Pharmacokinetics and pharmacodynamics. *Pharm. Genom.* **2012**, *22*, 820–827. [CrossRef]
12. Scheen, A.J. Clinical pharmacokinetics of metformin. *Clin. Pharmacokinet.* **1996**, *30*, 359–371. [CrossRef] [PubMed]
13. Hermann, L.S. Clinical Pharmacology of Biguanides (*Oral antidiabetes*). In *Handbook of Experimental Pharmacology*; Kuhlmann, J., Puls, W., Eds.; Springer: New York, NY, USA, 1996; pp. 373–407.
14. Snorgaard, O.; Kober, L.; Carlsen, J. The effect of metformin on blood pressure and metabolism in nondiabetic hypertensive patients. *J. Intern. Med.* **1997**, *242*, 407–412. [CrossRef] [PubMed]

15. Nies, A.T.; Koepsell, H.; Winter, S.; Burk, O.; Klein, K.; Kerb, R.; Zanger, U.M.; Keppler, D.; Schwab, M.; Schaeffeler, E. Expression of organic cation transporters OCT1 (SLC22A1) and OCT3 (SLC22A3) is affected by genetic factors and cholestasis in human liver. *Hepatology* **2009**, *50*, 1227–1240. [CrossRef]
16. Nies, A.T.; Hofmann, U.; Resch, C.; Schaeffeler, E.; Ruis, M.; Schwab, M. Proton pump inhibitors inhibit metformin uptake by organic cation transporters (OCTs). *PLoS ONE* **2011**, *6*, e22163. [CrossRef] [PubMed]
17. Choi, Y.H.; Kim, S.G.; Lee, M.G. Dose-independent pharmacokinetics of metformin in rats: Hepatic and gastrointestinal first-pass effects. *J. Pharm. Sci.* **2006**, *95*, 2543–2552. [CrossRef] [PubMed]
18. Kimura, N.; Masuda, S.; Tanihara, Y.; Ueo, H.; Okuda, M.; Katsura, T.; Inui, K.I. Metformin is a superior substrate for renal organic cation transporter OCT2 rather than hepatic OCT1. *Drug Metab. Pharmacokinet.* **2005**, *20*, 379–386. [CrossRef]
19. Yang, S.; Dai, Y.; Liu, Z.; Wang, C.; Meng, Q.; Huo, X.; Sun, H.; Ma, X.; Peng, J.; Liu, K. Involvement of organic cation transporter 2 in the metformin-associated increased lactate levels caused by contrast-induced nephropathy. *Biomed. Pharmacother.* **2018**, *106*, 1760–1766. [CrossRef]
20. Abbasi, M.M.; Valizadeh, H.; Hamishehkar, H.; Zakeri-Milani, P. Inhibition of P-glycoprotein expression and function by anti-diabetic drugs gliclazide, metformin, and pioglitazone in vitro and in situ. *Res. Pharm. Sci.* **2016**, *11*, 177–186.
21. Krausova, L.; Stejskalova, L.; Wang, H.; Vrzal, R.; Dvorak, Z.; Mani*f*, S.; Pavek, P. Metformin suppresses pregnane X receptor (PXR)-regulated transactivation of CYP3A4 gene. *Biochem. Pharmacol.* **2011**, *82*, 1771–1780. [CrossRef]
22. Khodneva, Y.; Shalev, A.; Frank, S.J.; Carson, A.P.; Safford, M.M. Calcium channel blocker use is associated with lower fasting serum glucose among adults with diabetes from the REGARDS study. *Diabetes Res. Clin. Pract.* **2016**, *115*, 115–121. [CrossRef] [PubMed]
23. Yin, T.; Kuo, S.C.; Chang, Y.Y.; Chen, T.T.; Wang, K.W.K. Verapamil use is associated with reduction of newly diagnosed diabetes mellitus. *J. Clin. Endocrinol. Metab.* **2017**, *102*, 2604–2610. [CrossRef] [PubMed]
24. Andersson, D.E.H.; Rojdmark, S. Improvement of glucose tolerance by verapamil in patients with non insulin dependent diabetes mellitus. *Acta Med. Scandina.* **2009**, *210*, 27–33. [CrossRef]
25. Cooper-Dehoff, R.; Cohen, J.D.; Bakris, G.L.; Messerli, F.H.; Erdine, S.; Hewkin, A.C.; Kupfer, S.; Pepine, C.J. Predictors of development of diabetes mellitus in patients with coronary artery disease taking antihypertensive medications (findings from the International Verapamil SR-Trandolapril Study [INVEST]). *Am. J. Cardiol.* **2006**, *98*, 890–894. [CrossRef] [PubMed]
26. Cooper-DeHoff, R.M.; Aranda, J.M., Jr.; Gaxiola, E.; Cangiano, J.L.; Garcia-Barreto, D.; Conti, C.R.; Hewkin, A.; Pepine, C.J. Blood pressure control and cardiovascular outcomes in high-risk Hispanic patients–findings from the International Verapamil SR/Trandolapril Study (INVEST). *Am. Heart J.* **2006**, *151*, 1072–1079. [CrossRef]
27. Hamann, S.R.; Blouin, R.A.; McAllister, R.G. Clinical pharmacokinetics of verapamil. *Clin. Pharmacokinet.* **1984**, *9*, 26–41. [CrossRef]
28. Hanada, K.; Ikemi, Y.; Kkita, K.; Mihara, K.; Ogata, H. Stereoselective first-pass metabolism of verapamil in the small intestine and liver in rats. *Drug Metab. Dispos.* **2008**, *36*, 2037–2042. [CrossRef]
29. Hong, S.P.; Chang, K.S.; Koh, Y.Y.; Choi, D.H.; Choi, J.S. Effects of lovastatin on the pharmacokinetics of verapamil and its active metabolite, norverapamil in rats: Possible role of p-glycoprotein inhibition by lovastatin. *Arch. Pharm. Res.* **2009**, *32*, 1447–1452. [CrossRef]
30. Uchida, Y.; Ohtsuki, S.; Terasaki, T. Pharmacoproteomics-based reconstruction of in vivo P-glycoprotein function at blood-brain barrier and brain distribution of substrate verapamil in pentylenetetrazole-kindled epilepsy, spontaneous epilepsy, and phenytoin treatment models. *Drug Metab. Dispos.* **2014**, *42*, 1719–1726. [CrossRef]
31. Zolk, O.; Solbach, T.F.; Konig, J.; Fromm, M.F. Functional characterization of the human organic cation transporter 2 Variant p.270Ala>Ser. *Drug Metab. Dispos.* **2009**, *37*, 1312–1318. [CrossRef]
32. Cho, S.K.; Kim, C.O.; Park, E.S.; Chung, J.-Y. Verapamil decreases the glucose-lowering effect of metformin in healthy volunteers. *Br. J. Clin. Pharmacol.* **2014**, *78*, 1426–1432. [CrossRef] [PubMed]
33. Han, S.Y.; Chae, H.S.; You, B.H.; Chin, Y.W.; Kim, H.; Choi, H.S.; Choi, Y.H. Lonicera japonica extract increases metformin distribution in the liver without change of systemic exposed metformin in rats. *J. Ethnopharmacol.* **2019**, *238*, 111892. [CrossRef] [PubMed]

34. You, B.H.; Chin, Y.W.; Kim, H.; Choi, H.S.; Choi, Y.H. Houttuynia cordata extract increased exposure and liver concentrations of metformin through OCTs and MATEs in rats. *Phytother. Res.* **2018**, *32*, 1004–1013. [CrossRef]
35. Liang, X.; Giacomini, K.M. Transporters involved in metformin pharmacokinetics and treatment response. *J. Pharm. Sci.* **2017**, *106*, 2245–2250. [CrossRef]
36. Tornio, A.; Filppula, A.M.; Niemi, M.; Backman, J.T. Clinical studies on drug-drug interactions involving metabolism and transport: Methodology, pitfalls, and interpretation. *Clin. Pharmacol. Ther.* **2019**, *105*, 1345–1361. [CrossRef]
37. Iwersen, S.; Schmoldt, A. A specific hydroxysteroid UGT is responsible for the conjugation of aliphatic alcohols in rats: An estimation of the importance of glucuronidation versus oxidation. *Alcohol* **1998**, *15*, 185–192. [CrossRef]
38. Peng, J.Z.; Remmel, R.P.; Sawchuk, R.J. Inhibition of murine cytochrome P4501A by tacrine: In vitro studies. *Drug Metab. Dispos.* **2004**, *32*, 805–812. [CrossRef]
39. Bradford, M.M. A rapid and sensitive method for the quantitation of microgram quantities of protein utilizing the principle of protein–dye binding. *Anal. Biochem.* **1976**, *72*, 248–254. [CrossRef]
40. Duggleby, R.G. Analysis of enzyme progress curves by nonlinear regression. *Methods Enzymol.* **1995**, *249*, 61–90.
41. Gibaldi, M.; Perrier, D. *Pharmacokinetics*, 2nd ed.; Marcel Dekker: New York, NY, USA, 1982.
42. Manitpisitkul, P.; Chiou, W.L. Intravenous verapamil kinetics in rats: Marked arteriovenous concentration difference and comparison with humans. *Biopharm. Drug Dispos.* **1993**, *14*, 555–566. [CrossRef]
43. US Food and Drug Administration, Center for Drug Evaluation and Research. Clinical Drug Interaction Studies-Study Design, Data Analysis, and Clinical Implications Guideline for Industry. 2017. Available online: https://www.fda.gov/downloads/drugs/guidances/ucm292362.pdf (accessed on 31 October 2017).
44. Davies, B.; Morris, T. Physiological parameters in laboratory animals and humans. *Pharm. Res.* **1993**, *10*, 1093–1095. [CrossRef] [PubMed]
45. Burt, H.J.; Neuhoff, S.; Almond, L.; Gaohua, L.; Harwood, M.D.; Jamei, M.; Rostami-Hodjegan, A.; Tucker, G.T.; Rowland-Yeo, K. Metformin and cimetidine: Physiologically based pharmacokinetic modelling to investigate transporter mediated drug-drug interactions. *Eur. J. Pharm. Sci.* **2016**, *88*, 70–82. [CrossRef] [PubMed]
46. Higgins, J.W.; Bedwell, D.W.; Zamek-Gliszczynski, M.J. Ablation of both organic cation transporter (Oct)1 and Oct2 alters metformin pharmacokinetics but has no effect on tissue drug exposure and pharmacodynamics. *Drug Metab. Dispos.* **2012**, *40*, 1170–1177. [CrossRef]
47. Zamek-Gliszczynski, M.J.; Bao, J.Q.; Day, J.S.; Higgins, J.W. Metformin sinusoidal efflux from the liver is consistent with negligible biliary excretion and absence of enterohepatic cycling. *Drug Metab. Dispos.* **2013**, *41*, 1967–1971. [CrossRef] [PubMed]
48. Lee, M.G.; Chiou, W.L. Evaluation of potential causes for the incomplete bioavailability of furosemide: Gastric first-pass metabolism. *J. Pharmacokinet. Biopharm.* **1983**, *11*, 623–640. [CrossRef] [PubMed]
49. Eichelbaum, M.; Mikus, G.; Vog Dunn, D.J.; Peters Elgesang, B. Pharmacokinetics of (+)-, (−)- and (+/−)-verapamil after intravenous administration. *Br. J. Clin. Pharmacol.* **1984**, *17*, 453–458. [CrossRef]
50. Wilkinson, G.R.; Shand, D.G. A physiological approach to hepatic drug clearance. *Clin. Pharmacol. Ther.* **1975**, *18*, 377–390. [CrossRef]
51. Scarpello, J.H.; Howlett, H.C. Metformin therapy and clinical uses. *Diabetes Vasc. Dis. Res.* **2008**, *5*, 157–167. [CrossRef]
52. US Food and Drug Administration, Center for Drug Evaluation and Reserach. Guidance for Industry: Estimating the Maximum Safe Starting Dose in Initial Clinical Trials for Therapeutics in Adult Healthy Volunteers. *Center Drug Eval. Res.* **2005**, *7*, 42346.

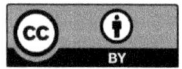

© 2020 by the authors. Licensee MDPI, Basel, Switzerland. This article is an open access article distributed under the terms and conditions of the Creative Commons Attribution (CC BY) license (http://creativecommons.org/licenses/by/4.0/).

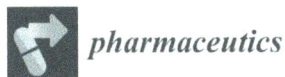

Article

Quercetin Is a Flavonoid Breast Cancer Resistance Protein Inhibitor with an Impact on the Oral Pharmacokinetics of Sulfasalazine in Rats

Yoo-Kyung Song [1,2,†], Jin-Ha Yoon [3,†], Jong Kyu Woo [3], Ju-Hee Kang [3], Kyeong-Ryoon Lee [2], Seung Hyun Oh [3], Suk-Jae Chung [1,*] and Han-Joo Maeng [3,*]

1. College of Pharmacy, Seoul National University, Seoul 08826, Korea; yksong777@gmail.com
2. Laboratory Animal Resource Center, Korea Research Institute of Bioscience and Biotechnology, Ochang 28116, Korea; Kyeongrlee@kribb.re.kr
3. College of Pharmacy, Gachon University, Incheon 21936, Korea; jinha89@daum.net (J.-H.Y.); apoptosis@snu.ac.kr (J.K.W.); applekjh0503@hanmail.net (J.-H.K.); eyeball@gachon.ac.kr (S.H.O.)
* Correspondence: sukjae@snu.ac.kr (S.-J.C.); hjmaeng@gachon.ac.kr (H.-J.M.); Tel.: +82-2-880-9176 (S.-J.C.); +82-32-820-4935 (H.-J.M.)
† These authors contributed equally to this work.

Received: 17 March 2020; Accepted: 23 April 2020; Published: 26 April 2020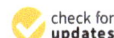

Abstract: The potential inhibitory effect of quercetin, a major plant flavonol, on breast cancer resistance protein (BCRP) activity was investigated in this study. The presence of quercetin significantly increased the cellular accumulation and associated cytotoxicity of the BCRP substrate mitoxantrone in human cervical cancer cells (HeLa cells) in a concentration-dependent manner. The transcellular efflux of prazosin, a stereotypical BCRP substrate, was also significantly reduced in the presence of quercetin in a bidirectional transport assay using human BCRP-overexpressing cells; further kinetic analysis revealed IC_{50} and Ki values of 4.22 and 3.91 µM, respectively. Moreover, pretreatment with 10 mg/kg quercetin in rats led to a 1.8-fold and 1.5-fold increase in the AUC_{8h} (i.e., 44.5 ± 11.8 min·µg/mL vs. 25.7 ± 9.98 min·µg/mL, $p < 0.05$) and C_{max} (i.e., 179 ± 23.0 ng/mL vs. 122 ± 23.2 ng/mL, $p < 0.05$) of orally administered sulfasalazine, respectively. Collectively, these results provide evidence that quercetin acts as an in vivo as well as in vitro inhibitor of BCRP. Considering the high dietary intake of quercetin as well as its consumption as a dietary supplement, issuing a caution regarding its food–drug interactions should be considered.

Keywords: quercetin; breast cancer resistance protein; inhibitor; prazosin; sulfasalazine; kinetic analysis; pharmacokinetics; food–drug interactions

1. Introduction

Flavonoids are a large group of polyphenolic antioxidants present in various human foods, such as vegetables, fruits, and tea. Quercetin is a major plant flavonol, a subclass of flavonoids with a 3-hydroxyflavone structure; it is present in high levels in onions, kale, broccoli, and tea [1,2]. Quercetin is mostly present in foods in the form of glycosides, which are efficiently hydrolyzed in the small intestine to release quercetin aglycone when ingested [3]. Dietary consumption of quercetin is estimated to be between 25 and 50 mg per day, accounting for approximately 70% of the total dietary flavonol and flavonone intake [4–6]. Moreover, it is well recognized that quercetin has diverse biological effects, including antioxidative, antiviral, antiulcer, and anticancer activities [7–10]. These activities have led to its consumption in various dosages and forms (e.g., 200–1000 mg aglycone per capsule/tablet [11]) as dietary supplements.

However, a recent analysis reported that the increased demand and consumption of dietary supplements is likely associated with a risk of adverse events. Indeed, a high number of adverse events (i.e., 23,000 emergency department visits per year in the United States) are attributed to dietary supplements [12]. In particular, flavonoids can modulate the activity of major ATP-binding cassette (ABC) efflux transporters [13]. For example, several studies have consistently shown that quercetin interacts with both P-glycoprotein (P-gp) [14–16] and multidrug resistance-associated protein 1 (MRP1) [17], inhibiting the efflux of substrates in the specific transporter-overexpressing cells in vitro or increasing the bioavailability/brain accumulation of substrate drugs in vivo by affecting the transporters' activity. Moreover, our research group recently reported that repeated pretreatment with quercetin could upregulate the human multidrug resistance protein 1 (MDR1) gene via a vitamin D receptor-dependent pathway in Caco-2 cells [18]. Therefore, the increasing use of dietary supplements containing quercetin emphasizes the need to investigate the potential clinical interactions that can be induced by the flavonoid.

Among ABC transporters, breast cancer resistance protein (BCRP; encoded by the ABCG2 gene) is a major efflux transporter abundantly expressed at the apical membrane of intestinal/kidney epithelial cells and hepatocytes. The transporter functions as a physiological barrier against oral absorption as well as a determinant of the disposition of substrate drugs [19]. Recently, several studies have attempted to determine whether quercetin interacts with BCRP. Sesink et al. reported that the flavonoid can be transported by the mouse Bcrp1 transporter in MDCKII/mBcrp1 cells [20]; moreover, its presence was shown to inhibit the cellular accumulation of the BCRP substrates Hoechst 33342 and mitoxantrone in BCRP-overexpressing MCF-7 cells [21,22]. However, such observations in cell systems cannot be directly translated to substantial effects on efflux transporter activity in vivo. For example, a study reported that coadministration of topotecan (a BCRP substrate) with the flavonoids chrysin or 7,8-benzoflavone (potent inhibitors of the transporter in BCRP-overexpressing MCF-7 cells) resulted in no significant effects on the pharmacokinetics of the substrate in rats or P-gp-knockout mice [23]. Therefore, considering that no apparent in vitro to in vivo association regarding BCRP inhibition by flavonoids was found [23], a more pharmacokinetic-based understanding of the interaction of quercetin with BCRP is needed. To our knowledge, the in vivo pharmacokinetic inhibition of BCRP by quercetin has not been previously reported.

Therefore, the objective of this study was to conduct an integrated study including in vitro and in vivo pharmacokinetic assessments on the inhibition of BCRP by quercetin. Here, we showed that quercetin can increase the cellular accumulation and associated cytotoxicity of the BCRP substrate mitoxantrone in human cervical cancer HeLa cells. Importantly, the high inhibitory potency of quercetin in limiting transporter-mediated efflux was demonstrated using the kinetic parameters (e.g., IC_{50} and K_i) associated with the efflux. Finally, the in vivo pharmacokinetics of the possible inhibition were studied in rats using sulfasalazine, a selective BCRP probe that was previously proven to show increased absorption by impaired BCRP function [24–26].

2. Materials and Methods

2.1. Materials

Quercetin (Figure 1), mitoxantrone (MX), Ko143, and sulfasalazine were purchased from Sigma-Aldrich (St Louis, MO, USA). Prazosin was purchased from Tokyo Chemical Industry (Tokyo, Japan). High-performance liquid chromatography-grade methanol and formic acid were purchased from Fisher Scientific (Pittsburgh, PA, USA) and Fluka (Cambridge, MA, USA), respectively.

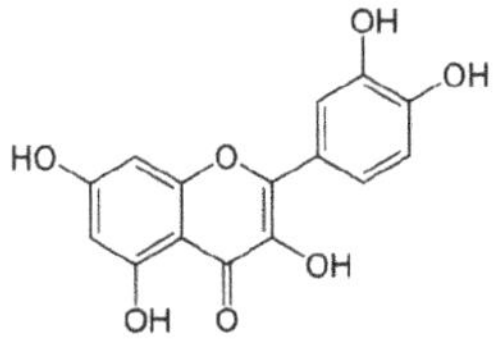

Figure 1. Chemical structure of quercetin.

2.2. Cell Culture

For the cellular accumulation and cytotoxicity studies, HeLa (human cervical cancer) cells were cultured in Dulbecco's modified Eagle's medium (DMEM; Welgene Inc., Daegu, Korea) supplemented with 10% fetal bovine serum (FBS; Welgene Inc., Daegu, Korea) and 100 U/mL penicillin–100 µg/mL streptomycin at 37 °C in a humidified incubator with 5% CO_2. For the bi-directional transport study, previously established human BCRP-overexpressing MDCKII cells [27] were used. Briefly, a plasmid construct containing cDNA for human BCRP was transfected into wildtype MDCKII cells to functionally express the transporter. MDCKII cells were grown in DMEM containing 10% FBS, 1% nonessential amino acid solution, 100 units/mL penicillin, and 0.1 mg/mL streptomycin under a humidified atmosphere containing 5% CO_2 at 37 °C.

2.3. RT-PCR Analysis

To measure the gene expression levels at the RNA level of BCRP, reverse-transcription polymerase chain reaction (RT-PCR) was performed. Total RNA was isolated from Hela, Caco-2, MCF-7, and SW620 cells using TRIzol reagent (Invitrogen, Carlsbad, CA, USA); complementary DNA (cDNA) was synthesized from 2 µg of the RNA extracted from cells, using the PrimeScript RT reagent Kit (TaKaRa, Shiga, Japan). cDNA was then amplified by PCR using human-specific primers: BCRP, 5′-TTC TCC ATT CAT CAG CCT CG-3′ (forward) and 5′-TGGTTGGTCGTCAGGAAGA-3′ (reverse); GAPDH 5′-GAA GGT GAA GGT CGG AGT C-3′ and 5′-GAAGATGGTGATGGGATTTC-3′ (reverse). Reverse transcription PCR (RT-PCR) was performed in a T-100TM thermal cycler (Bio-Rad, Hercules, CA, USA) using AccuPower PCR Premix (Bioneer, Daejeon, Korea), according to the manufacturer's protocol. The thermocycler conditions used for amplification were 95 °C for 5 min (hot start), 94 °C for 45 s, 55 °C for 30 s, and 72 °C for 30 s in 30 (BCRP) or 26 (GAPDH) cycles. Subsequently, the resultant products were analyzed by separation on a 1.5% agarose gel in tris-acetate/ethylenediaminetetraacetic acid (EDTA) buffer.

2.4. FACS-Cellular Accumulation Study

The cellular accumulation of quercetin was measured by FACSCalibur flow cytometry (Becton Dickinson, San Jose, CA, USA). For FACScan analysis, 2×10^5 HeLa cells/well were seeded into 6-well cell culture plates on the day before the experiment. On the following day, cells were treated with vehicle or quercetin and 1 µM MX. A time course experiment was conducted on HeLa cells following treatment with quercetin (1 and 100 µM) for 2, 4, and 6 h. After treatment, the cells were harvested by trypsinization and transferred to a fluorescence-activated cell sorting (FACS) tube, pelleted by centrifugation (1500 rpm, 5 min), and then resuspended in 200 µL of PBS. Flow cytometry analysis was performed using red fluorescence. A minimum of 10,000 cells were acquired per sample.

2.5. Cytotoxicity Assay

To determine the cytotoxic efficacy (i.e., the anticancer activity) of mitoxantrone associated with its intracellular accumulation, we performed the Cell Counting Kit-8 assay (CCK-8 assay kit; Dojindo Molecular Technologies, Kumamoto, Japan) following the manufacturer's instructions. HeLa cells (at a density of 1×10^4 cells per well) were seeded and cultured overnight in 96-well plates. Then, the medium was replaced with fresh medium containing the test drugs (mitoxantrone alone, mitoxantrone with 1 μM or 100 μM quercetin); the antiproliferation potential was examined at different drug concentrations after 24 h of incubation [28]. Additionally, 1 μM Ko143 was used as a positive control for BCRP inhibition. The absorbance was measured at a wavelength of 450 nm using a microplate reader (BioTeK, Highland Park, WI, USA).

2.6. Bi-Directional Transport Study

For the evaluation of the in vitro inhibitory potential of human BCRP by quercetin, the basolateral-to-apical (B-to-A) and apical-to-basolateral (A-to-B) permeability coefficients (P_{app}) of prazosin (the stereotypical substrate of BCRP) were determined in BCRP-overexpressing MDCKII cells in the presence of various concentrations of quercetin. Briefly, MDCKII cells were seeded on Transwell® filters (12 mm diameter, 0.4 μm pore size; Corning, NY, USA) at a density of 0.5×10^6 cells·mL^{-1} and then cultured for 5 days before being used in the transport assays. The confluence and integrity of the tight junctions were confirmed via microscopic observations as well as the measurement of transepithelial resistance [29]. The cells were washed twice and pre-incubated with transport buffer (9.7 g/L Hanks' balanced salt solution, 2.38 g/L HEPES, and 0.35 g/L sodium bicarbonate, pH adjusted to 7.4) for 30 min at 37 °C. Transport was initiated by adding transport buffer containing 10 μM prazosin in the presence or absence of quercetin (in a final concentration range of 0.1–300 μM) to the donor compartment (500 μL for the apical chamber or 1.5 mL for the basolateral chamber), followed by incubation at 37 °C for 120 min. At the end of the incubation, aliquots (300 μL for the apical chamber and 500 μL for the basolateral chamber) of the incubation mixture were collected from the donor and receiver chambers and subjected to LC-MS/MS assays.

2.7. Experimental Animals

Eight male Sprague-Dawley rats weighing 230–270 g (Orient Bio Inc., Seongnam, Korea) were used in the in vivo studies. The experimental protocols involving animals were reviewed and approved by the Seoul National University Institutional Animal Care and Use Committee, according to the National Institutes of Health Principles of Laboratory Animal Care (publication number 85-23, revised in 1985). The animal protocol number was SNU-180521-4; this protocol was approved on 9 October 2018.

2.8. Oral Pharmacokinetic Study in Rats

To determine whether quercetin affects the intestinal efflux mediated by BCRP, we divided the male rats into two groups: A sulfasalazine (a substrate of BCRP) control group and a quercetin pretreatment plus sulfasalazine group ($n = 4$, each). Considering the similar expression levels of intestinal BCRP between male and female rats, male rats were used in this study [30,31]. Briefly, overnight fasted male SD rats were anesthetized by intramuscular administration of 50 mg/kg tiletamine HCl/zolazepam HCl (Zoletil®) (Vibrac, TX, USA) and 10 mg/kg xylazine HCl (Rompun®, Bayer, Puteaux, France). While the rats were anesthetized, the femoral artery (for blood sampling) and vein (for supplementing body fluids) were catheterized using polyethylene tubing (PE 50; Clay Adams, Parsippany, NJ, USA). Upon recovery from anesthesia (i.e., after 4 h), quercetin was administered by oral gavage at 10 mg/kg (or 0 mg/kg in the case of the sulfasalazine control group; DMSO/polyethylene glycol 400/saline [1:4:5 (v/v/v)]). The pretreatment dose of quercetin was determined based on the compound solubility in the dosing vehicle and the likely daily dose of human dietary supplement. Fifteen minutes after the pretreatment, a dosing solution containing sulfasalazine at 2 mg/kg was administered by oral gavage. Blood samples (150 μL) were collected at 5, 15, 30, 60, 120, 240, 360, and 480 min after the sulfasalazine administration. Immediately after each blood collection, an identical volume of saline was intravenously provided to the animal to compensate for fluid loss. To prevent blood clotting during blood collection, the cannula was filled with 25 IU/mL heparinized saline. The plasma fraction was separated from the blood samples by centrifugation ($16{,}100 \times g$ for 5 min at 4 °C) and stored at −80 °C until the LC-MS/MS assay.

2.9. Quantification Using LC-MS/MS

Chromatographic quantification of sulfasalazine and prazosin was carried out using an LC-tandem mass spectrometry (LC-MS/MS) system equipped with a Waters e2695 high-performance liquid chromatography system (Milford, MA, USA) and an API 3200 QTRAP mass spectrometer (Applied Biosystems, Foster City, CA, USA). Briefly, an aliquot (50 µL) of a sample was vortex-mixed with an acetonitrile solution containing glipizide (300 ng/mL, internal standard); this was followed by centrifugation (16,100 × g for 5 min at 4 °C). An aliquot (5 µL) of the supernatant was directly injected into the LC-MS/MS system. Separations were carried out using a gradient of 0.1% formic acid in acetonitrile and 0.1% formic acid in water at a flow rate of 0.7 mL/min using a reversed-phase high-performance LC column (Agilent Poroshell 120, EC-C18 2.7 µm, 4.6 × 50 mm). The following transitions were used for analyte detection: m/z 399.0 → m/z 380.8 for sulfasalazine and m/z 384.1 → m/z 95.0 for prazosin. For the internal standard glipizide, the transition m/z 445.8 → m/z 320.9 was used. The limits of quantification were 10 ng/mL for sulfasalazine and 50 nM for prazosin.

2.10. Data Analysis

2.10.1. In Vitro Kinetic Analysis

The apparent permeability coefficient (P_{app}) of prazosin was estimated using the following equation (Equation (1)):

$$P_{app} = \frac{1}{A} \times \frac{1}{C_0} \times \frac{dQ}{dt} \tag{1}$$

where dQ/dt, A, and C_0 represent the transport rate, the surface area of the insert, and the initial concentration of the compound in the donor compartment, respectively. The efflux ratio (ER) was calculated by dividing the B-to-A apparent permeability coefficient ($P_{app, B\text{-to-}A}$) by the A-to-B apparent permeability coefficient ($P_{app, A\text{-to-}B}$). In the inhibition studies, the percentage of the control efflux ratio (%ER) was also calculated by dividing the value for ER in the presence of the inhibitor by that in the absence of the inhibitor (i.e., in the control). When necessary, the half maximal inhibitory concentration (IC_{50}) was determined by nonlinear regression analysis using WinNonlin Professional 5.0.1 software (Pharsight Corporation, Mountain View, CA, USA) and the following equation (Equation (2)):

$$V = V_{max} - (V_{max} - V_0) \times \left[\frac{[I]^n}{[I]^n + (IC_{50})^n}\right] \tag{2}$$

where V, V_{max}, V_0, [I], and n represent the rate of transport in the presence of the inhibitor, the maximal rate of transport, the basal rate of transport, the concentration of the inhibitor, and the Hill coefficient, respectively. When it was necessary to convert the IC_{50} to the inhibitory constant (K_i), the following equation (Equation (3)) [32] was used under the assumption that competitive inhibition existed between the substrate and the inhibitor:

$$K_i = \frac{IC_{50}}{1 + \frac{[S]}{K_m}} \tag{3}$$

where [S] is the concentration of the substrate and K_m represents the Michaelis–Menten constant.

2.10.2. Non-Compartmental Pharmacokinetic Analysis

Standard non-compartmental pharmacokinetic analysis was carried out using WinNonlin Professional 5.0.1 software (Pharsight, Cary, NC, USA) to calculate the pharmacokinetic parameters, including the peak concentration (C_{max}), time of the peak concentration (t_{max}), elimination half-life ($t_{1/2}$), area under the plasma concentration–time curve from time zero to the last sampling point, 8 h (AUC_{8h}), and elimination clearance (CL/F).

2.11. Statistical Analysis

For the comparison of means among the groups, one-way ANOVA (analysis of variance; for cytotoxicity and bi-directional transport studies) followed by Tukey's post hoc test were used. In these in vitro studies, a value of $p < 0.05$ was considered statistically significant. For the comparison of means between the groups for in vivo studies, the two-tailed/unpaired Student's t-test was used and a value of $p < 0.05$ with a statistical power more than 0.8 (Minitab 19.2, Minitab Inc., State College, PA, USA) was considered statistically significant.

3. Results

3.1. FACS-Cellular Accumulation Study

The expression of BCRP in Hela cells was confirmed by RT-PCR and compared with other cells, which were known to express high (Caco-2 and MCF-7) or low (SW620) levels of BCRP (Supplementary Figure S1) [33,34]. In the FACS-cellular accumulation study, the potential of quercetin to inhibit BCRP was first investigated by observing the cellular uptake of mitoxantrone (MX). The cellular uptake of MX with or without quercetin was analyzed by flow cytometry. The fluorescence intensity of a single cell measured by flow cytometry can be a good indication of the amount of MX internalized by each cell. As shown in Figure 2A, the peak fluorescence intensity of MX uptake was shifted to a higher level when MX was co-administered with quercetin, suggesting the promotion of MX internalization in HeLa cells. In the MX single treatment group, the percentage of cells with a significant uptake of MX was higher by 17.2% at 4 h of treatment and 27.1% at 6 h of treatment than at 2 h of treatment with MX alone as a control. In contrast, the cellular uptake of MX in the presence of quercetin was considerably higher by 30.2% at 4 h of treatment and 35.9% at 6 h of treatment (co-treatment with 1 µM quercetin) and by 45.3% at 4 h of treatment and 67.4% at 6 h of treatment (co-treatment with 100 µM quercetin) than at 2 h of treatment with MX alone. We also tested the internalization of MX when co-administered with 1 µM Ko143, a BCRP inhibitor. The results showed a considerably high number of cells that internalized MX when 1 µM Ko143 was co-administered with MX (Figure 2B). Thus, quercetin significantly promoted the cellular uptake of MX in HeLa cells likely via the inhibition of BCRP-mediated efflux.

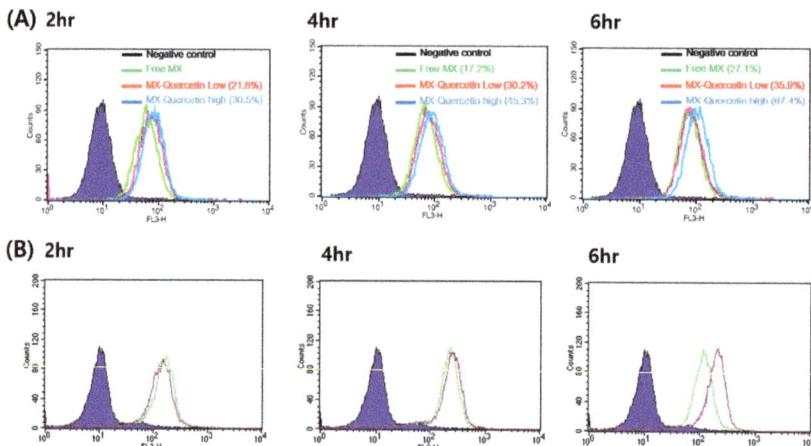

Figure 2. Representative histogram of mitoxantrone (MX) uptake in HeLa cells. (**A**) Flow cytometry measurement of MX fluorescence in HeLa cells incubated with MX alone (green line) or MX with 1 (red line) or 100 µM quercetin (blue line) for 2, 4, and 6 h. (**B**) Flow cytometry measurement of MX fluorescence in HeLa cells incubated with MX alone (green) or MX with 1 µM Ko143, a specific breast cancer resistance protein (BCRP) inhibitor (purple line), for 2, 4, and 6 h.

3.2. Cytotoxicity of Mitoxantrone in the Presence of Quercetin

To further confirm the effect of quercetin on the reversal of BCRP-mediated chemoresistance in HeLa cells, we examined the cytotoxicity (i.e., anticancer activity) of mitoxantrone in the absence and presence (1 or 100 µM) of quercetin. In this study, CCK-8 was used for the examination of mitoxantrone-associated cytotoxicity. As shown in Figure 3, mitoxantrone displayed concentration-dependent cytotoxicity in HeLa cells, which was further boosted in the presence of 1 µM Ko143, a stereotypical BCRP inhibitor. Likewise, the presence of 1 or 100 µM quercetin effectively enhanced the cytotoxicity associated with mitoxantrone as the IC_{50} decreased to 19.3% (1.13 µM) or 8.2% (0.478 µM), respectively, which differed from that observed with mitoxantrone alone (5.83 µM; Figure 3A). In addition, the cytotoxicity of quercetin alone without mitoxantrone was also examined. Treatment with 100 µM quercetin alone led to no significant changes in cell viability in comparison with the control (0.1% DMSO), demonstrating that the increased cytotoxicity observed in mitoxantrone-treated cells was not likely associated with the toxicity of quercetin (Supplementary Figure S2).

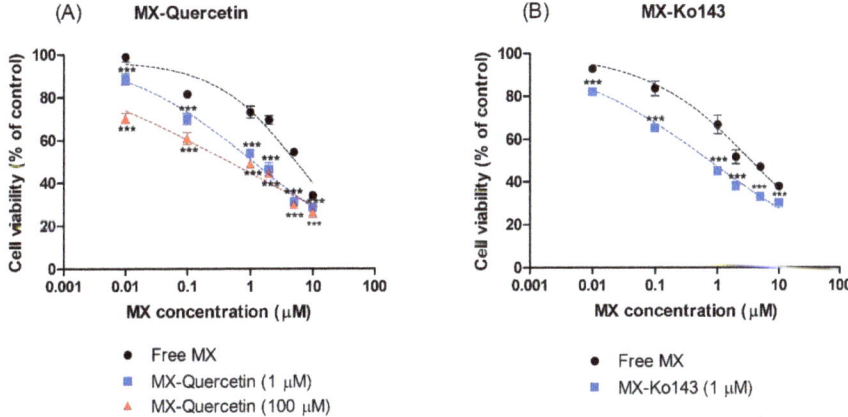

Figure 3. Effect of co-incubation of mitoxantrone (MX) with (**A**) quercetin (1 or 100 µM) and (**B**) Ko143 (1 µM) on the cell viability of HeLa cells. The Cell Counting Kit-8 (CCK-8) assay was used to determine the cytotoxicity associated with the cellular accumulation of MX after 24 h of incubation. Asterisks indicate statistical differences (* $p < 0.05$; ** $p < 0.01$; and *** $p < 0.001$) from the control group (i.e., without the quercetin or Ko143) according to one-way ANOVA, followed by Tukey's post hoc test. Data are presented as the mean ± SD of quintuplicate runs.

3.3. Bi-Directional Transport Study in MDCKII/BCRP Cells

We performed bi-directional transport studies in MDCKII cells expressing human BCRP (MDCKII/BCRP) to investigate the in vitro inhibitory potency of quercetin against BCRP in a concentration-dependent manner. Co-incubation with quercetin increased the $P_{app, A-to-B}$ of prazosin (Figure 4A) while simultaneously decreasing the $P_{app, B-to-A}$ (Figure 4B) with an increasing concentration of quercetin, leading to a concentration-dependent decrease in the overall ER (Figure 4C). Additionally, the functional expression of the efflux transporter in MDCKII/BCRP cells was also confirmed in this study, with an ER of 5.4 for prazosin (the stereotypical substrate of BCRP [27,35,36]), which decreased to 0.9 in the presence of the known inhibitor Ko143 (Figure 5C). Notably, the inhibitory effect of 10 µM quercetin on the B-to-A transport and efflux ratio was comparable to 1 µM Ko143 (Figure 5; $p > 0.05$). At quercetin concentrations higher than 10 µM, the ERs were less than 1.2, indicating the nearly complete inhibition of prazosin efflux (the complete inhibition of efflux would theoretically result in an ER of ~1, Figure 5). Kinetic analysis of the transport process yielded an estimated IC_{50} value of 4.22 µM for quercetin. Assuming the mechanism of inhibition to be competitive, the inhibitory constant (Ki) value was then estimated to be 3.91 µM using the K_m value of 128 µM [27] for prazosin.

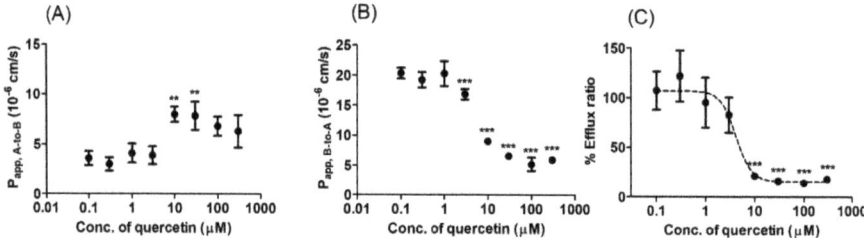

Figure 4. Bi-directional transport of prazosin in BCRP-overexpressing Madin-Darby Canine Kidney-II (MDCKII/BCRP) cells under various concentrations of quercetin (0.1–300 µM). (**A**) Apical-to-basolateral apparent permeability coefficient ($P_{app, A\text{-}to\text{-}B}$) and (**B**) basolateral-to-apical apparent permeability coefficient ($P_{app, B\text{-}to\text{-}A}$) of prazosin. (**C**) The percentage of the control efflux ratio (%ER, compared to the value without inhibitor) is shown together with the best-fit values generated from the nonlinear regression analysis based on Equation (2). Asterisks indicate statistical differences (* $p < 0.05$; ** $p < 0.01$; and *** $p < 0.001$) from the control (i.e., without quercetin) according to one-way ANOVA, followed by Tukey's post hoc test. Data are presented as the mean ± SD of triplicate runs. Data are presented as the mean ± SD of triplicate runs.

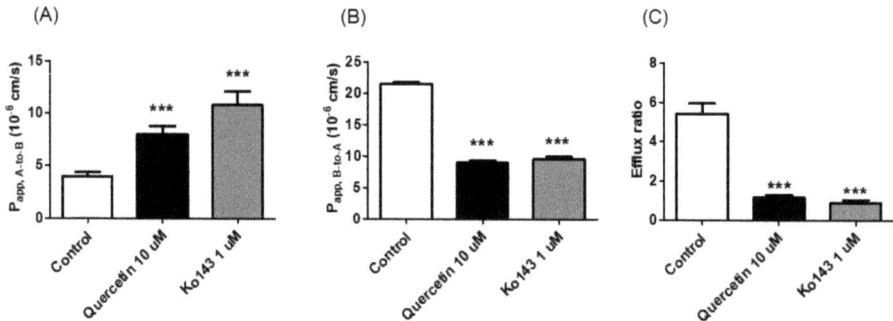

Figure 5. Effect of 10 µM quercetin or 1 µM Ko143 on the apparent permeability coefficient and efflux ratio of prazosin, a BCRP substrate, in MDCKII/BCRP cells. (**A**) Apical-to-basolateral apparent permeability coefficient ($P_{app, A\text{-}to\text{-}B}$), (**B**) basolateral-to-apical apparent permeability coefficient ($P_{app, B\text{-}to\text{-}A}$), and (**C**) efflux ratios of prazosin in the absence of inhibitor (i.e., the control) or in the presence of quercetin (10 µM) or Ko143 (the standard inhibitor of BCRP; 1 µM). Asterisks indicate statistical differences (* $p < 0.05$; ** $p < 0.01$; and *** $p < 0.001$) from the control group (i.e., without the inhibitor) according to one-way ANOVA, followed by Tukey's post hoc test. Data are presented as the mean ± SD of triplicate runs.

3.4. Oral Pharmacokinetic Study in Rats with or without Quercetin

To investigate the possible pharmacokinetic impact of quercetin as a BCRP inhibitor, we performed an oral pharmacokinetic study with sulfasalazine, a BCRP substrate, in rats. In this study, the change in the plasma concentration of sulfasalazine was used as an indicator of the in vivo interaction of BCRP with quercetin. To our knowledge, sulfasalazine has only limited interactions with other efflux transporters, including P-gp and MRP2 [34], whereas prazosin (the substrate used in the bi-directional transport study) is a dual substrate of P-gp and BCRP in vivo [37]. Thus, sulfasalazine is considered a relatively selective in vivo probe substrate of BCRP [25,26]. The mean plasma concentration–time profiles following the oral administration of 2 mg/kg sulfasalazine with or without pretreatment with 10 mg/kg quercetin in rats are shown in Figure 6. The pharmacokinetic parameters, as estimated using non-compartmental analysis, are summarized in Table 1. The plasma AUC_{8h} of sulfasalazine with or without quercetin pretreatment was 44.5 ± 11.8 min·µg/mL and 25.7 ± 9.98 min·µg/mL, respectively; this value was higher by 1.8-fold in the quercetin pretreatment group than in the control group, but it was not significantly different ($p < 0.05$, power < 0.8). More importantly, the C_{max} was significantly higher by 1.5-fold ($p < 0.05$, power > 0.8) in the quercetin pretreatment group (179 ± 23.0 ng/mL) than in the control group (i.e., 122 ± 23.2 ng/mL), whereas there was no significant change in the elimination half-life ($t_{1/2}$) of sulfasalazine. Collectively, these results suggest that pretreatment with quercetin led to the increased oral absorption of sulfasalazine in vivo.

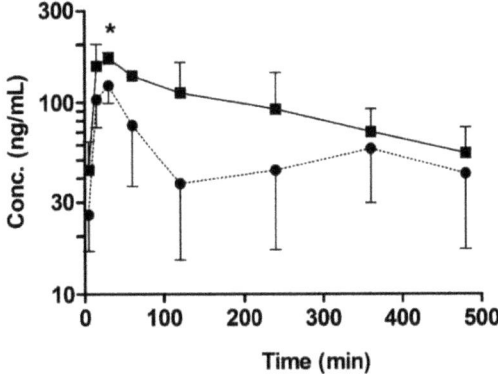

Figure 6. Temporal profiles of orally administered sulfasalazine (2 mg/kg) with or without the pre-administration of quercetin (10 mg/kg). Key: Control (●; without quercetin), quercetin pre-administration (■). Asterisks indicate statistical differences from the control (i.e., without quercetin) according to a two-tailed/unpaired Student's t-test (* $p < 0.05$, power > 0.8). Data are expressed as the mean ± SD of quadruplicate runs.

Table 1. Pharmacokinetic parameters of sulfasalazine after its oral administration (2 mg/kg dose) with and without pretreatment with quercetin (10 mg/kg) in rats. Data are expressed as the mean ± SD ($n = 4$ per group).

Parameter	Control	Pre-Administration Group (10 mg/kg Quercetin)
$t_{1/2}$ (min)	383 ± 111	242 ± 80.7
t_{max} (min)	30 ± 0	22.5 ± 8.70
C_{max} (ng/mL)	122 ± 23.2	179 ± 23.0 *
AUC_{8h} (min·ng/mL)	25700 ± 9980	44500 ± 11800
CL/F (mL/min/kg)	52.5 ± 33.5	33.2 ± 10.2

* significantly different from the control (i.e., without the pre-administration of quercetin) ($p < 0.05$, power > 0.8).

4. Discussion

Increasing lines of evidence from animal and human studies regarding food–drug interactions have indicated that a wide range of flavonoids can interact with ABC transporters, thereby leading to overexposure or underexposure of clinically important substrate drugs [13]. However, the accurate prediction of such interactions has been found to be difficult owing to limited in vitro data. The objective of this study was to investigate the inhibitory potential of quercetin against BCRP in vitro and in vivo. This study, which integrated the in vitro and in vivo effects of quercetin, was indeed necessary because a thorough understanding of the pharmacokinetic influence of this flavonoid is needed because of its high dietary intake as well as the lack of clear corresponding pharmacokinetic data.

Here, we demonstrated that the presence of quercetin can effectively enhance the cellular accumulation and associated cytotoxicity of mitoxantrone in HeLa cells (Figures 2 and 3), consistent with previous reports [38]. In the current study, the efficacy of quercetin as a BCRP inhibitor was quantitatively demonstrated via a significant reduction in the IC_{50} of mitoxantrone even in the presence of quercetin at a concentration as low as 1 µM (i.e., it decreased to 19.3% of the control value; from 5.83 to 1.13 µM). When the concentration of quercetin increased to 100 µM, the IC_{50} of mitoxantrone was further decreased (i.e., to 8.23% of the control value; 0.48 µM), similar to that in the presence of Ko143 (i.e., 0.62 µM), a stereotypical BCRP inhibitor. In addition, pharmacokinetically relevant parameters were obtained in a bi-directional transport study using MDCKII/BCRP cells, where the IC_{50} values of quercetin for the inhibition of BCRP-mediated efflux were estimated to be 4.22 µM. Assuming the mechanism of inhibition to be competitive, the IC_{50} value was further transformed to a Ki value of 3.91 µM, using the K_m value of 128 µM [27] for prazosin. The values obtained in the bi-directional transport studies were comparable to those previously observed in MCF-7/MX and MDCKII/BCRP cells using Hoechst 33342 accumulation (IC_{50} values of 7.6 and 6.9 µM, respectively) [21]. In both assays, it was shown that while quercetin is a less potent inhibitor compared to Ko143, it can show a similar inhibitory effect compared to 1 µM Ko143 in higher concentrations (Figures 3 and 5).

The US Food and Drug Administration recommends that orally administered compounds with an [I_{gut}] value (the maximal gastrointestinal concentration; defined as the dose divided by 250 mL) divided by the Ki value greater than 10 be evaluated for potential in vivo interactions [36]. For quercetin, the estimated [I_{gut}] value (662 µM, assuming a dietary quercetin intake of 50 mg/day) or even the estimated intestinal concentration (86.2 µM, when the intestinal fluid volume is assumed to be 1.92 L [39]) divided by the Ki (3.91 µM) value is far greater than 10. Thus, although the bioavailability of quercetin is somewhat low [40] and the daily dietary intake reportedly results in sub-micromolar concentrations in circulation [3], the substantially higher concentration in the gut is likely to result in the inhibition of intestinal BCRP and thereby an increase in the intestinal absorption of BCRP transporter substrates.

Consequently, the in vivo inhibitory potency of quercetin was further assessed to clarify its interaction with intestinal BCRP. In this study, the pharmacokinetic profile of orally administered sulfasalazine was used as an indicator of any alterations in intestinal BCRP activity. While sulfasalazine has been reported to be effluxed by P-gp and MRP2 to a low extent, previous studies have consistently demonstrated that the intestinal absorption of the compound following its oral administration was essentially unaffected in P-gp- or MRP2-knockout rats in contrast to the significantly higher AUC_{8h} and C_{max} values observed in BCRP-knockout rats [24], strongly suggesting that sulfasalazine is a good probe for observing intestinal BCRP activity. In this study, higher AUC_{8h} and C_{max} values of sulfasalazine (1.8-fold ($p < 0.05$, power < 0.8) and 1.5-fold ($p < 0.05$, power > 0.8), respectively) were observed in the presence of 10 mg/kg quercetin than in its absence (Table 1). The increased absorption in the presence of quercetin is clearly significant, but the degree is somewhat lower than that expected considering the approximately 20-fold increase observed in knockout rats [24] and, especially, the low Ki value of the flavonoid obtained in the current study. One possible reason for this discrepancy might be the rapid conjugation of quercetin to quercetin-3-glucuronide that occurs in the small intestine [20]. Once quercetin enters the intestinal cells by passive diffusion or uptake by the uptake transporters, it is subjected to glucuronidation by a UDP-glucuronosyltransferase present in both rat and human intestines [41–43], which results in the rapid clearance of quercetin from sites adjacent to the efflux transporter. Indeed, the oral bioavailability of quercetin was only 5.3% and the C_{max} value was the sub-micromolar range (i.e., 0.21 µg/mL) following 10 mg/kg oral administration to rats [44]. Another possibility that might result in relatively limited alterations in sulfasalazine absorption is the involvement of OATP2B1 in the intestinal absorption of sulfasalazine [25]. Sulfasalazine is a high-affinity substrate of OATP2B1 [25,45], whereas quercetin has been reported to be an inhibitor of OATP2B1 [46]. Therefore, the relatively low increase in sulfasalazine exposure in the presence of quercetin may be attributed to complex interactions between the simultaneous inhibition of the efflux by BCRP and the uptake by OATP2B1. In addition, considering that we only observed a single dosing of quercetin on the sulfasalazine pharmacokinetics, further studies regarding multiple dosing of quercetin are likely needed.

In a previous study by Zhang et al., an apparent discrepancy between the in vitro and in vivo inhibition of BCRP by the flavonoids chrysin and 7,8-benzoflavone was reported. In their investigation, the flavonoids were demonstrated to be potent inhibitors of human BCRP but weak inhibitors of mouse BCRP [23]; one possible explanation for this discrepancy may be species differences between the human and rodent transporters. Although a further study regarding food–drug interaction is required in humans, this may also be true for quercetin, in which case the clinical impact of the modulation of BCRP activity in humans may be much greater than that estimated from pharmacokinetic studies performed in rats.

5. Conclusions

The in vitro and in vivo inhibitory potencies of quercetin against BCRP were examined focusing on functional and/or kinetic aspects. Quercetin significantly increased the cellular accumulation and associated cytotoxicity of mitoxantrone in HeLa cells in a concentration-dependent manner. The transcellular efflux of prazosin was significantly reduced in the presence of quercetin as observed in a bi-directional transport assay using MDCKII/BCRP cells. These modulations in BCRP activity were consistent with the in vivo results, where pretreatment with quercetin led to not very dramatically different but still significantly higher intestinal absorption of sulfasalazine compared to that in the control group. Collectively, these results provide evidence that quercetin acts as a potent inhibitor of BCRP both in vitro and in vivo. Considering the high dietary intake of quercetin as well as its consumption as a dietary supplement, careful attention should be paid to potential flavonoid–drug interactions.

Supplementary Materials: The following are available online at http://www.mdpi.com/1999-4923/12/5/397/s1, Figure S1: mRNA expression levels of BCRP in HeLa, Caco-2, MCF-7 and SW620 cell lines using RT-PCR, Figure S2: Effect of 100 µM quercetin alone on the cell viability of HeLa cells.

Author Contributions: Conceptualization, H.-J.M. and Y.-K.S.; methodology, investigation and formal analysis, Y.-K.S., J.-H.Y., J.K.W., J.-H.K., K.-R.L., S.H.O. and H.-J.M.; resources, S.-J.C. and H.-J.M.; writing—original draft preparation and visualization, Y.-K.S., J.K.W. and H.-J.M.; writing—review and editing, S.-J.C. and H.-J.M.; supervision, S.-J.C. and H.-J.M; project administration, H.-J.M.; funding acquisition, H.-J.M. All authors have read and agreed to the published version of the manuscript.

Funding: This research was supported by Basic Science Research Program through the National Research Foundation of Korea (NRF) funded by the Ministry of Science, ICT & Future Planning (2019R1F1A1058103).

Conflicts of Interest: The authors declare that they have no conflicts of interests.

References

1. Hertog, M.; Hollman, P.; Katan, M. Flavonol and flavone content of vegetables and fruits. In *Flavonols and Flavones in Foods and Their Relation with Cancer and Coronary Heart Disease Risk*; CIP-Data Koninklijke Bibliotheek: The Hague, The Netherlands, 1994.
2. Hertog, M.G.L.; Hollman, P.C.H.; Van De Putte, B. Content of potentially anticarcinogenic flavonoids of tea infusions, wines, and fruit juices. *J. Agric. Food Chem.* **1993**, *41*, 1242–1246. [CrossRef]
3. Kelly, G.S. Quercetin. *Altern. Med. Rev.* **2011**, *16*, 172–195. [PubMed]
4. Sampson, L.; Rimm, E.; Hollman, P.C.; De Vries, J.H.; Katan, M.B. Flavonol and flavone intakes in US health professionals. *J. Am. Diet. Assoc.* **2002**, *102*, 1414–1420. [CrossRef]
5. De Vrie, J.H.; Janssen, P.; Hollman, P.C.; Van Staveren, W.A.; Katan, M.B. Consumption of quercetin and kaempferol in free-living subjects eating a variety of diets. *Cancer Lett.* **1997**, *114*, 141–144. [CrossRef]
6. Formica, J.; Regelson, W. Review of the biology of quercetin and related bioflavonoids. *Food Chem. Toxicol.* **1995**, *33*, 1061–1080. [CrossRef]
7. Takahama, U. Inhibition of lipoxygenase-dependent lipid peroxidation by quercetin: Mechanism of antioxidative function. *Phytochemistry* **1985**, *24*, 1443–1446. [CrossRef]
8. Lamson, D.W.; Brignall, M.S. Antioxidants and cancer, part 3: Quercetin. *Altern. Med. Rev. J. Clin. Ther.* **2000**, *5*, 196–208.
9. Ohnishi, E.; Bannai, H. Quercetin potentiates TNF-induced antiviral activity. *Antivir. Res.* **1993**, *22*, 327–331. [CrossRef]
10. De La Lastra, A.; Martin, M.; Motilva, V. Antiulcer and Gastroprotective Effects of Quercetin: A Gross and Histologic Study. *Pharmacology* **1994**, *48*, 56–62. [CrossRef] [PubMed]

11. Vida, R.G.; Fittler, A.; Somogyi-Végh, A.; Poór, M. Dietary quercetin supplements: Assessment of online product informations and quantitation of quercetin in the products by high-performance liquid chromatography. *Phytother. Res.* **2019**, *33*, 1912–1920. [CrossRef]
12. Geller, A.I.; Shehab, N.; Weidle, N.J.; Lovegrove, M.C.; Wolpert, B.J.; Timbo, B.B.; Mozersky, R.P.; Budnitz, D.S. Emergency Department Visits for Adverse Events Related to Dietary Supplements. *N. Engl. J. Med.* **2015**, *373*, 1531–1540. [CrossRef] [PubMed]
13. Alvarez, A.; Real, R.; Pérez, M.; Mendoza, G.; Prieto, J.G.; Merino, G. Modulation of the activity of ABC transporters (P-glycoprotein, MRP2, BCRP) by flavonoids and drug response. *J. Pharm. Sci.* **2010**, *99*, 598–617. [CrossRef] [PubMed]
14. Reddy, D.R.; Khurana, A.; Bale, S.; Ravirala, R.; Reddy, V.S.S.; Mohankumar, M.; Godugu, C. Natural flavonoids silymarin and quercetin improve the brain distribution of co-administered P-gp substrate drugs. *SpringerPlus* **2016**, *5*, 1618. [CrossRef] [PubMed]
15. Choi, J.-S.; Piao, Y.-J.; Kang, K.-W. Effects of quercetin on the bioavailability of doxorubicin in rats: Role of CYP3A4 and P-gp inhibition by quercetin. *Arch. Pharmacal Res.* **2011**, *34*, 607–613. [CrossRef]
16. Wang, Y.; Cao, J.; Zeng, S. Involvement of P-glycoprotein in regulating cellular levels of Ginkgo flavonols: Quercetin, kaempferol, and isorhamnetin. *J. Pharm. Pharmacol.* **2005**, *57*, 751–758. [CrossRef]
17. Van Zanden, J.J.; Wortelboer, H.M.; Bijlsma, S.; Punt, A.; Usta, M.; Van Bladeren, P.J.; Rietjens, I.M.C.M.; Cnubben, N.H. Quantitative structure activity relationship studies on the flavonoid mediated inhibition of multidrug resistance proteins 1 and 2. *Biochem. Pharmacol.* **2005**, *69*, 699–708. [CrossRef]
18. Chae, Y.-J.; Cho, K.H.; Yoon, I.-S.; Noh, C.-K.; Lee, H.-J.; Park, Y.; Ji, E.; Seo, M.-D.; Maeng, H.-J. Vitamin D Receptor-Mediated Upregulation of CYP3A4 and MDR1 by Quercetin in Caco-2 cells. *Planta Medica* **2015**, *82*, 121–130. [CrossRef]
19. Ni, Z.; Bikadi, Z.; Rosenberg, M.F.; Mao, Q. Structure and function of the human breast cancer resistance protein (BCRP/ABCG2). *Curr. Drug Metab.* **2010**, *11*, 603–617. [CrossRef]
20. Sesink, A.L.; Arts, I.C.; De Boer, V.C.; Breedveld, P.; Schellens, J.H.; Hollman, P.C.; Russel, F.G. Breast cancer resistance protein (Bcrp1/Abcg2) limits net intestinal uptake of quercetin in rats by facilitating apical efflux of glucuronides. *Mol. Pharmacol.* **2005**, *67*, 1999–2006. [CrossRef]
21. Pick, A.; Müller, H.; Mayer, R.; Haenisch, B.; Pajeva, I.; Weigt, M.; Bönisch, H.; Müller, C.E.; Wiese, M. Structure–activity relationships of flavonoids as inhibitors of breast cancer resistance protein (BCRP). *Bioorg. Med. Chem.* **2011**, *19*, 2090–2102. [CrossRef]
22. Zhang, S.; Yang, X.; Morris, M.E. Flavonoids Are Inhibitors of Breast Cancer Resistance Protein (ABCG2)-Mediated Transport. *Mol. Pharmacol.* **2004**, *65*, 1208–1216. [CrossRef] [PubMed]
23. Zhang, S.; Wang, X.; Sagawa, K.; Morris, M.E. Flavonoids chrysin and benzoflavone, potent breast cancer resistance protein inhibitors, have no significant effect on topotecan pharmacokinetics in rats or mdr1a/1b (-/-) mice. *Drug Metab. Dispos.* **2004**, *33*, 341–348. [CrossRef] [PubMed]
24. Zamek-Gliszczynski, M.J.; Bedwell, D.W.; Bao, J.Q.; Higgins, J.W. Characterization of SAGE Mdr1a (P-gp), Bcrp, and Mrp2 Knockout Rats Using Loperamide, Paclitaxel, Sulfasalazine, and Carboxydichlorofluorescein Pharmacokinetics. *Drug Metab. Dispos.* **2012**, *40*, 1825–1833. [CrossRef] [PubMed]
25. Kusuhara, H.; Furuie, H.; Inano, A.; Sunagawa, A.; Yamada, S.; Wu, C.; Fukizawa, S.; Morimoto, N.; Ieiri, I.; Morishita, M.; et al. Pharmacokinetic interaction study of sulphasalazine in healthy subjects and the impact of curcumin as an in vivo inhibitor of BCRP. *Br. J. Pharmacol.* **2012**, *166*, 1793–1803. [CrossRef] [PubMed]
26. Zaher, H.; Khan, A.A.; Palandra, J.; Brayman, T.G.; Yu, L.; Ware, J.A. Breast Cancer Resistance Protein (Bcrp/abcg2) Is a Major Determinant of Sulfasalazine Absorption and Elimination in the Mouse. *Mol. Pharm.* **2006**, *3*, 55–61. [CrossRef]
27. Song, Y.-K.; Park, J.E.; Oh, Y.; Hyung, S.; Jeong, Y.-S.; Kim, M.-S.; Lee, W.; Chung, S.-J. Suppression of Canine ATP Binding Cassette ABCB1 in Madin-Darby Canine Kidney Type II Cells Unmasks Human ABCG2-Mediated Efflux of Olaparib. *J. Pharmacol. Exp. Ther.* **2018**, *368*, 79–87. [CrossRef]
28. Kang, J.-W.; Cho, H.-J.; Lee, H.J.; Jin, H.-E.; Maeng, H.-J. Polyethylene glycol-decorated doxorubicin/carboxymethyl chitosan/gold nanocomplex for reducing drug efflux in cancer cells and extending circulation in blood stream. *Int. J. Boil. Macromol.* **2019**, *125*, 61–71. [CrossRef]
29. Irvine, J.D.; Takahashi, L.; Lockhart, K.; Cheong, J.; Tolan, J.W.; Selick, H.E.; Grove, J.R. MDCK (Madin-Darby Canine Kidney) Cells: A Tool for Membrane Permeability Screening. *J. Pharm. Sci.* **1999**, *88*, 28–33. [CrossRef]

30. Merino, G.; Van Herwaarden, A.E.; Wagenaar, E.; Jonker, J.W.; Schinkel, A.H. Sex-Dependent Expression and Activity of the ATP-Binding Cassette Transporter Breast Cancer Resistance Protein (BCRP/ABCG2) in Liver. *Mol. Pharmacol.* **2005**, *67*, 1765–1771. [CrossRef]
31. Tanaka, Y.; Slitt, A.L.; Leazer, T.M.; Maher, J.M.; Klaassen, C.D. Tissue distribution and hormonal regulation of the breast cancer resistance protein (Bcrp/Abcg2) in rats and mice. *Biochem. Biophys. Res. Commun.* **2004**, *326*, 181–187. [CrossRef]
32. Yung-Chi, C.; Prusoff, W.H. Relationship between the inhibition constant (KI) and the concentration of inhibitor which causes 50 per cent inhibition (I50) of an enzymatic reaction. *Biochem. Pharmacol.* **1973**, *22*, 3099–3108. [CrossRef]
33. To, K.K.; Robey, R.; Zhan, Z.; Bangiolo, L.; Bates, S.E. Upregulation of ABCG2 by romidepsin via the aryl hydrocarbon receptor pathway. *Mol. Cancer Res.* **2011**, *9*, 516–527. [CrossRef] [PubMed]
34. Ikai, A.; Watanabe, M.; Sowa, Y.; Kishimoto, M.; Yanagisawa, A.; Fujiwara, H.; Otsuji, E.; Sakai, A.T. Phosphorylated retinoblastoma protein is a potential predictive marker of irinotecan efficacy for colorectal cancer. *Int. J. Oncol.* **2016**, *48*, 1297–1304. [CrossRef] [PubMed]
35. Lepist, E.-I.; Phan, T.K.; Roy, A.; Tong, L.; MacLennan, K.; Murray, B.; Ray, A.S. Cobicistat Boosts the Intestinal Absorption of Transport Substrates, Including HIV Protease Inhibitors and GS-7340, In Vitro. *Antimicrob. Agents Chemother.* **2012**, *56*, 5409–5413. [CrossRef]
36. FDA. In Vitro Metabolism and Transporter Mediated Drug-Drug Interaction Studies: Guidance for Industry; US Department of Health and Human Services, Food and Drug Administration, Center for Drug Evaluation and Research (CDER). 2017. Available online: https://www.fda.gov/media/108130/download (accessed on 24 October 2017).
37. Zhou, L.; Schmidt, K.; Nelson, F.R.; Zelesky, V.; Troutman, M.D.; Feng, B. The effect of breast cancer resistance protein (Bcrp) and P-glycoprotein (Mdr1a/1b) on the brain penetration of flavopiridol, Gleevec, prazosin and PF-407288 in mice. *Drug Metab. Dispos.* **2009**, *37*, 946–955. [CrossRef]
38. Cooray, H.C.; Janvilisri, T.; Van Veen, H.W.; Hladky, S.B.; A Barrand, M. Interaction of the breast cancer resistance protein with plant polyphenols. *Biochem. Biophys. Res. Commun.* **2004**, *317*, 269–275. [CrossRef]
39. Tachibana, T.; Kato, M.; Watanabe, T.; Mitsui, T.; Sugiyama, Y. Method for predicting the risk of drug–drug interactions involving inhibition of intestinal CYP3A4 and P-glycoprotein. *Xenobiotica* **2009**, *39*, 430–443. [CrossRef]
40. Khaled, K.A.; El-Sayed, Y.M.; Al-Hadiya, B.M. Disposition of the Flavonoid Quercetin in Rats After Single Intravenous and Oral Doses. *Drug Dev. Ind. Pharm.* **2003**, *29*, 397–403. [CrossRef]
41. Murota, K.; Terao, J. Antioxidative flavonoid quercetin: Implication of its intestinal absorption and metabolism. *Arch. Biochem. Biophys.* **2003**, *417*, 12–17. [CrossRef]
42. Radominska-Pandya, A.; Little, J.M.; Pandya, J.T.; Tephly, T.R.; King, C.D.; Barone, G.W.; Raufman, J.-P. UDP-glucuronosyltransferases in human intestinal mucosa. *Biochim. Biophys. Acta (BBA)-Lipids Lipid Metab.* **1998**, *1394*, 199–208. [CrossRef]
43. Crespy, V.; Morand, C.; Manach, C.; Besson, C.; Demigne, C.; Remesy, C. Part of quercetin absorbed in the small intestine is conjugated and further secreted in the intestinal lumen. *Am. J. Physiol. Content* **1999**, *277*, G120–G126. [CrossRef] [PubMed]
44. Chen, X.; Yin, O.Q.P.; Zuo, Z.; Chow, M.S. Pharmacokinetics and Modeling of Quercetin and Metabolites. *Pharm. Res.* **2005**, *22*, 892–901. [CrossRef] [PubMed]
45. Tomaru, A.; Morimoto, N.; Morishita, M.; Takayama, K.; Fujita, T.; Maeda, K.; Kusuhara, H.; Sugiyama, Y. Studies on the intestinal absorption characteristics of sulfasalazine, a breast cancer resistance protein (BCRP) substrate. *Drug Metab. Pharmacokinet.* **2012**, *28*, 71–74. [CrossRef] [PubMed]
46. Mandery, K.; Bujok, K.; Schmidt, I.; Keiser, M.; Siegmund, W.; Balk, B.; Koenig, J.; Fromm, M.F.; Glaeser, H. Influence of the flavonoids apigenin, kaempferol, and quercetin on the function of organic anion transporting polypeptides 1A2 and 2B1. *Biochem. Pharmacol.* **2010**, *80*, 1746–1753. [CrossRef]

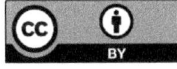

© 2020 by the authors. Licensee MDPI, Basel, Switzerland. This article is an open access article distributed under the terms and conditions of the Creative Commons Attribution (CC BY) license (http://creativecommons.org/licenses/by/4.0/).

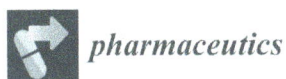

Article

Pharmacokinetic Evaluation of Metabolic Drug Interactions between Repaglinide and Celecoxib by a Bioanalytical HPLC Method for Their Simultaneous Determination with Fluorescence Detection

Dong-Gyun Han [1,†], Jinsook Kwak [1,†], Seong-Wook Seo [1], Ji-Min Kim [1], Jin-Wook Yoo [1], Yunjin Jung [1], Yun-Hee Lee [2], Min-Soo Kim [1], Young-Suk Jung [1], Hwayoung Yun [1,*] and In-Soo Yoon [1,*]

1. Department of Manufacturing Pharmacy, College of Pharmacy, Pusan National University, Busan 46241, Korea
2. Department of Pharmacy, College of Pharmacy, Seoul National University, Seoul 08826, Korea
* Correspondence: hyun@pusan.ac.kr (H.Y.); insoo.yoon@pusan.ac.kr (I.-S.Y.); Tel.: +82-51-510-2810 (H.Y.); +82-51-510-2806 (I.-S.Y.)
† These authors contributed equally to this work.

Received: 15 May 2019; Accepted: 29 July 2019; Published: 2 August 2019

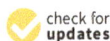

Abstract: Since diabetes mellitus and osteoarthritis are highly prevalent diseases, combinations of antidiabetic agents like repaglinide (REP) and non-steroidal anti-inflammatory drugs (NSAID) like celecoxib (CEL) could be commonly used in clinical practice. In this study, a simple and sensitive bioanalytical HPLC method combined with fluorescence detector (HPLC-FL) was developed and fully validated for simultaneous quantification of REP and CEL. A simple protein precipitation procedure and reversed C18 column with an isocratic mobile phase (mixture of ACN and pH 6.0 phosphate buffer) were employed for sample preparation and chromatographic separation. The fluorescence detector was set at a single excitation/emission wavelength pair of 240 nm/380 nm. The linearity (10–2000 ng/mL), accuracy, precision, extraction recovery, matrix effect, and stability for this method were validated as per the current FDA guidance. The bioanalytical method was applied to study pharmacokinetic interactions between REP and CEL in vivo, successfully showing that concurrent administration with oral REP significantly altered the pharmacokinetics of oral CEL. Furthermore, an in vitro metabolism and protein binding study using human materials highlighted the possibility of metabolism-based interactions between CEL and REP in clinical settings.

Keywords: celecoxib; drug–drug interaction; fluorescence; HPLC; metabolism; repaglinide

1. Introduction

Arthritis and diabetes mellitus are highly prevalent diseases with a total of over 350 million patients worldwide [1,2]. The most common types of arthritis and diabetes mellitus are osteoarthritis (OA) and type 2 diabetes mellitus (T2DM), respectively [3]. OA affects 14% of adults aged ≥25 years, and 34% of these patients are aged >65 years [4]; similarly, T2DM affects 12% of adults aged ≥20 years, and 26% of these are aged >65 years [5]. A recent survey estimated that the prevalence of OA was higher in individuals with T2DM than in those without T2DM [6]. Thus, T2DM is generally recognized as a comorbidity of arthritis [7], while some previous studies have focused on diabetes as a risk factor of arthritis [8,9]. Anyway, it is evident that T2DM is closely associated with an increased incidence and prevalence of OA, though the reasons remain unclear.

Repaglinide (REP), as shown in Figure 1, is a short-acting oral antidiabetic drug belonging to the class of meglitinides and is used to lower postprandial blood glucose levels in T2DM patients [10]. It stimulates insulin release from the pancreas, depending on the residual function of β-cells in the pancreatic islets [11]. REP is eliminated primarily by CYP2C8- and CYP3A4-mediated oxidative metabolism [12]. Systemic exposure to REP has been reported to be altered by co-administration of trimethoprim (inhibitor of CYP2C8) [13], itraconazole (inhibitor of CYP3A4) [14], or rifampicin (inducer of CYP3A4) [11]. Celecoxib (CEL), as shown in Figure 1, is a cyclooxygenase-2 (COX-2) selective non-steroidal anti-inflammatory drug (NSAID) and is used to treat pain and inflammation associated with OA and rheumatoid arthritis (RA) [15]. Because gastrointestinal mucosal integrity is compromised by COX-1 inhibition, traditional nonselective NSAIDs such as aspirin, ibuprofen, and indomethacin that inhibit both COX-1 and COX-2 may cause serious side effects in the gastrointestinal tract [16]. Thus, CEL exhibits distinctly reduced gastrointestinal toxicity as compared to conventional NSAIDs, thereby becoming a blockbuster drug for treating OA and RA [17]. CEL is eliminated primarily by extensive metabolism through methyl hydroxylation to form hydroxycelecoxib, which is catalyzed by CYP2C9 and CYP3A4 [18].

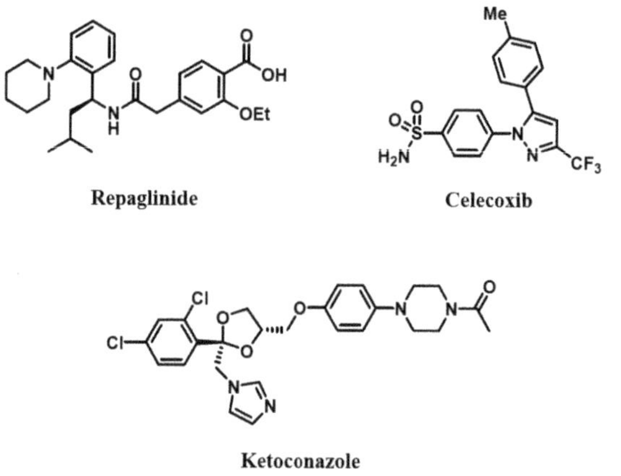

Figure 1. Chemical structures of repaglinide, celecoxib, and ketoconazole (internal standard, IS).

Because T2DM frequently co-exists with OA, there is a possibility of concurrent administration of REP and CEL. Hence, a bioanalytical method of simultaneous determination of REP and CEL could be useful and efficient for further pharmaceutical development and therapeutic optimization. To date, several bioanalytical methods have been developed and validated for quantitative determination of REP or CEL individually using HPLC with UV/Vis detection [19–23] or using liquid chromatography with tandem mass spectrometry (LC-MS/MS) systems [24–26]. However, these methods are associated with a few limitations, such as an insufficient sensitivity, relatively large sample volume, and/or time-consuming liquid–liquid extraction procedures with volatile solvents that are potentially hazardous to health. Moreover, LC-MS/MS methods require relatively complex and/or expensive instrumentation, which may not be affordable for small-sized laboratories and companies in resource-limited settings. To the best of our knowledge, there have been no reported methods of simultaneous quantification of REP and CEL in biological samples using HPLC coupled with a fluorescence detector (HPLC-FL). Furthermore, a previous in vitro study reported that CEL inhibited REP metabolism in pooled human liver microsomes (HLM) with a K_i of 3.1 μM [27]. This suggests the possibility of pharmacokinetic drug interaction between REP and CEL, but no information is currently available regarding this issue. Therefore, further investigation of the pharmacokinetic drug interaction between REP and CEL is necessary to prevent adverse effects in the use of these drugs.

In the current study, a sensitive and simple HPLC-FL method was developed and fully validated for simultaneous quantification of REP and CEL in rat plasma. The linearity, sensitivity, precision, accuracy, recovery, matrix effect, and stability of this HPLC-FL method were determined. Next, the potential for the pharmacokinetic drug interactions between REP and CEL was investigated in vivo using Sprague-Dawley rats and in vitro using rat liver microsomes (RLM) and HLM.

2. Materials and Methods

2.1. Materials

CEL (purity ≥98%), ketoconazole (as internal standard [IS]; purity ≥98%), as shown in Figure 1, and REP (purity >98%) were purchased from Tokyo Chemical Industry Co. (Tokyo, Japan). DMSO, ethanol, potassium phosphate monobasic/dibasic, and polyethylene glycol 400 were purchased from Sigma-Aldrich Co. (St. Louis, MO, USA). β-nicotinamide adenine dinucleotide phosphate (NADPH), HLM, and RLM were purchased from BD-Genetech (Woburn, MA, USA). ACN and methanol of HPLC grade were purchased from Thermo Fisher Scientific, Inc. (Waltham, MA, USA).

2.2. Animals

Male Sprague-Dawley rats (nine-week-old; approximately 300 g) were purchased from Samtako Bio Korea Co. (Gyeonggi-do, Korea). They were kept in a clean room of the Laboratory Animal Center of Pusan National University (Busan, Korea) at a relative humidity of 50 ± 5% and temperature of 20–23 °C with 12 h dark (19:00–07:00) and light (07:00–19:00) cycles. They were housed in metabolic cages (Tecniplast USA Inc., West Chester, PA, USA) with tap water and standard chow diet (Agribrands Purina Canada Inc., Levis, QC, Canada) provided ad libitum. The present animal study protocols were approved by the Pusan National University-Institutional Animal Care and Use Committee (PNU-IACUC, Busan, South Korea) for ethical procedures and scientific care (approval number: PNU-2018-1848; approval date: 01/05/2018).

2.3. Calibration Standards and Quality Control Samples

Stock solutions of REP, CEL, and IS (1000 µg/mL in DMSO) were prepared. The stock solutions of the mixture of REP and CEL were diluted with mobile phase for the preparation of working standard solutions with concentrations ranging from 1 to 200 µg/mL. The working solution of IS (final concentration of 5 µg/mL in ACN) was prepared by diluting the stock solution of IS with ACN. Calibration standard samples were prepared by spiking blank rat plasma with each working solution, yielding final plasma concentrations of 10, 20, 50, 100, 200, 500, 1000, and 2000 ng/mL. Quality control (QC) samples were prepared from separate stocks of REP and CEL in an identical manner to the preparation of calibration standards. The concentration levels of QC samples were 10 (lower limit of quantification; LLOQ), 30 (low; LQC), 120 (middle; MQC), and 1200 ng/mL (high; HQC).

2.4. Sample Preparation

For deproteinization, 400 µL ice-cold ACN containing IS (50 ng/mL) was added to 120 µL plasma samples. The resultant mixture was vortex-mixed for 5 min, followed by centrifugation at 15,000× g for 5 min. Next, 400 µL supernatant was transferred to another microtube and dried by N_2 gas stream. For reconstitution, 60 µL mobile phase was added to the resultant residue, and after sufficient vortex-mixing, 20 µL finally prepared sample solution was injected to the HPLC system.

2.5. Chromatographic Conditions

In this study, we used a Shimadzu HPLC system (Shimadzu Co., Kyoto, Japan) equipped with a fluorescence detector (RF-20A), column oven (CTO-20A), autosampler (SIL-20AC), and pump (LC-20AT). A Kinetex C18 column (250 × 4.6 mm, 5 µm, 100 Å; Phenomenex, Torrance, CA, USA) protected by a C18 guard column (SecurityGuard HPLC Cartridge System; Phenomenex) at 40 °C was used for chromatographic separation. Isocratic elution of mobile phase consisting of 10 mM phosphate buffer (pH 6.0) and ACN (53.6:46.4, v/v) was performed at a flow rate of 1 mL/min. The injection volume and total run time were 20 µL and 23 min, respectively. The fluorescence excitation and emission wavelengths for REP, CEL, and IS were 240 and 380 nm, respectively.

2.6. Method Validation

This new bioanalytical method for simultaneous determination of REP and CEL was validated based on the US-FDA guidelines [28]. The selectivity was assessed based on the comparison among chromatograms of REP, CEL, and IS in blank rat plasma; blank rat plasma spiked with REP, CEL, and IS; and rat plasma sample obtained from a pharmacokinetic study in rats. The presence of endogenous interferences at the acquisition windows of the analytes was examined.

The linearity was determined by the addition of increasing amounts of REP and CEL to a blank biological matrix. Calibration curves ($n = 5$) were constructed by plotting the peak area ratios of analytes to IS (y-axis) versus the concentration ratios of REP and CEL (10–2000 ng/mL) to IS (50 ng/mL) in plasma (x-axis), and linear regression analysis was conducted using the least squares method with a weighting factor of $1/x$ (x = concentration). The sensitivity was assessed based on LLOQ, defined as the lowest quantifiable concentration levels of REP and CEL in calibration curves (signal-to-noise [S/N] ratio of more than 5). REP and CEL peaks at the LLOQ level should be identifiable, reproducible, and discrete with acceptable accuracy (within 80–120%) and precision (<20%).

The precision and accuracy were estimated by comparison between the measured concentrations and their respective nominal concentrations in the QC samples, which were prepared as five separate sets on one day (intra-day) and five different days (inter-day). Precision was expressed as a coefficient of variation (CV) of the mean values of the measured concentration. Accuracy was expressed as a relative error between the measured and nominal concentrations. They determined with plasma samples spiked with REP and CEL at the four different QC levels in five replicates.

The extraction recovery and matrix effect were determined by comparison among the analytical signals (peak area) obtained from (A) the extracted sample, (B) the post-extracted spiked sample (extracts of blanks spiked with the analyte post extraction), and (C) non-extracted neat sample (diluted stock solution). The recovery was calculated as 'A/B × 100', and the matrix effect was calculated as 'B/C × 100'. Five replicates were assessed at the four different QC levels.

The stability was assessed by comparison of the analytical signals (peak area) obtained from plasma samples exposed to various handling and storage conditions with those obtained from plasma samples. Bench-top stability was determined by exposing spiked plasma samples to room temperature for 180 min. Freeze–thaw stability was determined by exposing spiked plasma samples to freeze–thaw cycles (from −20 °C to room temperature) three times on consecutive days. Long-term stability was determined by storing spiked plasma samples at −20 °C for 30 days. Autosampler stability (post-preparative stability) was determined by exposing extracted plasma samples to 25 °C for 1 day in an autosampler. The stability was determined at the four different QC levels.

2.7. In Vivo Pharmacokinetic Study in Rats

Rats were fasted for 12 h prior to the pharmacokinetic experiment and then anesthetized with zoletil (intramuscular, 20 mg/kg). The femoral artery and vein of the rats were cannulated with a polyethylene tube (BD Medical; Franklin Lakes, NJ, USA) at 240 min prior to drug dosing. A single oral dose of REP alone (0.4 mg/kg), CEL alone (2 mg/kg), or REP and CEL at the same doses was administered to the rats ($n = 5$ per group). Drugs were dissolved in a vehicle that is a clear mixture of DMSO, ethanol, polyethylene glycol 400, and saline at a ratio of 1:5:30:64 ($v/v/v/v$). Approximately 300 µL aliquots of blood were collected in heparin pre-treated microcentrifuge tubes via the femoral artery at 0, 10, 20, 30, 45, 60, 90, 120, 180, 240, 360, and 480 min after the oral dosing. Following centrifugation of blood samples at 2000× g at 4 °C for 10 min, 120 µL aliquots of plasma were stored at −80 °C until HPLC analysis.

2.8. In Vitro Metabolism and Protein Binding Study

An in vitro microsomal metabolism study was conducted using Corning® Gentest™ pooled male RLM (from Sprague-Dawley rats) and HLM (from more than 5 male donors) as previously described [29,30], with slight modifications and in accordance with the manufacturer's protocol. To assess the possibility of metabolic interaction between REP and CEL, a microsomal reaction mixture was prepared as follows (total volume: 0.2 mL): RLM or HLM (0.5 mg/mL), 50 mM phosphate buffer, 1 mM NADPH, 10 mM $MgCl_2$, 1 µM substrate, and various concentrations of inhibitor (1–100 µM). The disappearance rates of REP (as a substrate) in the absence or presence of CEL (as an inhibitor), and vice versa, were determined. At 0 and 15 min (REP) or 0 and 45 min (CEL) after starting the metabolic reaction, a 50 µL aliquot of microsomal incubation mixture was sampled and transferred into a clean 1.5 mL microcentrifuge tube containing 100 µL cold ACN containing IS (50 ng/mL) to stop the metabolic reaction. After vortex mixing and centrifugation at 15,000× g for 10 min, a 100 µL aliquot of the supernatant was stored at −80 °C until HPLC analysis.

The fractions of unbound REP and CEL (f_u) in rat and human plasma were measured using the rapid equilibrium dialysis (RED) device (Thermo Fisher Scientific, Inc.) as previously described [31]. The plasma was spiked with REP alone, CEL alone, and both drugs, yielding final concentration of 10 µM. A 0.2-mL spiked plasma was placed into the 'sample' chamber, and a 0.35 mL isotonic phosphate buffered saline was placed into the adjacent 'buffer' chamber. The fraction unbound was calculated as the ratio of the drug concentrations in the 'buffer' compartment to those in the 'sample' compartment.

2.9. Data Analysis

The IC_{50} of CEL for the inhibition of the metabolism of REP was determined by GraphPad Prism 5.01 (GraphPad Software, San Diego, CA, USA) according to the following Hill equation:

$$y = \text{Min} + \frac{\text{Max} - \text{Min}}{1 + (\frac{x}{IC_{50}})^{-P}}.$$

Analytical data were acquired and processed using the LC Solution Software (Version 1.25; Shimadzu Co.). Non-compartmental analysis was conducted to estimate pharmacokinetic parameters such as total area under plasma concentration versus time curve from time zero to infinity (AUC_{inf}), total area under plasma concentration versus time curve from time zero to time of last sampling (AUC_{last}), and terminal half-life ($t_{1/2}$) using the NCA200 and 201 models of WinNonlin software (Version 3.1; Certara USA Inc., Princeton, NJ, USA) [32]. Peak plasma concentration (C_{max}) and time to reach C_{max} (T_{max}) were directly read from the observed data.

2.10. Statistical Analysis

A p-value below 0.05 was considered statistically significant by using t-test for comparison between two unpaired means or by using analysis of variance (ANOVA) with post-hoc Tukey's honestly significant difference test for comparison among three unpaired means. Unless indicated otherwise, all data except T_{max} were expressed as mean ± standard deviation (median (ranges) for T_{max}). All data numbers were rounded to three significant figures.

3. Results and Discussion

3.1. Method Development

In this study, various chromatographic conditions were evaluated for sufficient sensitivity and good separation of analytes from endogenous substances of biological matrix within an appropriate run time. Several experiments were performed to choose suitable stationary phase, mobile phase, sample preparation procedure, and IS.

To choose a stationary phase, several types of HPLC columns including Accucore™ HILIC LC column (150 × 4.6 mm, 2.6 µm; Thermo Fisher Scientific, Waltham, MA, USA), XTerra Shield RP18 column (150 × 3.9 mm, 5 µm; Waters Co., Milford, MA, USA), and Kinetex® C8 and C18 columns (250 × 4.6 mm, 5 µm; Phenomenex) were tested. Our analysis found that Kinetex® C18 column showed higher peak resolution and intensity than other columns (data not shown). Therefore, Kinetex® C18 column was chosen as a stationary phase for the analytes.

The composition of mobile phase was optimized with different buffer types, such as citrate buffer (pH 3–5) and phosphate buffer (pH 6–7), and various ACN contents. Changes in the pH of mobile phase considerably influenced the peak retention times of REP (acidic compound) and endogenous interferences; however, it exerted little influence on those of CEL and ketoconazole that are neutral compounds. As a result, the mobile phase of pH 6.0 containing 46.4% ACN achieved good separation from endogenous interference in plasma with acceptable peak resolution. Thus, we settled for this mobile phase in developing the present HPLC-FL method.

Sample preparation was performed using a solvent precipitation-reconstitution method which is an efficient and economical sample pretreatment procedure compared with a solid phase or liquid–liquid extraction method. For optimization, several organic solvents, such as acetone, methanol, trichloroacetic acid, ACN, and their mixtures, were evaluated. Among them, ACN yielded the lowest matrix effect and highest recovery for analytes following centrifugation at 15,000× g for a relatively short precipitation time of 5 min.

Several fluorescent compounds, such as diclofenac, diflunisal, doxorubicin, metoprolol, naproxen, propranolol, and quinidine, were tested as a potential IS. However, these were unsuitable as IS, due to poor separation from analytes and endogenous substances in biological matrix. As a result, ketoconazole was finally chosen, because it exhibited good separation with acceptable retention time, peak resolution, and fluorescence intensity at the same wavelength as REP and CEL.

3.2. Method Validation: Selectivity, Linearity, Sensitivity, Precision, and Accuracy

As shown in Figure 2, the analyte peaks were well separated from each other and from endogenous matrix peaks in the blank plasma. Thus, it appears that the present bioanalytical method could offer acceptable selectivity without endogenous interferences occurring at the retention times of the analytes. The calibration curves (REP-to-IS or CEL-to-IS peak area ratio versus REP or CEL concentration, respectively) for REP and CEL were observed to be linear from 10 to 2000 ng/mL in rat plasma samples. A representative equation for the calibration curves was constructed, as follows: $y = 1.018x - 3.029$ for REP and $y = 2.093x - 0.723$ for CEL, where y represents the ratio of the peak area of REP or CEL to that of IS, and x represents the ratio of nominal concentration of REP or CEL. The correlation coefficients (r^2) were over 0.999, showing good linearity of this method. Generally, the sensitivity of a bioanalytical method is represented by the LLOQ value, which, in the present study, was determined to be 10 ng/mL for both REP and CEL. Moreover, the present method offered good sensitivity for CEL, with LLOQ comparable to those reported by previous LC-MS/MS methods in human plasma (LLOQ: 5–10 ng/mL; plasma volume: 100–200 µL) [25,26,33]. The intra- and inter-day precision and accuracy of this method were determined for REP and CEL at the four different QC levels, as shown in Table 1. The precision was estimated to be 8.30% or less, and the accuracy ranged from 98.6% to 112%. These values are within a generally acceptable range, showing that the present method was precise, accurate, and reproducible.

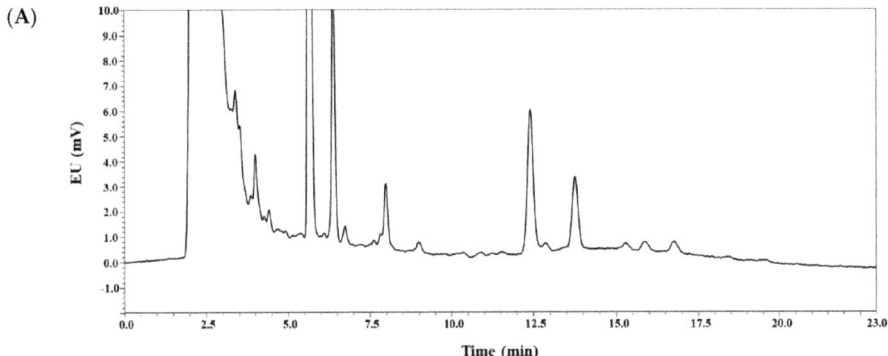
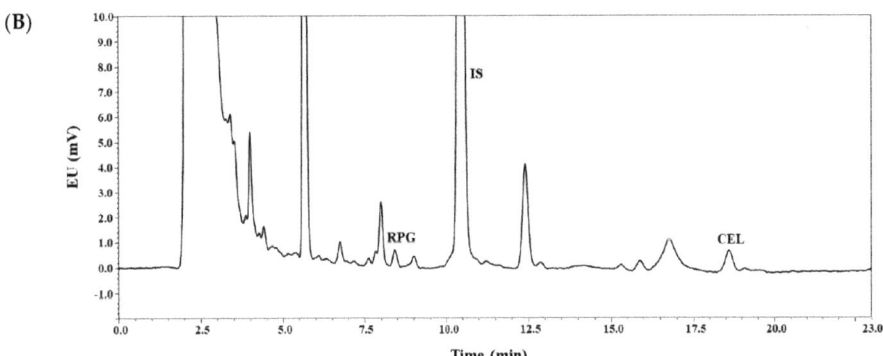
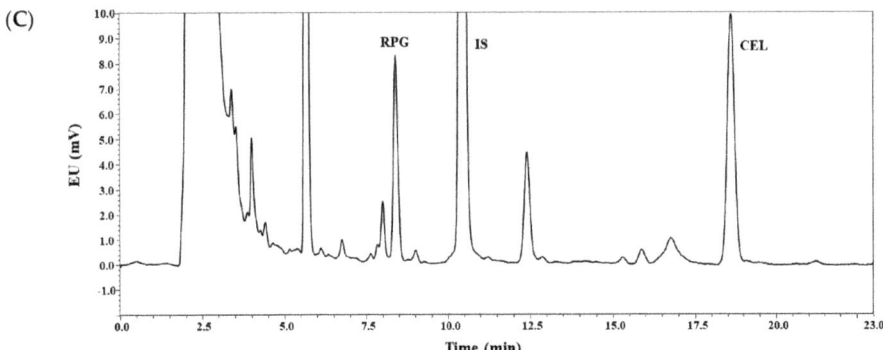

Figure 2. *Cont.*

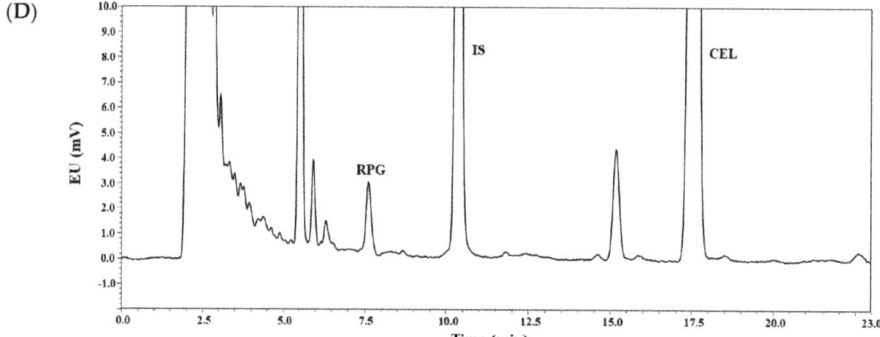

Figure 2. Representative chromatograms of repaglinide (REP), celecoxib (CEL), and ketoconazole (IS) in rat plasma: blank rat plasma (**A**); blank rat plasma spiked with REP, CEL (10 ng/mL, lower limit of quantification (LLOQ)), and IS (**B**); blank rat plasma spiked with REP, CEL (120 ng/mL, middle quality control (MQC)), and IS (**C**); plasma sample collected 120 min after concurrent oral administration of REP and CEL solution in rats, where calculated concentrations of REP and CEL were 53 and 968 ng/mL, respectively (**D**). EU: emission unit.

Table 1. Intra- and inter-day precision and accuracy of REP and CEL in rat plasma ($n = 5$). HQC: high quality control.

Nominal Concentration (ng/mL)	Precision (%)		Accuracy (%)	
	Intra-Day	Inter-Day	Intra-Day	Inter-Day
Repaglinide (REP)				
LLOQ (10)	2.69	6.21	112	101
LQC (30)	1.20	3.99	104	99.4
MQC (120)	1.16	0.70	102	101
HQC (1200)	0.79	1.43	99.2	99.8
Celecoxib (CEL)				
LLOQ (10)	4.06	8.30	111	103
LQC (30)	0.79	2.15	104	103
MQC (120)	1.19	2.18	100	102
HQC (1200)	1.55	1.63	98.6	100

3.3. Method Validation: Recovery, Matrix Effect, and Stability

As shown in Table 2, we assessed the recovery and matrix effect of the method for REP and CEL at the four different QC levels and for IS at 50 ng/mL. The mean recovery of REP and CEL was observed to be 98.5–104% with CV values of ≤2.57%. There were no significant differences in recovery values among the four different QC levels ($p = 0.066$ for REP and 0.502 for CEL), indicating concentration-independent recovery for both drugs. The mean matrix effect for REP and CEL was observed to be 92.1–102% with CV values of ≤5.25%. The stability was assessed under various handling and storage conditions relevant to this HPLC-FL method. Bench-top stability, autosampler stability, freeze–thaw stability, and long-term stability were determined for REP and CEL at the four different QC levels. The extent of bias in the concentration was within ±15% of the corresponding nominal value, while the remaining fraction of REP and CEL was observed to be 89.2–106% with CV values of ≤6.04%, as shown in Table 3. These data clearly indicate that the sample preparation procedure employed in the bioanalytical method proposed herein offered sufficient extraction recovery with minimal matrix effect, and that REP and CEL remained stable under several conditions related to the present bioanalytical procedures.

Table 2. Recovery and matrix effect of REP, CEL, and IS in rat plasma ($n = 5$).

Nominal Concentration (ng/mL)	Recovery (%)	Matrix Effect (%)
Repaglinide (REP)		
LLOQ (10)	98.5 ± 5.3	101 ± 6
LQC (30)	98.6 ± 1.1	102 ± 4
MQC (120)	103 ± 2	95.6 ± 3.0
HQC (1200)	101 ± 1	92.1 ± 2.5
Celecoxib (CEL)		
LLOQ (10)	104 ± 3	97.6 ± 3.0
LQC (30)	102 ± 4	98.5 ± 3.5
MQC (120)	104 ± 2	93.8 ± 1.8
HQC (1200)	103 ± 2	90.7 ± 2.4
IS (Ketoconazole, 50)	96.7 ± 1.2	99.4 ± 1.3

Table 3. Stability (%) of REP and CEL in rat plasma ($n = 5$).

Nominal Concentration (ng/mL)	Bench-Top [a]	Autosampler [b]	Freeze-Thaw [c]	Long-Term [d]
Repaglinide (REP)				
LLOQ (10)	102 ± 6	106 ± 3	106 ± 6	96.4 ± 3.4
LQC (30)	92.7 ± 4.2	102 ± 4	98.1 ± 3.7	97.6 ± 3.7
MQC (120)	92.9 ± 1.4	104 ± 0	102 ± 2	95.1 ± 1.8
HQC (1200)	90.6 ± 0.7	101 ± 1	100 ± 1	93.3 ± 0.8
Celecoxib (CEL)				
LLOQ (10)	98.3 ± 2.4	95.2 ± 2.6	90.3 ± 2.4	92.7 ± 3.0
LQC (30)	89.2 ± 2.7	97.8 ± 1.8	97.9 ± 2.1	92.7 ± 3.5
MQC (120)	93.1 ± 2.2	103 ± 1	101 ± 2	92.9 ± 1.2
HQC (1200)	89.6 ± 1.9	101 ± 1	99.6 ± 0.4	91.7 ± 0.7

[a] Room temperature for 3 h. [b] 10 °C for 1 day in the autosampler. [c] Three freezing and thawing cycles. [d] −20 °C for 30 days.

3.4. Pharmacokinetic Drug Interaction Studies

Rats received oral REP (0.4 mg/kg) and CEL (2 mg/kg) either alone or in combination. Then, plasma concentration versus time profiles of REP and CEL were evaluated as shown in Figure 3. The relevant pharmacokinetic parameters are listed in Table 4. The oral doses used were selected based on previous rat pharmacokinetic studies on REP or CEL [34–36]. After oral dosing of REP, plasma REP levels increased for 20 to 45 min and then declined in a multi-exponential fashion. The AUC_{last}, AUC_{inf}, and $t_{1/2}$ of REP were not significantly changed by concurrent administration with oral CEL, as shown in Table 4. After oral administration of CEL, its plasma concentration profiles markedly fluctuated during the whole period of blood collection (480 min). Thus, the AUC_{inf} and $t_{1/2}$ of CEL could not be determined in this study because there was no discernible linear terminal phase observed in the plasma concentration versus time curves of CEL. The multiple peaks in the plasma concentration profiles of CEL may be caused by slow and variable gastrointestinal absorption, which warrants further investigation. Notably, the AUC_{last} of CEL was significantly higher (by 76.2%) after co-administration of CEL and REP than after administration of CEL alone ($p = 0.0213$). Because CEL is eliminated primarily by extensive metabolism [15], the increased systemic exposure of oral CEL could be attributable to a reduction of hepatic first-pass and/or systemic metabolism of CEL caused by concurrent administration of REP.

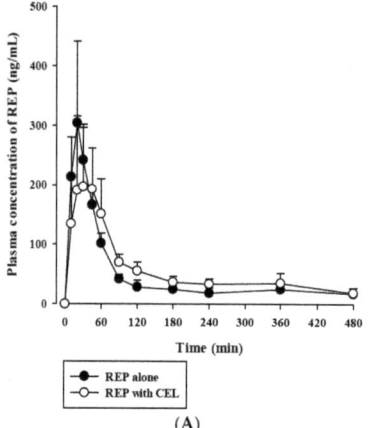
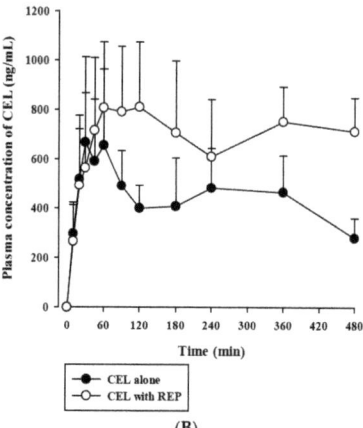

Figure 3. Plasma concentration versus time profiles of REP (**A**) and CEL (**B**) after oral administration of 0.4 mg/kg REP and 2 mg/kg CEL either alone (closed circle) or in combination (open circle) to rats. The circles and vertical bars represent means and standard deviations, respectively ($n = 5$).

Table 4. Pharmacokinetic parameters of REP and CEL in rats after oral administration of 0.4 mg/kg REP and 2 mg/kg CEL either alone or in combination ($n = 5$).

Parameter	REP		CEL	
	Single	Combined	Single	Combined
AUC_{last} (×10³ ng·min/mL)	21.1 ± 5.1	25.9 ± 2.8	189 ± 70	333 ± 89 *
AUC_{inf} (×10³ ng·min/mL)	30.5 ± 5.5	35.4 ± 8.3	ND	ND
C_{max} (ng/mL)	297 ± 103	224 ± 102	741 ± 299	954 ± 196
T_{max} (min)	20 (20–45)	45 (20–60)	180 (30–240)	120 (45–360)
$t_{1/2}$ (min)	374 ± 45	290 ± 123	ND	ND

* Significantly different from the single group ($p < 0.05$).

Previously reported pharmacokinetic parameters of intravenous REP and CEL in rats are listed in Table S1. Because the blood-to-plasma concentration ratio (R_B) was 0.61 for REP and 2.66 for CEL in rat blood (our in-house data), the blood CL (CL_B) was determined to be 8.52 mL/min/kg for REP and 2.92 mL/min/kg for CEL (calculated as plasma CL/R_B). Because the urinary excretion of the unchanged drug was reported to be negligible for both drugs, as shown in Table S1, it is plausible to assume that the CL_B of REP and CEL could represent their hepatic clearance, which is far below the reported hepatic blood flow rate in rats (Q_H; ranging from 50 to 80 mL/min/kg) [37]. This indicates that REP and CEL are drugs with low hepatic extraction ratios of 0.037 to 0.170 (calculated as CL_H/Q_H). Based on the well-stirred model, the CL_H of a drug with a low hepatic extraction ratio primarily depends on its intrinsic metabolic clearance (CL_{int}) and fraction unbound in blood (f_B) [30]. Thus, the hepatic metabolism and plasma protein binding of the drugs were further investigated using an in vitro rat and human liver microsomes and plasma. As shown in Figure 4, dose-response curves for the inhibitory effect of REP on the metabolism of CEL were constructed in RLM and HLM. REP significantly inhibited the metabolic reaction of CEL with IC_{50} values of 16.1 ± 4.5 µM in RLM and 14.4 ± 0.6 µM in HLM. However, the metabolism of REP in RLM and HLM was not significantly altered by CEL (data not shown). Additionally, protein binding interactions between the two drugs in rat and human plasma were assessed. As shown in Figure 5, there were no significant differences in fractions of unbound drugs either alone or in combination, suggesting the minimal possibility of protein binding-based interactions between the two drugs.

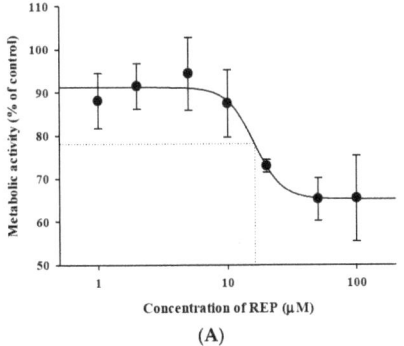
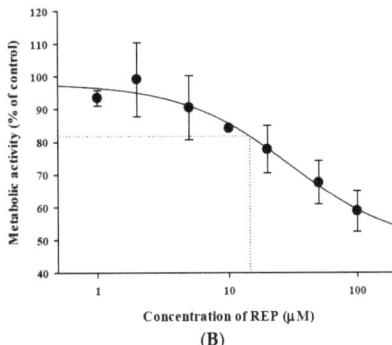

Figure 4. Dose-response curves for the inhibitory effect of REP on metabolic reactions of CEL in RLM (**A**) and HLM (**B**). The circles and vertical bars represent the means and standard deviations, respectively ($n = 4$).

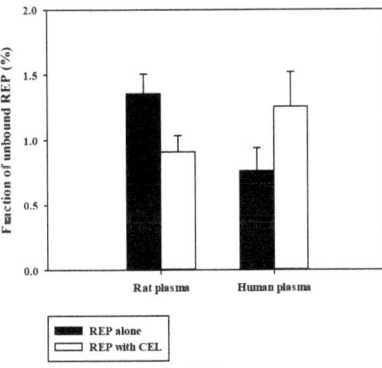
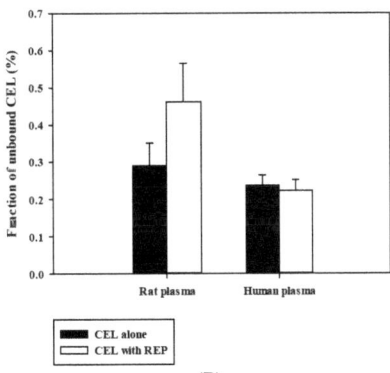

Figure 5. Fraction of unbound REP (**A**) and CEL (**B**) either alone or in combination in rat and human plasma ($n = 3$).

Since oral AUC is calculated as F × D/CL (F, oral bioavailability; D, dose; CL, total clearance), an increase in F and/or decrease in CL result in an increase in AUC. Moreover, hepatic metabolism is the major elimination route for both REP and CEL that are drugs with a low hepatic extraction ratio. Thus, the inhibition of hepatic metabolism of the two drugs can reduce their hepatic first-pass effect (increase in F) and hepatic systemic clearance (decrease in CL), consequently leading to an increase in AUC. In our present in vitro metabolism study in RLM and HLM, as shown in Figure 4, the metabolism of REP was not significantly changed by CEL, while the metabolism of CEL was inhibited by REP with a mean IC_{50} of 16.1 µM in RLM and 14.4 µM in HLM. Assuming that the in vivo concentration levels of REP in the rat liver after oral dosing are high enough to inhibit the metabolism of CEL, the increased oral systemic exposure of CEL by concurrent administration of REP (AUC_{last} in Table 4) could be attributable to a reduction of hepatic first-pass effect and/or hepatic systemic clearance of CEL caused by the inhibitory activity of REP on the hepatic metabolism of CEL.

The present rat study highlighted the possibility for metabolism-based interactions between CEL and REP in clinical settings. As shown in Figure 4, REP significantly inhibited the metabolic reaction of CEL with comparable IC_{50} values between RLM and HLM. The C_{max} of REP administered orally to rats was reported to be 297 ± 103 ng/mL (dose: 0.4 mg/kg) in this study, as shown in Table 4, and 105.1 ± 30 ng/mL (dose: 0.5 mg/kg) in a previous study [35], which are roughly comparable to the reported C_{max} of 65.8 ± 30.1 ng/mL (dose: 4 mg; converted to 0.41 mg/kg in rats based on the human equivalent dose concept proposed by the FDA) in humans (FDA drug label information). Moreover, there were no significant differences in the unbound fraction of REP between rat and human plasma, as shown in Figure 5. Based on these findings, it is plausible that the increased systemic exposure of CEL by co-administration of REP in the present rat pharmacokinetic study could have some clinical relevance, depending on species differences in hepatic distribution profiles of REP between rats and humans.

Additionally, there have been no reported studies on the relationships between the AUC and toxicity of CEL. However, the FDA drug label of CEL indicates that the steady-state AUC of CEL is increased about 40% and 180% by mild (Child-Pugh Class A) and moderate (Child-Pugh Class B) hepatic impairment, respectively. Thus, the daily recommended dose of CEL should be reduced by approximately 50% in patients with moderate (Child-Pugh Class B) hepatic impairment. In our present study, the AUC_{last} of CEL in rats was observed to be 189 (ranging from 113 to 285) µg·min/mL after administration of CEL alone and 333 (ranging from 458) µg·min/mL after administration of CEL and REP in combination. If these rat data could be extrapolated to humans, it is plausible that careful toxicity monitoring and/or dose modification may be needed for the combined dose of CEL and REP in clinical practice. Despite intrinsic limitations associated with nonclinical studies, our present in vivo rat and in vitro HLM data warrant further clinical study on drug interactions between REP and CEL.

4. Conclusions

This study successfully developed a simple, sensitive, and validated HPLC-FL method for simultaneous determination of REP and CEL in rat plasma. The new bioanalytical method provided several merits, including good sensitivity, high extraction recovery, negligible matrix effect, and simplicity of sample preparation procedures. The application of this method in the study of pharmacokinetic interactions between REP and CEL revealed that the pharmacokinetics of oral CEL were significantly altered by concurrent administration with oral REP. Furthermore, an in vitro metabolism and protein binding study using HLM and human plasma highlighted the possibility of metabolism-based interactions between CEL and REP in clinical settings. Therefore, the bioanalytical method proposed herein could become a promising tool for preclinical pharmacokinetic studies and, by extension, clinical use after partial modification and validation.

Supplementary Materials: The following is available online at http://www.mdpi.com/1999-4923/11/8/382/s1, Table S1. pharmacokinetic parameters of intravenous repaglinide (REP) and celecoxib (CEL) reported in previous studies on rats.

Author Contributions: Conceptualization, D.-G.H., H.Y., and I.-S.Y.; Formal analysis, D.-G.H., J.K., S.-W.S., J.-M.K., and I.-S.Y.; Funding acquisition, H.Y. and I.-S.Y.; Investigation, D.-G.H., J.K., S.-W.S., J.-M.K., H.Y., and I.-S.Y.; Methodology, D.-G.H., J.K., J.-W.Y., Y.J., Y.-H.L., M.-S.K., Y.-S.J., H.Y., and I.-S.Y.; Software, H.Y. and I.-S.Y.; Supervision, I.-S.Y.; Validation, D.-G.H.; Writing—original draft, D.-G.H., J.K., H.Y., and I.-S.Y.; Writing—review & editing, J.-W.Y., Y.J., Y.-H.L., M.-S.K., Y.-S.J., H.Y., and I.-S.Y.

Funding: This research was supported by PNU-RENovation (2018–2019) and by the National Research Foundation of Korea (NRF) grants funded by the Ministry of Education (NRF-2017R1D1A3B03030252) and by the Bio & Medical Technology Development Program of the National Research Foundation of Korea (NRF) funded by the Korean government (MSIT) (NRF-2017M3A9G7072568).

Conflicts of Interest: The authors have declared no conflict of interest.

References

1. Centers for Disease Control and Prevention (CDC). Prevention Prevalence of doctor-diagnosed arthritis and arthritis-attributable activity limitation-United States, 2010–2012. *MMWR Morb. Mortal. Wkly. Rep.* **2013**, *62*, 869–873.
2. Cefalu, W.T.; Buse, J.B.; Tuomilehto, J.; Fleming, G.A.; Ferrannini, E.; Gerstein, H.C.; Bennett, P.H.; Ramachandran, A.; Raz, I.; Rosenstock, J.; et al. Update and next steps for real-world translation of interventions for type 2 diabetes prevention: Reflections from a diabetes care editors' expert forum. *Diabetes Care* **2016**, *39*, 1186–1201. [CrossRef] [PubMed]

3. March, L.; Smith, E.U.; Hoy, D.G.; Cross, M.J.; Sanchez-Riera, L.; Blyth, F.; Buchbinder, R.; Vos, T.; Woolf, A.D. Burden of disability due to musculoskeletal (MSK) disorders. *Best Pract. Res. Clin. Rheumatol.* **2014**, *28*, 353–366. [CrossRef] [PubMed]
4. Lawrence, R.C.; Felson, D.T.; Helmick, C.G.; Arnold, L.M.; Choi, H.; Deyo, R.A.; Gabriel, S.; Hirsch, R.; Hochberg, M.C.; Hunder, G.G.; et al. Estimates of the prevalence of arthritis and other rheumatic conditions in the United States. Part II. *Arthritis Rheum.* **2008**, *58*, 26–35. [CrossRef] [PubMed]
5. Piva, S.R.; Susko, A.M.; Khoja, S.S.; Josbeno, D.A.; Fitzgerald, G.K.; Toledo, F.G. Links between osteoarthritis and diabetes: Implications for management from a physical activity perspective. *Clin. Geriatr. Med.* **2015**, *31*, 67–87. [CrossRef] [PubMed]
6. Centers for Disease Control and Prevention (CDC). Prevention Arthritis as a potential barrier to physical activity among adults with diabetes-United States, 2005 and 2007. *MMWR Morb. Mortal. Wkly. Rep.* **2008**, *57*, 486–489.
7. Dong, Q.; Liu, H.; Yang, D.; Zhang, Y. Diabetes mellitus and arthritis: Is it a risk factor or comorbidity? A systematic review and meta-analysis. *Medicine (Baltimore)* **2017**, *96*, e6627. [CrossRef] [PubMed]
8. Tam, L.S.; Tomlinson, B.; Chu, T.T.; Li, M.; Leung, Y.Y.; Kwok, L.W.; Li, T.K.; Yu, T.; Zhu, Y.E.; Wong, K.C.; et al. Cardiovascular risk profile of patients with psoriatic arthritis compared to controls-the role of inflammation. *Rheumatology* **2008**, *47*, 718–723. [CrossRef]
9. Boyer, J.F.; Gourraud, P.A.; Cantagrel, A.; Davignon, J.L.; Constantin, A. Traditional cardiovascular risk factors in rheumatoid arthritis: A meta-analysis. *Joint Bone Spine* **2011**, *78*, 179–183. [CrossRef]
10. Kajosaari, L.I.; Niemi, M.; Backman, J.T.; Neuvonen, P.J. Telithromycin, but not montelukast, increases the plasma concentrations and effects of the cytochrome P450 3A4 and 2C8 substrate repaglinide. *Clin. Pharmacol. Ther.* **2006**, *79*, 231–242. [CrossRef]
11. Hatorp, V.; Hansen, K.T.; Thomsen, M.S. Influence of drugs interacting with CYP3A4 on the pharmacokinetics, pharmacodynamics, and safety of the prandial glucose regulator repaglinide. *J. Clin. Pharmacol.* **2003**, *43*, 649–660. [CrossRef] [PubMed]
12. Bidstrup, T.B.; Bjornsdottir, I.; Sidelmann, U.G.; Thomsen, M.S.; Hansen, K.T. CYP2C8 and CYP3A4 are the principal enzymes involved in the human in vitro biotransformation of the insulin secretagogue repaglinide. *Br. J. Clin. Pharmacol.* **2003**, *56*, 305–314. [CrossRef] [PubMed]
13. Niemi, M.; Kajosaari, L.I.; Neuvonen, M.; Backman, J.T.; Neuvonen, P.J. The CYP2C8 inhibitor trimethoprim increases the plasma concentrations of repaglinide in healthy subjects. *Br. J. Clin. Pharmacol.* **2004**, *57*, 441–447. [CrossRef] [PubMed]
14. Niemi, M.; Backman, J.T.; Neuvonen, M.; Neuvonen, P.J. Effects of gemfibrozil, itraconazole, and their combination on the pharmacokinetics and pharmacodynamics of repaglinide: Potentially hazardous interaction between gemfibrozil and repaglinide. *Diabetologia* **2003**, *46*, 347–351. [CrossRef] [PubMed]
15. Oh, H.A.; Kim, D.; Lee, S.H.; Jung, B.H. Simultaneous quantitative determination of celecoxib and its two metabolites using liquid chromatography-tandem mass spectrometry in alternating polarity switching mode. *J. Pharm. Biomed. Anal.* **2015**, *107*, 32–39. [CrossRef] [PubMed]
16. Wallace, J.L.; McKnight, W.; Reuter, B.K.; Vergnolle, N. NSAID-induced gastric damage in rats: Requirement for inhibition of both cyclooxygenase 1 and 2. *Gastroenterology* **2000**, *119*, 706–714. [CrossRef]
17. Ma, Y.; Gao, S.; Hu, M. Quantitation of celecoxib and four of its metabolites in rat blood by UPLC-MS/MS clarifies their blood distribution patterns and provides more accurate pharmacokinetics profiles. *J. Chromatogr. B* **2015**, *1001*, 202–211. [CrossRef] [PubMed]
18. Gong, L.; Thorn, C.F.; Bertagnolli, M.M.; Grosser, T.; Altman, R.B.; Klein, T.E. Celecoxib pathways: Pharmacokinetics and pharmacodynamics. *Pharmacogenet. Genom.* **2012**, *22*, 310–318. [CrossRef]
19. Venkatesh, P.; Harisudhan, T.; Choudhury, H.; Mullangi, R.; Srinivas, N.R. Simultaneous estimation of six anti-diabetic drugs-glibenclamide, gliclazide, glipizide, pioglitazone, repaglinide and rosiglitazone: Development of a novel HPLC method for use in the analysis of pharmaceutical formulations and its application to human plasma assay. *Biomed. Chromatogr.* **2006**, *20*, 1043–1048.
20. Ruzilawati, A.B.; Wahab, M.S.; Imran, A.; Ismail, Z.; Gan, S.H. Method development and validation of repaglinide in human plasma by HPLC and its application in pharmacokinetic studies. *J. Pharm. Biomed. Anal.* **2007**, *43*, 1831–1835. [CrossRef]

21. Guirguis, M.S.; Sattari, S.; Jamali, F. Pharmacokinetics of celecoxib in the presence and absence of interferon-induced acute inflammation in the rat: Application of a novel HPLC assay. *J. Pharm. Pharm. Sci.* **2001**, *4*, 1–6.
22. Stormer, E.; Bauer, S.; Kirchheiner, J.; Brockmoller, J.; Roots, I. Simultaneous determination of celecoxib, hydroxycelecoxib, and carboxycelecoxib in human plasma using gradient reversed-phase liquid chromatography with ultraviolet absorbance detection. *J. Chromatogr. B* **2003**, *783*, 207–212. [CrossRef]
23. Jalalizadeh, H.; Amini, M.; Ziaee, V.; Safa, A.; Farsam, H.; Shafiee, A. Determination of celecoxib in human plasma by high-performance liquid chromatography. *J. Pharm. Biomed. Anal.* **2004**, *35*, 665–670. [CrossRef]
24. Zhang, J.; Gao, F.; Guan, X.; Sun, Y.-T.; Gu, J.-K.; Fawcett, J.P. Determination of repaglinide in human plasma by high-performance liquid chromatography–tandem mass spectrometry. *Acta Pharm. Sin. B* **2011**, *1*, 40–45. [CrossRef]
25. Ptacek, P.; Klima, J.; Macek, J. Determination of celecoxib in human plasma by liquid chromatography-tandem mass spectrometry. *J. Chromatogr. B* **2012**, *899*, 163–166. [CrossRef]
26. Park, M.S.; Shim, W.S.; Yim, S.V.; Lee, K.T. Development of simple and rapid LC-MS/MS method for determination of celecoxib in human plasma and its application to bioequivalence study. *J. Chromatogr. B* **2012**, *902*, 137–141. [CrossRef]
27. VandenBrink, B.M.; Foti, R.S.; Rock, D.A.; Wienkers, L.C.; Wahlstrom, J.L. Evaluation of CYP2C8 inhibition in vitro: Utility of montelukast as a selective CYP2C8 probe substrate. *Drug Metab. Dispos.* **2011**, *39*, 1546–1554. [CrossRef]
28. US-FDA Guidance for Industry: Bioanalytical Method Validation. Center for Drug Evaluation and Research 2018. Available online: https://www.fda.gov/downloads/drugs/guidances/ucm070107.pdf (accessed on 24 May 2018).
29. Kim, S.B.; Kim, K.S.; Kim, D.D.; Yoon, I.S. Metabolic interactions of rosmarinic acid with human cytochrome P450 monooxygenases and uridine diphosphate glucuronosyltransferases. *Biomed. Pharmacother.* **2019**, *110*, 111–117. [CrossRef]
30. Kim, S.B.; Kim, K.S.; Ryu, H.M.; Hong, S.H.; Kim, B.K.; Kim, D.D.; Park, J.W.; Yoon, I.S. Modulation of rat hepatic CYP1A and 2C activity by honokiol and magnolol: Differential effects on phenacetin and diclofenac pharmacokinetics in vivo. *Molecules* **2018**, *23*, 1470. [CrossRef]
31. Kim, S.B.; Lee, T.; Lee, H.S.; Song, C.K.; Cho, H.J.; Kim, D.D.; Maeng, H.J.; Yoon, I.S. Development and validation of a highly sensitive LC-MS/MS method for the determination of acacetin in human plasma and its application to a protein binding study. *Arch. Pharm. Res.* **2016**, *39*, 213–220. [CrossRef]
32. Avery, B.A.; Pabbisetty, D.; Li, L.; Sharma, A.; Gundluru, M.K.; Chittiboyina, A.G.; Williamson, J.S.; Avery, M.A. A pharmacokinetic comparison of homodimer ARB-92 and heterodimer ARB-89: Novel, potent antimalarial candidates derived from 7β-hydroxyartemisinin. *J. Pharm. Investig.* **2018**, *48*, 585–593. [CrossRef]
33. Werner, U.; Werner, D.; Pahl, A.; Mundkowski, R.; Gillich, M.; Brune, K. Investigation of the pharmacokinetics of celecoxib by liquid chromatography-mass spectrometry. *Biomed. Chromatogr.* **2002**, *16*, 56–60. [CrossRef]
34. Choi, J.S.; Choi, I.; Choi, D.H. Effects of nifedipine on the pharmacokinetics of repaglinide in rats: Possible role of CYP3A4 and P-glycoprotein inhibition by nifedipine. *Pharmacol. Rep.* **2013**, *65*, 1422–1430. [CrossRef]
35. Xu, Y.; Zhou, D.; Wang, Y.; Li, J.; Wang, M.; Lu, J.; Zhang, H. CYP2C8-mediated interaction between repaglinide and steviol acyl glucuronide: In vitro investigations using rat and human matrices and in vivo pharmacokinetic evaluation in rats. *Food Chem. Toxicol.* **2016**, *94*, 138–147. [CrossRef]
36. Paulson, S.K.; Zhang, J.Y.; Breau, A.P.; Hribar, J.D.; Liu, N.W.; Jessen, S.M.; Lawal, Y.M.; Cogburn, J.N.; Gresk, C.J.; Markos, C.S.; et al. Pharmacokinetics, tissue distribution, metabolism, and excretion of celecoxib in rats. *Drug Metab. Dispos.* **2000**, *28*, 514–521.
37. Lee, J.Y.; Kim, S.B.; Chun, J.; Song, K.H.; Kim, Y.S.; Chung, S.J.; Cho, H.J.; Yoon, I.S.; Kim, D.D. High body clearance and low oral bioavailability of alantolactone, isolated from *Inula helenium*, in rats: Extensive hepatic metabolism and low stability in gastrointestinal fluids. *Biopharm. Drug Dispos.* **2016**, *37*, 156–167. [CrossRef]

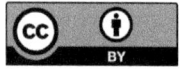

© 2019 by the authors. Licensee MDPI, Basel, Switzerland. This article is an open access article distributed under the terms and conditions of the Creative Commons Attribution (CC BY) license (http://creativecommons.org/licenses/by/4.0/).

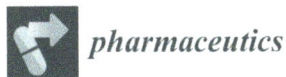

Review

Imbalance of Drug Transporter-CYP450s Interplay by Diabetes and Its Clinical Significance

Yiting Yang and Xiaodong Liu *

Center of Drug Metabolism and Pharmacokinetics, China Pharmaceutical University, Nanjing 210009, China; 1821010209@stu.cpu.edu.cn
* Correspondence: xdliu@cpu.edu.cn; Tel.: +86-25-3271006

Received: 9 March 2020; Accepted: 2 April 2020; Published: 11 April 2020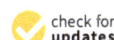

Abstract: The pharmacokinetics of a drug is dependent upon the coordinate work of influx transporters, enzymes and efflux transporters (i.e., transporter-enzyme interplay). The transporter–enzyme interplay may occur in liver, kidney and intestine. The influx transporters involving drug transport are organic anion transporting polypeptides (OATPs), peptide transporters (PepTs), organic anion transporters (OATs), monocarboxylate transporters (MCTs) and organic cation transporters (OCTs). The efflux transporters are P-glycoprotein (P-gp), multidrug/toxin extrusions (MATEs), multidrug resistance-associated proteins (MRPs) and breast cancer resistance protein (BCRP). The enzymes related to drug metabolism are mainly cytochrome P450 enzymes (CYP450s) and UDP-glucuronosyltransferases (UGTs). Accumulating evidence has demonstrated that diabetes alters the expression and functions of CYP450s and transporters in a different manner, disordering the transporter–enzyme interplay, in turn affecting the pharmacokinetics of some drugs. We aimed to focus on (1) the imbalance of transporter-CYP450 interplay in the liver, intestine and kidney due to altered expressions of influx transporters (OATPs, OCTs, OATs, PepTs and MCT6), efflux transporters (P-gp, BCRP and MRP2) and CYP450s (CYP3As, CYP1A2, CYP2E1 and CYP2Cs) under diabetic status; (2) the net contributions of these alterations in the expression and functions of transporters and CYP450s to drug disposition, therapeutic efficacy and drug toxicity; (3) application of a physiologically-based pharmacokinetic model in transporter–enzyme interplay.

Keywords: diabetes; transporter-enzyme interplay; influx transporter; efflux transporter; physiologically based pharmacokinetic model; pharmacokinetics; cytochrome P450 enzymes

1. Introduction

The pharmacokinetics of a drug is determined by absorption, distribution, excretion and metabolism. Drug absorption, distribution and excretion are mainly controlled by drug transporters, while drug metabolism is mediated by metabolic enzymes. These drug transporters are classified into the ATP binding cassette (ABC) family and the solute carrier (SLC) family. The main SLC transporters involved in drug transport are multidrug/toxin extrusions (MATEs), organic anion transporting polypeptides (OATPs), monocarboxylate transporters (MCTs), organic anion transporters (OATs), peptide transporters (PepTs), and organic cation transporters (OCTs). Most SLC transporters belong to influx transporters, except for MATEs. The identified ABC transporters related to drug efflux include P-glycoprotein (P-gp), multidrug resistance-associated proteins (MRPs) and breast cancer resistance protein (BCRP). These transporters are widely expressed in the intestine, liver and kidney. They affect drug therapeutic effects/toxicity via regulating drug uptake or secretion. Enzymes involved in drug metabolism mainly include cytochrome P450 enzymes (CYP450s) and UDP-glucuronosyltransferases (UGTs). These enzymes are also widely distributed in the liver, intestine and kidney. Drug disposition in tissues is highly dependent on the coordinate work of these influx transporters, enzymes and efflux transporters, termed as the "interplay of transporters and enzymes" [1–3]. Moreover, multiple SLC transporters, ABC transporters and enzymes often participate in the disposition of drugs. A typical example is atorvastatin. Atorvastatin is a substrate of P-gp, MRP2, BCRP, OATP1B1, OATP1B2, OATP2A1, CYP3A4/5 [4] and UGTs [5,6]. Sodium taurocholate co-transporting polypeptide (NTCP) also mediates hepatic uptake of atorvastatin [7]. In the liver, atorvastatin enters hepatocytes from portal blood mainly via influx transporters at the basolateral surface of hepatocytes. In hepatocytes, atorvastatin is metabolized via CYP3As or UGTs. Atorvastatin and its metabolites are excreted into bile via efflux transporters (MRP2, BCRP and P-gp) or returned to the blood via MRP3 [8]. The transporter–enzyme interplay also occurs in the intestine and kidney. Accumulating studies [9–12] have demonstrated that diabetes remarkably alters the expression and functions of drug transporters and CYP450s, disordering transporter-CYP450 interplay and in turning affecting the disposition of corresponding drugs, their therapeutic efficacy or drug toxicity. Here, we aimed to focus on (1) the imbalance of transporter-CYP450 interplay in the liver, intestine and kidney due to alterations in the expression of influx transporters, efflux transporters and CYP450s under diabetic status; (2) the net contributions of the altered expressions and functions of transporters and CYP450s to drug disposition, therapeutic efficacy and drug toxicity; (3) application of a physiologically based pharmacokinetic model (PBPK) in the imbalance of transporter–enzyme interplay under diabetic conditions.

2. Liver

Drugs are eliminated in the liver mainly via metabolism and biliary excretion. The liver highly expresses various drug transporters (such as P-gp, BCRP, MRPs, OATPs, OCTs, OATs and MATEs) (Figure 1A) and drug metabolic enzymes (such as CYP450s and UGTs). They work in series to control the disposition of drugs in the liver (Figure 1B).

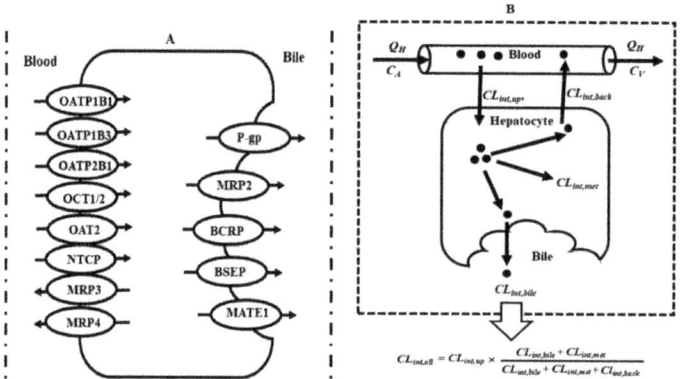

Figure 1. (**A**) Possible location of main transporters in liver. (**B**) Transporter–enzyme interplay in the elimination of drugs in the liver. Symbol: BCRP, breast cancer resistance protein; BSEP, bile salt export pump; C_A, concentrations of drug in arterial blood; $CL_{int,all}$, overall hepatic intrinsic clearance; $CL_{int,up}$, intrinsic uptake clearance; $CL_{int,back}$, intrinsic clearance of backflux to blood; $CL_{int,met}$, intrinsic metabolism clearances; $CL_{int,bile}$, biliary clearance of unbound drug; C_V, concentrations of drug in venous blood; MATEs, multidrug/toxin extrusion; MRPs, multidrug resistance-associated proteins; NTCP, sodium taurocholate co-transporting polypeptide; OATs, organic anion transporters; OATPs, organic anion transporting polypeptides; OCTs, organic cation transporters; Q_H, hepatic blood flow; P-gp, P-glycoprotein.

2.1. OATPs

OATPs, expressed at the basolateral membrane of hepatocytes, mediates hepatocyte uptake of many anions from the blood, which becomes a rate-limited process of hepatic clearances for some drugs [3]. It was found that in diabetic rats (type 2 diabetes) induced by a streptozocin (STZ) and high-fat diet (HFD) combination (termed as STZ/HFD), hepatic OATP1B2 (rodent orthologue of human OATP1B1 and OATP1B3) is remarkably induced, leading to increased hepatic uptake of repaglinide [9,10], atorvastatin [9,11] and simvastatin [12] as well as hepatic clearances [9,11]. In line with this, the diabetic rats showed lower plasma concentrations of atorvastatin [9,11], simvastatin [12] and pravastatin [13] compared with control rats. Clinical trials also showed that tuberculosis patients with diabetes showed significantly lower concentrations of rifampicin than non-diabetic patients [14,15], which may be attributed to the induction of hepatic OATPs by diabetes and rifampicin.

2.2. P-gp

P-gp, expressed at the canalicular membrane of hepatocytes, mediates biliary excretion of its substrates. Diabetes was reported to upregulate the expression of hepatic Mdr1b (ABCB1b) mRNA and P-gp protein in 8-day diabetic Wistar rats (type 1 diabetes) induced by STZ, which was associated with the activation of protein kinase C alpha (PKCα) and nuclear factor kappa-B (NF-κB) [16]. A similar increase in the expression of hepatic Mdr1b mRNA was found in STZ-induced diabetic rats [17]. The induction of hepatic P-gp protein expression was also observed in STZ/HFD-induced diabetic rats [11]. However, a report showed that in STZ-induced diabetic Sprague-Dawley rats, 5-week diabetes significantly increased Mdr1a (ABCB1a) and decreased Mdr1b mRNA expression, but significantly decreased expressions of both Mdr1a and Mdr1b mRNA were found in 8-week diabetic rats. Immunoblotting demonstrated that 5-week diabetes significantly reduced the expression of P-gp protein in rats, but the decreases were not found in 8-week diabetic rats, indicating that the regulation of P-gp protein occurred at post transcriptional level under diabetic status [18].

2.3. BCRP

BCRP, expressed at the canalicular membrane of hepatocytes, is also involved in the biliary excretion of its substrates. Altered expressions of hepatic BCRP under diabetic status are dependent on the type of diabetes, and diabetic progression. For example, expressions of hepatic BCRP mRNA in 5-week and 8-week diabetic rats induced by STZ were significantly downregulated, but expression of BCRP protein only showed a trend to decrease [19]. Similarly, He et al. reported that hepatic BCRP mRNA level was decreased in STZ-induced diabetic rats, whereas in type 2 diabetic patients and Goto-Kakizaki (GK) rats BCRP mRNA expression was significantly increased, although BCRP protein was unaltered [20]. Decreased expression of hepatic BCRP protein was observed in 10-day (but not 22-day) diabetic rats induced by STZ/HFD [11]. Interestingly, pregnancy also affected the expression of hepatic BCRP under diabetic status. For example, STZ treatment upregulated the expression of BCRP mRNA and protein in non-pregnant mice, but not in pregnant mice [21].

2.4. MRP2

MRP2 is co-expressed with P-gp and BCRP at the canalicular membrane of hepatocytes. Alterations in the expression of MRP2 by diabetes are also dependent on species. STZ-induced diabetic Donryu rats showed significantly lower expression of hepatic MRP2 mRNA, which was in line with lower biliary excretion of pravastatin [13]. A similar decrease in the protein (not mRNA) of hepatic MRP2 was found in STZ-induced diabetic male Wistar rats [22]. However, STZ-induced diabetic Sprague-Dawley rats showed higher expression of hepatic MRP2 protein, which was in line with higher biliary excretion of sulfobromophthalein compared with control rats [23]. Moreover, STZ treatment upregulated the expression of MRP2 in non-pregnant mice but not in pregnant mice [21]. The induction of hepatic MRP2 may partly explain the increased biliary excretions of cefoperazone and some anions (such as bengal, indocyanine green and bromcresol green) under diabetic status [24,25].

2.5. CYP450s

Growing evidence has demonstrated that diabetes increases the expression of some CYP450s (such as CYP2A1, CYP1A2, CYP2B1/2, CYP2C6, CYP2C7, CYP3A1/2 and CYP2E1) in rats [9,11,12,26–30], although opposite reports have also been shown [31,32]. The induction of CYP3A1/2 led to lower plasma exposure of simvastatin [12], atorvastatin [9,11], verapamil [27,29] and lidocaine [30] following intravenous dose to diabetic rats. The formation of 1,3-dimethyluric acid from theophylline is mainly mediated via CYP1A2 and CYP2E1. Both alloxan-induced diabetes and STZ-induced diabetes were reported to increase expressions of hepatic CYP2E1 and CYP3A2 by three-fold, leading to a lower area under the curve (AUC) of theophylline and a higher AUC of 1,3-dimethyluric acid following oral and intravenous administration to rats [28]. The induction of CYP1A2 (and CYP3A1/2) may contribute to a lower AUC of oltipraz [33], higher non-renal clearances of omeprazole [34] and systemic clearance of antipyrine [35] in diabetic rats. Diazinon is metabolized to toxic metabolite diethylphosphate via CYP3A2 and CYP1A2. The increases in diazinon toxicity and urinary recovery of its metabolite diethylphosphate in diabetic rats may be attributed to the enhancement of hepatic CYP1A2 (and CYP3A2)-mediated metabolism of diazinon [35]. A report showed that protein expression and activity of hepatic CYP2E1 in STZ-induced diabetic rats were increased by three- and 2.5-fold in comparison to control rats, respectively. The increases were in line with the increased oxidative stress, demonstrating crucial roles of CYP2E1 in stress-induced pathological processes under diabetic status [31,32,36].

Hyperketonemia (such as acetone) is considered as a reason for diabetes inducing CYP2E1. Data from primary cultured rat hepatocytes demonstrated that insulin decreased the expression of CYP2E1 and CYP2B protein and mRNA, inferring that a deficiency of insulin is also a reason that diabetes induces the expression of CYP2E1 and CYP2B [37]. Furthermore, data from both Fa2N-4 cells and HepG2 cells demonstrated that fatty acids (palmitic acid, oleic acid, stearic acid and linoleic acid), but not insulin, upregulated the activity and expression of CYP3A4 mRNA and protein, indicating that increased levels of fatty acids may be one of the reasons that diabetes elevated the function and expression of CYP3A4 [38]. Recent studies showed that diabetes reduced the expression of hepatic peroxisome proliferator activated receptor γ (PPARγ) protein [39,40] and PPARα protein [41]. The decreased expression of hepatic PPARα was attributed to the increased palmitic acid [41]. A report showed that PPARα agonist gemfibrozil in PPARα-null mice showed more induction of the mRNA, protein and activity of CYP3a, CYP2b and CYP2c than in wild-type mice, indicating that the induction of gemfibrozil on CYP450s was suppressed by PPARα activation [42]. The downregulation of PPARα protein expression by diabetes [41] might attenuate the inhibition of PPARα on the expression of CYP450s, leading to the induction of hepatic CYP450s, which needs further investigation. Moreover, diabetes was reported to increase the expression of hepatic glucocorticoid receptor and increase the circulating level of corticosterone [43,44]. The increased level of corticosterone might induce expressions of CYP2B [45] and CYP2C [46] via activating glucocorticoid receptor. All these results demonstrate that alterations in the expressions of hepatic CYP450s were involved in various mechanisms. In contrast to CYP2C6 induction, diabetes significantly lowered the expression of CYP2C11 [26,47–50], impairing the metabolism of diclofenac [49], glibenclamide [48] and nateglinide [47]. The increase in CYP2C6 expression and decrease in CYP2C11 expression may partly explain why the AUC values of both phenytoin and 4′-hydroxylphenytoin in diabetic rats were comparable to control rats [51].

Some contradictory results have also been reported. In Goto-Kakizaki rats, it was found that expressions of hepatic CYP reductase and CYP3A2 were significantly upregulated, accompanied by increases in the activities of midazolam 4-hydroxylase and CYP reductase. In contrast, hepatic expressions of CYP1A2 and CYP3A1 were downregulated, and the activities of 7-methoxyresorufin-O-demethylase and 7-ethoxyresorufin-O-deethylase were decreased. Expressions of other CYP450s, such as CYP1B1, CYP2B1, CYP2C11 and CYP2E1, were unaltered, inferring that diabetes regulates the expression of hepatic CYP450s in an isoform-specific manner [30,52]. Similarly, in 20-week-old male db/db mice, testosterone-6β-hydroxylation but not midazolam-1-

hydroxylation was significantly decreased, the intrinsic clearance (CL_{int}) value of testosterone-6β-hydroxylation (CYP3A11) was less than 46% of control mice. Other metabolic reactions such as dextromethorphan-O-demethylation (CYP2D), phenacetin-O-deethylation (CYP1A2), coumarin-7-hydroxylation (CYP2A4/5), tolbutamide-4-hydroxylation (CYP2C), bupropion-hydroxylation (CYP2B10) and omeprazole-5-hydroxylation (CYP2C29), chlorzoxazone-6-hydroxylation (CYP2E1) were unaltered [53]. Expressions and functions of hepatic CYP450s are dependent on diabetic progression. It was reported that 25-week-old db/db mice showed substantial decreases in mRNA expressions and functions of CYP2B10 and CYP2C29 compared with those of the 10-week-old db/db mice. But mRNA expressions of CYP3A11 and CYP2E1 in the 25-week-old db/db mice were comparable to those of the 10-week-old db/db mice [54]. In Zucker diabetic fatty (ZDF) rats, CYP1A1/2, and CYP3A1 levels were similar among the livers of 5 and 11-week-old ZDF rats and control rats, although 11-week-old ZDF rats possessed the higher serum glucose and glycated hemoglobin levels, but not 5-week-old ZDF rats. Moreover, 5-week-old ZDF rats, but not 11-week-old ZDF rats, showed lower levels of cytochrome b5, CYP2B1, CYP2C11, CYP2E1 and CYP3A2. Consistently, pentoxyresorufin O-depentylation, testosterone 2α- and 16α-hydroxylation, chlorzoxazone 6-hydroxylation, and midazolam 1'- and 4-hydroxylation were decreased only in 5-week-old ZDF rats [55]. Expressions (mRNA and proteins) of CYP3A11/13 and their activities were significantly increased in STZ-induced diabetic C57BLKS/J mice and db/db mice [56]. In contrast, Wang et al. reported that the levels of hepatic CYP3A11 mRNA in C57BL/6 mice diabetic mice induced by HFD/STZ were less than 30% of control mice [31]. All these results indicate that alterations in the expressions of hepatic CYP450s are highly dependent on the type of diabetes, diabetic progression and animal species.

Expressions of hepatic CYP450s in diabetes patients have been widely investigated, although some results are often in contrast to findings in diabetic mice. Gravel et al. [57] assessed the activities of seven major CYP450s (CYP1A2, CYP2B6, CYP2C9, CYP2C19, CYP2D6, CYP2E1, and CYP3A4/5) in 38 type 2 diabetic patients and 35 non-diabetic subjects following the oral administration of a cocktail of probes (caffeine, bupropion, tolbutamide, omeprazole, dextromethorphan, chlorzoxazone and midazolam). They found that the activities of CYP2C19, CYP2B6, and CYP3A in diabetic patients were decreased by about 46%, 45%, and 38%, respectively. CYP1A2 and CYP2C9 activities showed a trend to slightly increase in subjects with diabetes, but activities of CYP2D6 and CYP2E1 were unaltered [57]. Meanwhile, obese children showed higher oral clearance of chlorzoxazone and lower AUC of chlorzoxazone. The AUC was only 46% of nonobese peers, inferring the increased CYP2E1 activity [58].

In vitro data demonstrated that protein expressions and activities of CYP3A4 in hepatic microsomes of diabetic livers were significantly lower than those in non-diabetic donors, although a great variability (8.2-fold) in CYP3A4 protein levels was observed. However, the expression and activity of CYP2E1 were significantly increased [59]. The disposition of nisoldipine in humans was investigated. The results show that the disposition of nisoldipine is enantioselective and nisoldipine is preferentially metabolized. Compared with non-diabetes patients, AUC values of (+)-nisoldipine and (−)-nisoldipine in diabetes patients were increased by 94% and 143%, respectively. Similar increases were also found in their peak concentration (C_{max}). Lidocaine tests demonstrated a decrease in activity of CYP3A (and CYP1A2) [60]. Similarly, pregnant women with gestational diabetes showed significantly higher C_{max} and AUC of lidocaine following peridural anesthesia administration of lidocaine than non-diabetic patients [61]. However, oral plasma concentrations of nifedipine [62] and metoprolol [63] in pregnant women with gestational diabetes were comparable to those in non-diabetic pregnant women. Adith et al. [64] investigated phenytoin kinetics in 10 male type 1 and 10 type 2 diabetic patients. Age- and sex-matched epileptic patients receiving phenytoin alone served as control groups. They found that steady-state concentrations of phenytoin were significantly lower in both types of diabetic patients compared to the respective controls. In line with this, diabetes patients showed significantly increased V_{max}/K_m values of phenytoin. Similarly, the AUCs of cyclosporin A in kidney transplant recipients with diabetes mellitus were approximately 50%~60% that of non-diabetic patients [65,66], which was partly attributed to the delayed gastric emptying [66]. Moreover, no difference in cyclosporine A trough levels between renal transplant patients and renal transplant patients with diabetes was found [67]. Diabetes patients were also reported to show a trend to increase in the expression and activity of CYP3A4, although no statistical significance was observed. Importantly, significant decreases were found in diabetic patients with non-alcoholic fatty liver or non-alcoholic steatohepatitis. Furthermore, the decrease in activity and protein level of CYP3A4 continued with the severity of disease as it progressed from non-alcoholic fatty liver to non-alcoholic steatohepatitis [68]. Matzke et al. [69] also investigated the activities of CYP1A2 and CYP2D6 in type 1 diabetes and type 2 diabetes patients using the probes antipyrine, caffeine and dextromethorphan. The results show that compared with controls, oral clearance of antipyrine was increased 72% in type 1 diabetes patients. Formation clearances of 4-hydroxyantipyrine and 3-hydroxymethylantipyrine were increased by 74% and 137%, respectively. The caffeine metabolic index (paraxanthine/caffeine) was increased by 34%, but no statistical significance was obtained. These alterations did not occur in type 2 diabetes patients. Similarly, although plasma clearance of theophylline in diabetic patients was comparable to that in healthy subjects, there was a positive correlation between hemoglobin A1c values and formation clearances of both 1,3-dimethyluric acid and 1-methyluric acid [70], in line with inductions of CYP1A2 and CYP2E1.

Although antipyrine is widely used to assess the activity of CYP450s in diabetic patients, the results are often confusing [69,71–73]. Sotaniemi et al. [73] assessed the effects of diabetes on hepatic drug metabolism clearance in men using antipyrine in 298 diabetic patients, who were classified by type of the disease, age, gender, duration of therapy and liver involvement. They found that a 13-fold individual variation in antipyrine metabolism existed among all the diabetic patients. Antipyrine was eliminated faster in untreated type 1 patients, which was reversed by insulin treatment. Males aged 16–59 years, who responded insufficiently to insulin therapy, had a rapid antipyrine elimination, which could be normalized by the readjustment of insulin. The antipyrine elimination rate in women with insufficient glucose control on insulin therapy was comparable to controls. In type 2 diabetic patients, the clearance of antipyrine was unaltered in women, but men over 40 years of age showed a reduced antipyrine metabolism. Diet/drinking-habits also affect the expression of hepatic CYP450s. Urry et al. [74] investigated CYP1A2 activity in diabetic patients using coffee as a probe in 57 type 2 diabetes and 146 non-type 2 diabetes. They found that diabetes patients showed higher activity of CYP1A2 than control groups. Further studies showed that participants habitually consuming more caffeine showed higher CYP1A2 activity than participants with lower caffeine consumption. Several studies have demonstrated that CYP2D6 activity is unaltered by diabetes [43,69,75].

2.6. Interplay of Transporter-CYP450s in Liver

In the liver, drugs enter hepatocytes from portal blood through passive diffusion or transporter-mediated transport. In hepatocytes, drugs are metabolized by metabolic enzymes. Parent drugs and their metabolites are pumped out of hepatocytes to bile through efflux transporters (such as P-gp, BCRP or MRP2) and are exported to the blood through passive diffusion or efflux transporters (such as MRP3 and MRP4) (Figure 1B). Typical examples are statins. Most statins are substrates of CYP450s, MRPs, OATPs, BCRP and P-gp, characterizing transporter–enzyme interplay. The overall hepatic intrinsic clearance ($CL_{int,all}$) is a hybrid parameter which is composed of intrinsic influx clearances ($CL_{int,up}$) from portal blood, intrinsic metabolism clearance ($CL_{int,met}$), biliary excretion clearance ($CL_{int,bile}$) and intrinsic efflux clearance ($CL_{int,back}$) of unbound drugs from hepatocytes to the blood, i.e.,

$$CL_{intt,all} = CL_{int,up} \times \frac{CL_{int,bile} + CL_{int,met}}{CL_{int,bile} + CL_{int,met} + CL_{int,back}} \quad (1)$$

According to the relative values of $CL_{int,bile}$ and $CL_{int,met}$ to $CL_{int,back}$, the drugs are classified into three groups.

1. $CL_{int,back}$ is much smaller than the sum of $CL_{int,bile}$ and $CL_{int,met}$, thus, $CL_{int,all}$ is equal to $CL_{int,up}$; this is to say, $CL_{int,all}$ is only controlled by uptake clearance, which is mainly mediated by influx transporters. Typical drugs are statins.
2. Sum of $CL_{int,bile}$ and $CL_{int,met}$ is much less than $CL_{int,back}$. $CL_{int,all} = CL_{int,up} \times (CL_{int,bile} + CL_{int,met})/CL_{int,back}$, indicating that $CL_{int,all}$ is determined by the net effect of $CL_{int,up}$, $CL_{int,back}$, $CL_{int,bile}$ and $CL_{int,met}$.
3. Some drugs (such as midazolam) are not substrates of transporters. These drugs also rapidly penetrate the sinusoidal membrane, i.e., $CL_{int,up} = CL_{int,back}$, thus, $CL_{int,all} = CL_{int,bile} + CL_{int,met}$.

Diabetes significantly disorders transporter-CYP450 interplay via altering expressions and functions of transporters and CYP450s, finally affecting pharmacokinetics and activity/toxicity of drugs. For example, diabetes upregulated expressions and functions of hepatic CYP3A and OATP1B2, enhanced hepatic uptake and metabolism of simvastatin [12], atorvastatin [9,11], in turn, increasing hepatoxicity of atorvastatin [76]. Data from PBPK also showed that both hepatic OATP1B2 and CYP3A contribute to the clearance of atorvastatin, but the roles of hepatic OATP1B2 were much larger than that of CYP3A [11]. Another example is cyclosporin A. Cyclosporin A is also a substrate of CYP3A, MRP2, P-gp, OATP1B1 and BCRP. Significantly increased systemic clearance of cyclosporin A in diabetic rats [77] should be attributed to the net effect of alterations in these transporters and CYP3A. Methotrexate transport in the liver is mediated by various transporters such as OATP1B1, MRP2, BCRP and OAT2. Moreover, induction of CYP2E1 also enhanced methotrexate-induced hepatocytoxicity [78]. These results indicate that the regulation of hepatic OATPs and CYP2E1 expressions and functions may explain clinic findings that diabetic patients were particularly at increased risk of methotrexate hepatotoxicity [79].

3. Intestine

A series of transporters (such as P-gp, BCRP, OATPs, OCT1, PepTs, MRP2, MRP3 and MCTs) and enzymes (such as CYP450s and UGTs) have been expressed in enterocytes, implicating intestinal absorption of drugs and first-pass effects (Figure 2).

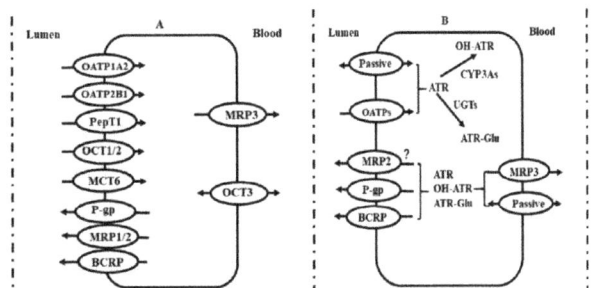

Figure 2. (**A**) Possible location of main transporters in human intestine and (**B**) roles of transporter-CYP3A interplay in disposition of atorvastatin in enterocytes. Symbol: ATR, atorvastatin; BCRP, breast cancer resistance protein; MCTs, monocarboxylate transporters; MRPs, multidrug resistance-associated proteins; OATPs, organic anion transporting polypeptides; OCTs, organic cation transporters; PepT1, peptide transporters; P-gp, P-glycoprotein; OH-ATR, hydroxyl atorvastatin; ATR-Glu, atorvastatin acyl glucuronide.

3.1. P-gp

P-gp is highly expressed at the apical membrane of the intestinal epithelium, pumping out of its substrates from enterocytes to the intestinal lumen. The expression of intestinal P-gp protein is region-dependent. P-gp protein progressively increases from proximal to distal regions. The highest expression of P-gp occurs at the ileum [80]. Several studies have demonstrated that diabetes impairs expression and function of intestinal P-gp, leading to the enhancement of intestinal absorption and increasing plasma exposure following oral administration of P-gp substrates such as arctigenin [81], protoberberine alkaloids [82], digoxin [83], grepafloxacin [84], paclitaxel [17] and morphine [85]. In line with the increased plasma levels of morphine, diabetic mice showed a stronger analgesic effect following an oral dose compared with control mice [85]. The decreased expression and function of intestinal P-gp under diabetes status may explain that clinic findings that diabetic patients also showed higher serum concentration of digoxin compared with non-diabetic patients following an oral dose of digoxin [86,87].

Downregulation of intestinal P-gp expression by diabetes was considered to be partly attributed to the acceleration of the ubiquitin-proteasome [88] via nitric oxide synthase (NOS) activation [89–91]. However, the role of NO in intestinal P-gp is time-dependent. In Caco-2 cells, it was reported that short-term exposure to sodium nitroprusside impaired P-gp function and expression, whereas long-term exposure stimulated P-gp function and expression [92]. Increased levels of short chain fatty acids (SCFAs) were also found in the intestinal content of diabetic rats [47]. A recent study showed that SCFAs downregulated the expression of intestinal P-gp via inhibiting histone deacetylase and NF-κB pathways [93].

3.2. MRP2

MRP2 (and MRP1) is co-located with phase II conjugating enzymes (such as UGTs and glutathione S-transferase) in the small intestine, pumping out of anions from enterocytes to the intestinal lumen. In contrast to P-gp, diabetes was reported to enhance the expression and function of intestinal MRP2 in rats [23]. Gliclazide is also a substrate of MRP2 [94]. C_{max} and AUC_{0-tn} of gliclazide following oral administration to diabetic rats were only 55% and 56% of those in control rats [94], respectively, which seemed to be attributed to the increased expression of intestinal MRP2. As expected, gliclazide administration significantly decreased glucose concentrations in healthy rats, but hypoglycemic effects of gliclazide were not observed in diabetic rats [95].

3.3. BCRP

Similarly to P-gp, BCRP is expressed at the luminal membrane of enterocytes. The BCRP protein gradually rises from proximal to distal regions. Diabetes-induced alterations in the expression of intestinal BCRP are dependent on the type of diabetes and duration of diabetes. STZ-induced diabetic rats showed significantly lowered expression and function of intestinal BCRP, accompanied by decreased intestinal clearance of glibenclamide and increased apparent intestinal effective permeability (P_{eff}) [48], leading to the increased oral plasma exposure of glibenclamide following oral administration to diabetic rats. However, in STZ/HFD-induced diabetic rats, 10-day diabetic rats showed significantly lowered expression and function of intestinal BCRP, but remarkable inductions of intestinal BCRP expression and function were found in 22-day diabetic rats [11]. The induction of intestinal BCRP was considered to be related to the increased levels of short chain fatty acids (SCFAs) via activating PPARγ [96].

3.4. PepT1

PepT1, located on the luminal membrane of enterocytes, is responsible for intestinal absorption of peptidomimetic drugs, dipeptides and tripeptides resulting from the dietary breakdown of proteins and bacterial peptidomimetics. Several investigations have demonstrated that diabetes downregulated the expression and function of intestinal PepT1 in experimental animals [47,97–99], decreasing oral plasma exposures of cephalexin and acyclovir following oral dose of cephalexin and valacyclovir [99]. Importantly, altered expression and function of intestinal PepT1 are also dependent on sex. For example, in Sprague-Dawley rats, it was reported that STZ-induced diabetes decreased the expression and function of intestinal PepT1 in male rats, but increased them in female rats [100]. Leptin and insulin deficiencies may contribute to the downregulation of intestinal PepT1 [101,102]. Dyshomeostasis of bile acid compositions was observed in intestinal content of diabetic rats. Bile acids downregulated the expression of intestinal PepT1 via activating farnesoid X receptor (FXR) [99].

3.5. MCT6

MCT6, located on the apical side of human intestinal villous epithelial cells, mediates intestinal absorption of nateglinide [103]. Loop diuretics such as furosemide, piretanide, azosemide, and torasemide may also be substrates of MCT6 [104]. Diabetes significantly decreased the expression of intestinal MCT6 and decreased plasma exposure of nateglinide following oral dose to rats. Further study demonstrated that SCFAs, especially butyrate, downregulated the expression of intestinal MCT6 via activating PPARγ [47]. The downregulation of intestinal MCT6 may also partly explain that diabetes significantly decreased plasma exposures of furosemide [105] and azosemide [106] following oral doses to rats.

3.6. CYP450s

Intestine also highly expresses CYP450s, especially CYP3As, which mediate drug metabolism, contributing to first-pass effects. In STZ-induced diabetes, it was found that diabetes significantly decreased CYP3A activity. In line with this, formations of norverapamil [27] and 6-β hydroxyltestosterone [107] were reduced to 21% and 50% that of control rats, respectively. Significant downregulation of intestinal CYP3A expression and function was also found in STZ/HFD-induced diabetic rats [11] and in Tsumura Suzuki obese diabetic (TSOD) mice [108]. Insulin treatment partly reversed the decreased CYP3A expression in STZ-induced diabetic rats [107], but not in TSOD mice [108]. However, the real mechanism leading to the decreased expression of intestinal CYP3A was unclear. In generally, expressions of CYP3A and P-gp were mainly controlled by pregnane X receptor (PXR). We recently reported upregulation of intestinal FXR [83]. A report showed that FXR agonist GW4064 remarkably induced expression of small heterodimer partner (SHP) [109], in turn, inhibiting the transcriptional activity of PXR [109,110]. Moreover, levels of bile acids, FXR agonist, were increased in intestinal contents of diabetic rats, which inhibited the expression of intestinal CYP3A and P-gp via the activation of FXR-SHP pathway.

3.7. Transporter-CYP450 Interplay in Intestine

Some drugs are often substrates of various transporters and CYP3As. Alterations in oral plasma exposure of drug should be attributed to common effects of the altered transporters and CYP3As. For example, atorvastatin is a substrate of intestinal P-gp, BCRP and OATPs, indicating that the P_{eff} of atorvastatin should be the integrated effects of passive diffusion, OATP1A5-mediated absorption, P-gp mediated efflux and BCRP-mediated efflux. Diabetes also downregulated the expression of intestinal OATP1A5 [11]. Thus, the P_{eff} of atorvastatin under diabetic status should be the net effects of these altered transporters. Downregulation of intestinal CYP3A expression by diabetes was also involved in the first-pass effect of atorvastatin. PBPK simulation demonstrated that contributions of intestinal transporters and CYP3A was intestinal BCRP > intestinal CYP3A > intestinal P-gp > intestinal OATP1A5 [11]. Cyclosporin A is also a substrate of BCRP, OATPs, CYP3A and P-gp, indicating that increased oral plasma exposure of cyclosporin A in diabetic rats [111] was also partly attributed to the common effects of the intestinal transporters and CYP3A. Verapamil is a substrate of P-gp and CYP3As. PBPK simulation also showed that the contribution of intestinal P-gp was much larger than that of intestinal CYP3A [93], indicating that increased oral plasma exposure of verapamil [27] was mainly attributed to downregulation of intestinal P-gp. Grepafloxacin [112] is also a substrate. Decreased expression of BCRP may partly explain why the decreased secretory transport of grepafloxacin was not in line with the decrease in expression of P-gp protein in diabetic rats [84]. Similarly, intestinal OATP1A5 also mediates intestinal absorption of glibenclamide [113], inferring that the increased P_{eff}

of glibenclamide by impairment of intestinal BCRP [48] may be partly weakened by the decreased expression of OATP1A5 protein.

4. Kidney

Drugs are eliminated in the kidney via urinary excretion. The process consists of glomerular filtration, secretion and reabsorption at the renal tubule. The secretion and reabsorption are mainly mediated by transporters. The identified renal transporters include OAT1/3, OCT1/2, PepT1/2, MATE1, MATE2/K, P-gp, BCRP, MCTs and urate transporter 1 (URAT1) (Figure 3A). Transporter interplay occurs at the kidney. For example, metformin, a substrate of OCTs and MATEs, is taken in renal epithelial cells via OCT1/2 at the basolateral membrane, then secreted into urine via MATEs at the brush-border membrane of renal tubular cells, mediating the renal excretion of metformin. The transporter interplay also participates in renal excretion of uric acid. URAT1, OAT1, OAT3, OAT4, OAT10, BCRP, sodium-dependent phosphate transport protein 1/4 (NPT1/4) and glucose transporter 9 (GLUT9) work together to regulate the excretion of uric acid via the kidney [114] (Figure 3B).

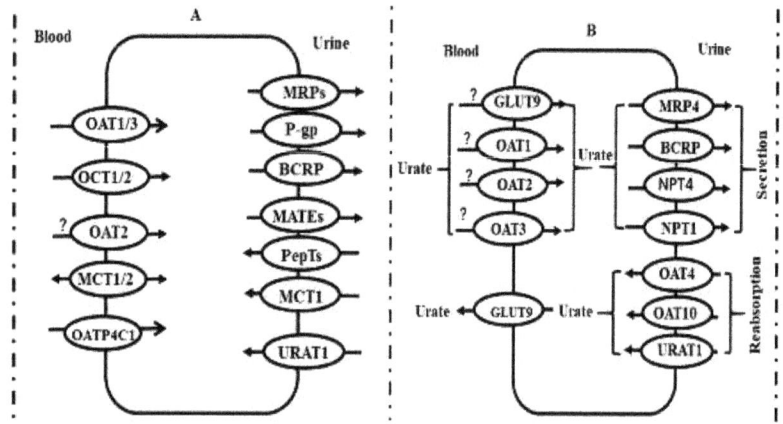

Figure 3. (A) Possible location of main transporters in human kidney and (B) roles of transporter interplay in renal excretion of uric acid. Symbol: OATPs, organic anion transporting polypeptides; OATs, organic anion transporters; OCTs, organic cation transporters; PepTs, peptide transporters; P-gp, P-glycoprotein; MRPs, multidrug resistance-associated proteins; BCRP, breast cancer resistance protein; MATEs, multidrug and toxin extrusion, NPTs, sodium-dependent phosphate transport proteins, GLUT9, glucose transporter 9, URAT1, urate transporter 1.

4.1. OAT1 and OAT3

The basolateral membrane of renal proximal tubule cells highly expresses OAT1 and OAT3, mediating the excretion of their substrates including ACE inhibitors, angiotensin II receptor blockers, diuretics, β-Lactam antibiotics, antiviral agents and endogenous compounds [3]. Several studies demonstrated that diabetes also impaired the function and expression of renal OATs. In STZ-induced diabetic rats, it was found that diabetes significantly decreased the membrane expression of renal OAT3, leading to lower uptake of [^{3}H] estrone sulfate in renal cortical slice. These decreases were in line with the activation of PKCα and NF-κB pathways, increased nuclear factor erythroid 2-related factor 2 (Nrf2) and oxidative stress [115,116]. Alteration in OATs by diabetes is dependent on sex. In lean and obese Zucker spontaneously hypertensive fatty (ZSF1) rats, it was found that the levels of renal OAT1 and OAT3 mRNA were higher in lean females than in lean males. Obesity remarkably reduced the expression of renal OAT1 and OAT3 in female ZSF1 rats but not in male ZSF1 rats [117]. Clinical trials showed that expressions of renal OAT1 and OAT3 in patients with diabetic kidney disease were less than 50% of the normal levels, which were in line with decreased urinary excretion of some organic acid metabolites and increased plasma levels of organic acid metabolites [118].

Diuretics show their diuretic effect via affecting proximal tubular epithelial cells. Some diuretics (such as torasemid and furosemide) are also substrates of OATs [3]. Several studies have showed that OAT1 or OAT3 deficiency damage the natriuretic effects of furosemide and bendroflumethiazide [119,120], inferring that the decreased expression of OATs by diabetes may impair the diuretic effect of diuretics. In line with the deduction, alloxan-induced diabetes significantly increased the plasma exposure of furosemide and decreased recovery from urine following intravenous dose to rats [105]. Importantly, diuretic efficiency, natriuretic efficiency, kaluretic efficiency and chloruretic efficiency of furosemide in diabetic rats showed a trend to decrease. Similarly, the diuretic efficiency, natriuretic efficiency, kaluretic efficiency and chloruretic efficiency of torasemide were significantly impaired both in alloxan-induced diabetic rats and STZ-induced diabetes, although its plasma exposure was unaltered [50]. These findings also may explain the clinical finding that diabetic patients need higher furosemide doses [121]. Moreover, sodium-glucose cotransporter (SGLT2) inhibitor empagliflozin is a substrate of OAT3. A report showed that OAT3 deficiency damaged the glucosuric effect of empagliflozin [122], indicating that the decreased expression of renal OAT3 by diabetes may attenuate the glucosuric effect of empagliflozin, which may also explain the clinic finding that compared with normal renal function and normal-to-mildly reduced renal function, diabetic patients with mild-to-moderately reduced renal function showed the lowest lowering glucose effect of luseogliflozin [123].

4.2. OCTs

Renal OCT1/2, mainly expressed at the basolateral membrane of tubule cells, transport a variety of organic cations, such as metformin, cisplatin, cephalexin and acyclovir. In STZ/HFD-induced diabetic rats, it was found that OCT2 protein expression was only 50% of control rats [124]. Similarly, in STZ-induced diabetic rats, the expressions of renal OCT1 and OCT2 were decreased by 50% and 70%, respectively [125]. The reduced mRNA and protein expressions of OCT1, OCT2 and OCT3 under diabetic status were also associated with a reduction in the clearance of N^1-methylnicotinamide [126,127]. The decreased mRNA and protein expressions of renal OCT2/3 were reported to be negatively correlated with the accumulation of renal and plasma advanced glycation end-products (AGEs) [127]. Insulin or AGE inhibitor aminoguanidine could reverse the decreased OCT2/3 by diabetes [125,127], inferring that the accumulation of AGEs may be involved in impaired expression of renal OCTs by diabetes [127]. Expressions of OCT1 and OCT2 are also be dependent on sex. In lean female ZSF1 rats, the mRNA expression level of OCT1 was significantly higher than that in their male counterparts. Obesity significantly reduced renal mRNA expressions of OCT1 and OCT2 in female ZSF1 rats, but not in male rats [117]. The decreased expression of renal OCTs by diabetes may affect pharmacokinetics of their substrates. For example, significantly higher AUC of metformin and lower renal clearance were observed in alloxan-induced diabetic rats than in normal rats following an intravenous dose [128]. A clinic trial [129] showed that renal clearance of metformin decreased along with diabetes progression. A report demonstrated the rank of the renal clearances of metformin in healthy subjects (525 ± 125 mL/min) > newly diagnosed maturity onset diabetic patients (322 ± 166 mL/min) > maturity onset diabetic patients (224 ± 38 mL/min). Interestingly, pregnancy seems to increase the functions of renal MATEs and OCTs [130]. Renal clearances of N^1-methylnicotinamide (endogenous probe for the renal OCTs and MATEs) in both mid (504 ± 293 mL/min) and late pregnancy (557 ± 305 mL/min) were reported to be higher than in postpartum (240 ± 106 mL/min). The renal secretion of N^1-methylnicotinamide was 3.5-fold higher in mid pregnancy and 4.5-fold higher in late pregnancy compared with postpartum [130]. In line, gestational diabetes mellitus pregnant women showed higher renal clearance and renal secretion [131], and lower plasma concentrations of metformin [131,132] compared with non-pregnant controls. Another example is cisplatin. Cisplatin is a substrate of OCTs. Its main toxicity is nephrotoxicity. Several studies have demonstrated that both insulin-dependent and insulin-independent diabetes show resistance against cisplatin-induced nephrotoxicity [133–135]. Animal experiments showed that diabetes prevented nephrotoxicity partly via decreasing the renal accumulation of cisplatin [136,137]. However, cisplatin treatment was not beneficial in diabetes due to its compromising its antitumor effect [136].

4.3. Other Transporters

Diabetes induced an approximately two-fold increase in renal PepT1 protein and slightly induced mRNA of PepT1 and PepT2 [138]. Reports on the expression of ABC transporters are often contradictory. For renal P-gp, it was reported that spontaneous type 1 and type 2 diabetic mice showed lower expressions of renal P-gp protein. The high glucose was considered to be a reason reducing the expression and function of P-gp [139]. However, the expression of P-gp protein was also reported to be unchanged [17,111,138], although level of Mdr1a mRNA was increased [17,138].

For MRP2, increased expression of renal MRP2 protein was found in STZ/HFD-diabetic rats [124] and in STZ-induced diabetic rats [23]. For BCRP, HFD/STZ-induced diabetes significantly increased the expression of BCRP protein in rats, but STZ-induced diabetes significantly decreased mRNA level of renal BCRP in rats [136]. These discrepancies may result from the duration of diabetes, sex and the type of diabetes. For example, in female rats, obesity decreased the expressions of MRP4 and Mdr1b mRNA, but the expression of MRP2 mRNA was unaltered. In male ZSF1 rats, expressions of MRP2, MRP4 and Mdr1b mRNA remained unchanged in obese rats compared to lean rats [117].

4.4. CYP450

The identified renal CYP450s include CYP2C, CYP2J, CYP2E1, CYP4As and CYP4Fs. They mainly mediate local biotransformation of endogenous compounds such as arachidonic acid. For example, arachidonic acid is metabolized by CYP4As and CYP4Fs to 20-hydroxyeicosatetraenoic acid (vasoconstrictor) and by CYP2C and CYP2J to epoxyeicosatrienoic acid (vasodilator), synergistically regulating renal vasoactivity. Several reports have shown that diabetes also affect the expressions of renal CYP450s. In mice, it was found that HFD feeding significantly decreased activities of CYP3A (1'-hydroxymidazolam), CYP2E1 (hydroxychlorzoxazone), CYP2J (ebastine hydroxylation) and CYP2B6 (hydroxybupropion) and CYP4A (12-hydroxydecanoic acid), but increased the activities of CYP2C (hydroxytolbutamide) and CYP2D (Hydroxybufuralol) [140]. Diabetes affects the expressions and activities of renal CYP450s in an isoform- and species-specific manner. In STZ-induced diabetic rats, formations of hydroxyandrostenedione and 2α-hydroxytestosterone were significantly increased by 250% and 300% compared to control rats, but formations of androstenedione and 6β-hydroxytestosterone were significantly decreased. The formations of 16α-hydroxytestosterone and 7α-hydroxytestosterone were unaltered [141]. Induction of CYP2E1, 4A2 and K-4 as well as increases in omega- and (omega-1) hydroxylation of lauric acid were also observed in kidney of STZ-induced rats [26]. Insulin treatment partly reversed these alterations by diabetes [26,141]. However, a recent report showed that expression of CYP4A protein in diabetic mice induced by HFD/STZ was downregulated by 29.16% of control mice [142]. The roles of altered renal CYP450s by diabetes in disposition of drugs needed further investigation.

4.5. Transporter Interplay in Kidney

Transporter interplay occurs in the kidney. For example, methotrexate is eliminated mainly via renal active excretion, which is involved in OAT1/3 at basolateral membrane of tubule and BCRP and MRP2 at brush-border membrane of tubule, these transporters in series work to regulate renal active excretion of methotrexate. Both higher plasma concentration of methotrexate and higher toxicity of methotrexate in STZ-diabetic rats [143] may partly be explained by the imbalance of expressions of renal OATs, BCRP and MRP2. Another example is β-lactam antibiotics. OATs mediate the uptake of β-lactam antibiotics into the tubule from the blood and PepT1/2 located in the brush-border membrane of the tubule, mediate reabsorption of antibiotics from the urine, and regulate urinary excretion of β-lactam antibiotics. Downregulation of renal OATs may partly contribute to a decrease in the renal clearance of DA-1131 (a carbapenem antibiotics) [144] and lower renal cortical cephaloridine accumulation in diabetic rats [145]. Creatinine is also substrate of OCT1/2, MATEs and OAT1/3, indicating that the decreased expressions of renal OATs and OCTs at least partly contribute to decreased clearance of creatinine under diabetic status.

5. Application of PBPK to Transporter-Enzyme Interplay

The above statements demonstrated that diabetes may simultaneously affect functions and expressions of transporters and enzymes in the intestine, liver and kidney. Their contributions to the disposition of drugs are often opposite. Moreover, some physiological parameters such as blood flow rates, intestinal transit and the free fraction of drug in plasma are often altered. Thus, the effects of diabetes on pharmacokinetics of drugs should be the integrated effects of these alterations, which may be accomplished using PBPK.

5.1. Atorvastatin

Atorvastatin is a substrate of P-gp, OATPs, BCRP and CYP3As. Diabetes reduced expressions of intestinal P-gp, CYP3A and OATP1A5, while induced expressions of liver OATP1B2 and CYP3A. Intestinal BCRP was highly dependent upon diabetes course, which was decreased at an early phase of diabetes (10-day) but induced at a late phase (22-day). A pharmacokinetic study showed that oral plasma exposure was increased in 10-day diabetic rats, but decreased in 22-day diabetic rats. PBPK simulation demonstrated that contributions of these targeted protein to altered oral plasma exposure of atorvastatin were intestinal BCRP > hepatic OATP1B2 > hepatic CYP3A > intestinal CYP3A > intestinal P-gp > intestinal OATP1A5. The increased oral plasma atorvastatin exposure in 10-day diabetic rats and the decreased oral plasma atorvastatin exposure in 22-day diabetic rats were attributed to the altered intestinal BCRP [11].

5.2. Verapamil

Verapamil is substrate of CYP3As and P-gp. Rat experiments showed that diabetes increased plasma exposure of verapamil following an oral dose but decreased plasma exposure of verapamil following an intravenous dose [29]. A semi-PBPK model (Figure 4) was successfully developed to simulate the pharmacokinetics of verapamil (Figure 5A,B) in rats using the parameters listed in Tables 1 and 2. Intestinal P-gp in diabetic rats was set to 60% of control rats [82]. The contributions of intestinal/hepatic CYP3A and intestinal P-gp to alterations in oral plasma concentration of verapamil in diabetic rats were investigated. The results demonstrate that increased oral plasma exposure of verapamil was mainly attributed to the impairment of intestinal P-gp (Figure 5E) and the role of intestinal CYP3As was minor (Figure 5D). Furthermore, the contribution of increased expression of hepatic CYP3As to the altered plasma concentration of verapamil following oral dose to rats was less than that of intestinal P-gp impairment, whose net effect was to increase oral plasma exposure of verapamil (Figure 5G).

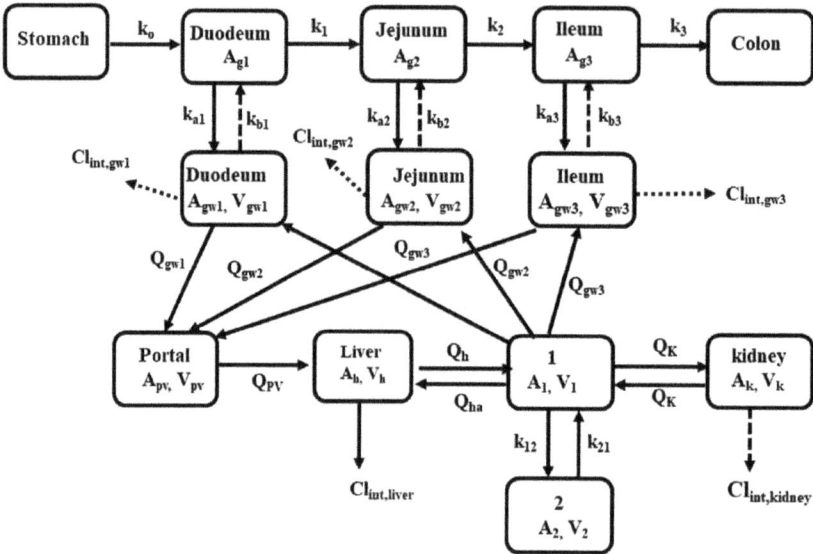

Figure 4. Schematic diagram of semi-physiologically based pharmacokinetic model (PBPK) model describing the pharmacokinetics of verapamil and furosemide in rats. A_i, Q_i and V_i indicate drug amount, blood flow and volume in corresponding compartment, respectively. k_i, $k_{a,i}$ and $k_{b,i}$ represent the transit rate constant, drug absorption rate constant and efflux rate constant from enterocytes to the gut lumen, respectively. $Cl_{int,gwi}$, $Cl_{int,liver}$ and $Cl_{int,kidney}$ mean the intrinsic clearance in enterocytes, hepatocytes and kidney, respectively.

Table 1. The physiological parameters of rats for the semi-PBPK model [11].

Parameters	Unit	Control Rats	Diabetic Rats
Gastric emptying rate	h^{-1}	20.8	20.8
Duodenum transit time	h^{-1}	28.74	28.74
Jejunum transit time	h^{-1}	4.2	4.2
Ileum transit time	h^{-1}	0.789	0.789
Intestinal radius	cm	0.2	0.2
Duodenum wall volume	mL	1.08	1.08
Jejunum wall volume	mL	9.94	9.94
Ileum wall volume	mL	0.32	0.32
Portal vein volume	mL	0.25	0.25
Liver volume	mL	10	10
Renal volume	mL	1.83 [146]	1.83
Duodenum wall blood flow	mL/min	0.972	2.223
Jejunum wall blood flow	mL/min	9.125	20.877
Ileum wall blood flow	mL/min	0.253	0.580
Portal vein blood flow	mL/min	16.043	23.68
Hepatic artery blood flow	mL/min	2.243	11.914
Liver blood flow	mL/min	18.286	35.594
Renal blood flow	ml/min	11.7 [146]	4.10[a]
Hepatic microsomal protein	mg/g liver	44.8	44.8
Intestinal microsomal protein	mg/g intestine	25.9	25.9
Liver weight	g/kg body weight	40	36

[a] Renal blood flow was reduced by 65% of control rats [147].

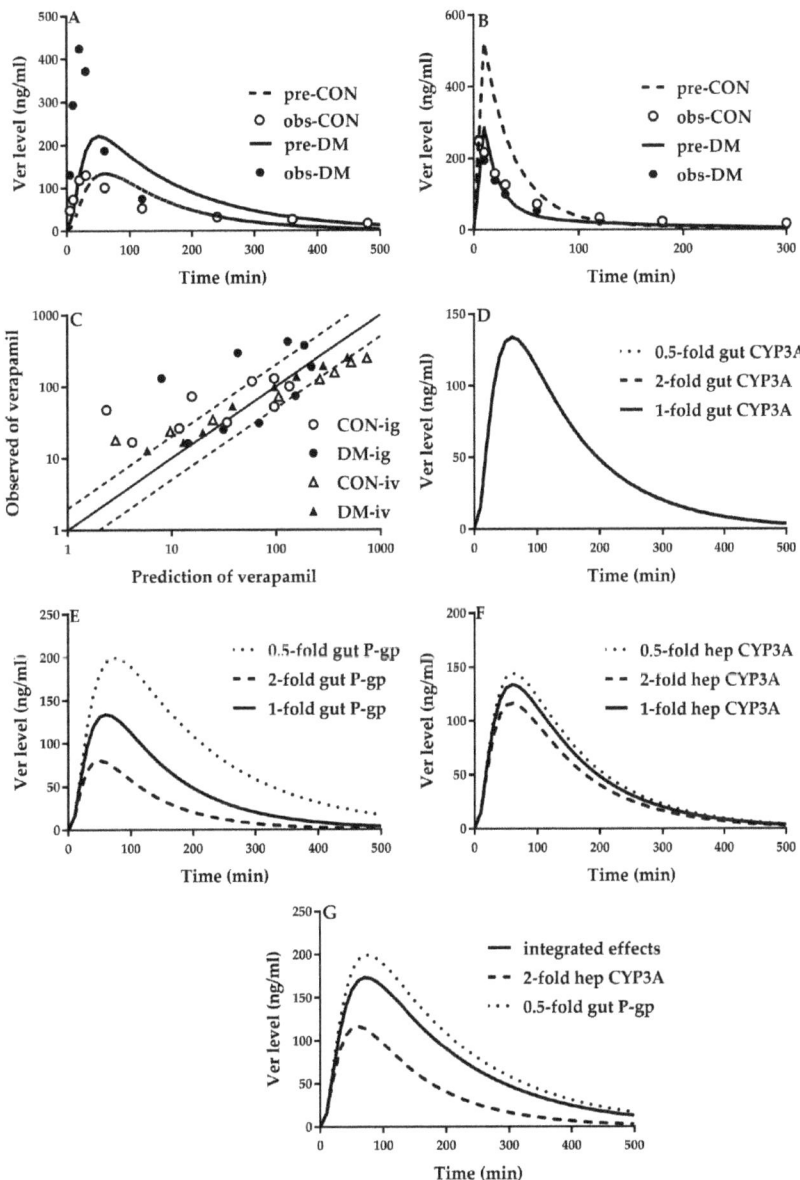

Figure 5. Observed (point) and predicted (line) plasma concentrations of verapamil (Ver) following (**A**) oral (10 mg/kg, ig) and (**B**) intravenous dose (1 mg/kg, iv) to diabetic rats (DM) and control rats (CON); (**C**) comparison of mean observed and predicted plasma concentrations of verapamil at each time point; (**D**) individual contributions of altered hepatic CYP3A, (**E**) intestinal CYP3A and (**F**) intestinal P-gp to oral plasma exposure of verapamil as well as (**G**) their integrated effects. The observations were obtained from the literature [27].

Table 2. Pharmacokinetic parameters of verapamil and furosemide for PBPK simulation in diabetic rats (DM) and control rats (CON).

Parameter	Unit	Furosemide		Verapamil	
		CON rats	DM rats	CON rats	DM rats
Vc	L/kg	0.127 [148]	0.127	0.505 [a]	0.505
k21	h^{-1}	0.835 [148]	0.835	11.880 [a]	11.88
k12	h^{-1}	0.989 [148]	0.989	10.740 [a]	10.74
fu	%	10.4 [105]	10.4 [89]	0.05 [93]	0.05
Kt:p Liver	Liver	0.33 [148]	0.33	8.20 [b]	8.20
Kt:p	Intestine	0.517 [148]	0.517	319.39 [b]	319.39
Kt:p	Kidney	1.36 [148]	1.36	/	/
$P_{app,A-B}$ (caco-2)	cm/s × 10^{-6}	6.90 [149]	3.45 [c]	13.8	13.8
$P_{app,B-A}$ (caco-2)	cm/s × 10^{-6}	/	/	24.84	14.90 [d]
CL_{kidney}	mL/min/kg	4.33 [105]	/	/	/
CL_{liver}	mL/min/kg	2.20 [105]	/	/	/
Fu × $CL_{int,liver}$	mL/min/250 g	0.60 [e]	0.75 [f]	/	/
Fu × $CL_{int,kidney}$	mL/min/250 g	1.19 [e]	0.48 [g]	/	/
Microsomes					
Liver					
V_{max}	nmol/(min/mg prot)	/	/	1.60 [27]	2.38 [27]
K_m	μM	/	/	13.21 [27]	16.09 [27]
Intestine					
V_{max}	pmol/(min/mg prot)	/	/	49.04 [27]	22.70 [27]
K_m	μM	/	/	34.06 [27]	55.37 [27]

[a] Estimated using the reported data [150]; [b] estimated according to a method [151] reported by Ruark et al. and physicochemical properties of verapamil; [c] function of intestinal MCT6 was set to be 50% that of control rats [47]; [d] level of intestinal P-gp protein was 60% that of control rats [82]; [e] fu × Clint were estimated using equation fu*Clint = Q × CL/(Q − CL); [f] contribution of CYP2C11 was 61.5% of the total metabolism [152], rests (38.5%) were assumed to attributed to CYP2E1 and CYP3As. Diabetes increased the expression of CYP2E1 and CYP3As by 3-fold [28] and expression of CYP2C11 mRNA was decreased to 16% that of control rats [47]; [g] function of renal OATs was decreased to 40% that of control rats [115].

5.3. Furosemide

Rat experiments demonstrated that diabetes decreased plasma furosemide exposure following oral dose but increased plasma furosemide exposure following intravenous dose [105]. Intestinal absorption of furosemide may be involved in MCT6 [84]. It was assumed that intestinal absorption of furosemide was mediated by MCT6. Function of intestinal MCT6 under diabetic status was set to be 50% according previous report [47]. Furosemide is eliminated mainly via renal secretion due to OAT1/2 [3]. Part of furosemide is metabolized by CYP2C11, CYP3As and CYP2E1 [152]. The contribution of CYP2C11 was 61.5% of the total metabolism [152], rests (38.5%) were assumed to attributed to CYP2E1 and CYP3As. Hepatic clearance (CL_{liver}) of furosemide was reported to be 2.20 mL/min/kg [105] and the estimated value of fu × $CL_{int,liver}$ was 0.75 mL/min/250g. Diabetes increased the expression of CYP2E1 and CYP3As by 3-fold [28] and the expression of CYP2C11 mRNA was decreased to 16% that of control rats [47]. Thus, fu × $CL_{int,liver}$ and CL_{liver} were estimated to be 0.75 mL/min/250g and 2.20 mL/min/kg. The estimated CL_{liver} of furosemide was near to observed data (2.98) in diabetic rats [105]. Diabetes altered expression of these targeted proteins (CYP2C11, CYP3As, CYP2E1 and OATs), intestinal blood, liver blood flow and renal blood flow. It was assumed that intestinal absorption of furosemide was mediated by MCT6. All these contribute to the altered furosemide pharmacokinetics, whose integrated effects (Figure 6) were predicted using PBPK model. The results demonstrate that the contribution of increases in CYP3A and CYP2E1 to hepatic clearance of furosemide was partly attenuated by decreases in CYP2C11, which may explain why non-renal clearance of furosemide was only slightly increased under diabetic status [105]. PBPK simulation demonstrated that decreases in renal excretion of furosemide due to downregulation of renal OATs and renal blood flow rates mainly contributed the increased plasma exposure of furosemide following an intravenous dose. Decreased oral exposure of furosemide was mainly attributed to the impairment of intestinal absorption due to the suppression of intestinal MCT6. The contribution of decreased expression of renal OATs to the altered oral plasma exposure of furosemide was less than that of intestinal MCT6 impairment, whose net effect was to decrease oral plasma of furosemide (Figure 6G).

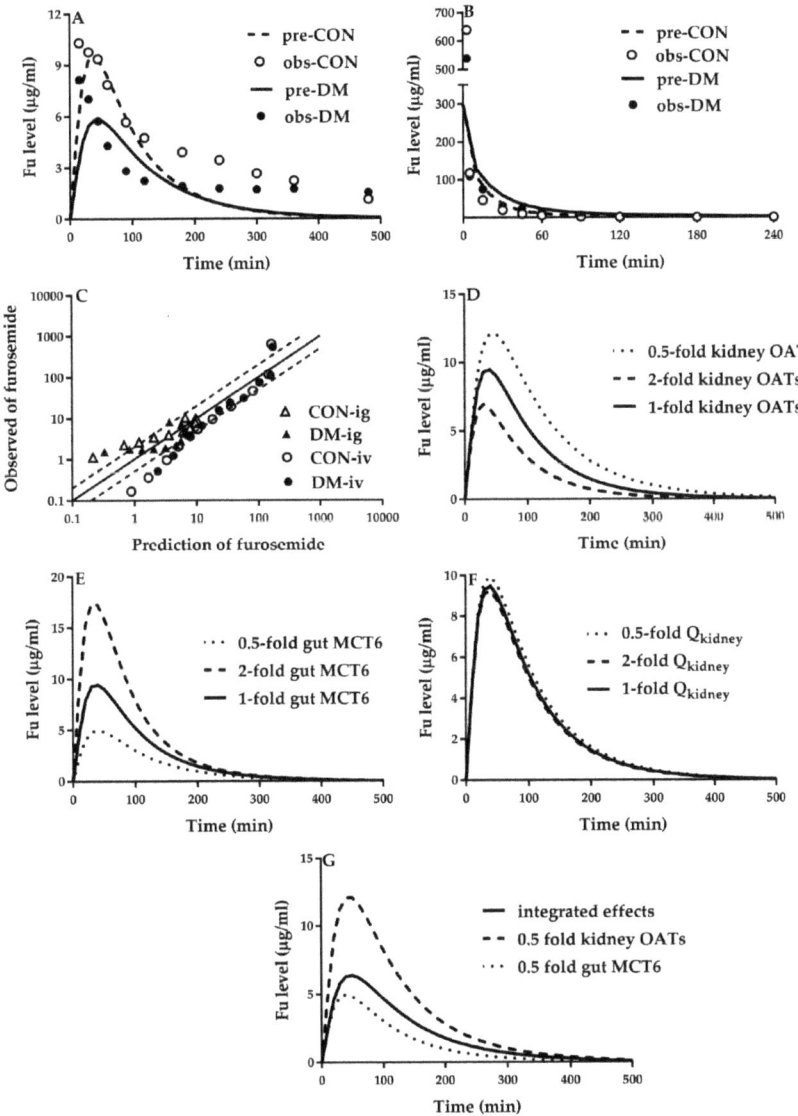

Figure 6. Observed (point) and predicted (line) plasma concentrations of furosemide (Fu) following (A) oral (6 mg/rat, ig) and (B) intravenous dose (6 mg/rat, iv) to diabetic rats (DM) and control rats (CON). Comparison of mean observed and predicted plasma concentrations of furosemide at each time point (C). Contributions of altered (D) renal OATs, (E) intestinal MCT6 and (F) renal blood flow (Q_{kidney}) to oral plasma exposure of furosemide as well as (G) integrated effects of intestinal MCT6 impairment and renal OATs impairment. The observations were obtained from the literature [89].

5.4. Metformin and Nisoldipine

A whole-body PBPK model was also used to predict the pharmacokinetics of metformin in diabetic patients [153]. The results show that increased plasma levels of metformin following oral dose mainly resulted from both the impairment of renal function and delaying gastrointestinal transit. The metabolism of nisoldipine is mediated by CYP3As. Decreased CYP3A activity may partly explain the increased oral plasma exposure. However, when nisoldipine, in controlled-release tablets, was given to diabetic patients, the roles of gastrointestinal transit were nonnegligible. PBPK simulation also demonstrated that delaying gastrointestinal transit increased the intestinal absorption of nisoldipine, indicating that increased oral plasma of nisoldipine following oral administration of nisoldipine controlled-release tablet in diabetes patients was mainly attributed to both decreased CYP3As and delaying gastrointestinal transit.

6. Future Perspective

Growing evidence has demonstrated that diabetes often simultaneously affects transporters and enzymes in the intestine, liver and kidney. Moreover, these alterations are dependent on tissue and diabetic progression. For example, diabetes induced the expression of hepatic CYP3A, but downregulated the expression of intestinal CYP3A. In STZ/HFD-induced diabetic rats, 10-day diabetes decreased the expression of both intestinal and hepatic BCRP, but 22-day diabetes induced the expression of intestinal BCRP not hepatic BCRP protein [11]. Moreover, mRNA levels are often indexed as the expression of targets, but mRNA levels do not always reflect the protein expression and activity. For example, a report showed that diabetes induced a five-fold increase in the expression of renal Mdr1a mRNA in rats, but the expression of renal P-gp protein was unaltered [138]. Similarly, mRNA expression of BCRP in the liver of GK rats was increased by 20-fold, but the expression of BCRP protein and function (biliary excretion of rosuvastatin) was unchanged [19]. In contrast, diabetes decreased the level of hepatic MRP2 protein by 80% in rats without affecting the mRNA expression of MRP2 [22]. Similarly, no correlation between the mRNA level and activity (chlorzoxazone 6-hydroxylation activity) of CYP2E1 was also found in human liver [154]. All these indicate that data based on mRNA sometimes give the wrong conclusion. Clinical trials [66,68,73,74,131,132] have also demonstrated that many factors such as type of diabetes, diabetic progression, gender, age, therapy/effectiveness, diet/drinking habits, complications and co-medicines affect expressions and functions of CYP450s and transporters, which may partly explain contradictory effects of diabetes on expressions of CYP450/transporters and pharmacokinetics. Alterations in expressions and functions of transporters and CYP450s by diabetes are dependent on specific isoforms (CYP450s and transporters) and tissues. Moreover, physiological parameters such as blood flow rates in tissues are altered. All these results indicate that alterations in the disposition of drugs under diabetes should be attributed to the integrated effect of these factors. We thought that PBPK model could be used to accomplish the prediction of drug disposition under diabetic status. Furthermore, the PBPK model could separately illustrate individual contributions of each factor to drug disposition and their integrated effects.

Author Contributions: Both authors shared in the searching for publication, preparation and editing of the manuscript. All authors have read and agreed to the published version of the manuscript.

Funding: This research was funded by National Natural Science Foundation of China (No. 81573490)

Conflicts of Interest: The authors declare no conflict of interest.

Abbreviations

ABC, ATP binding cassette; AGEs, advanced glycation end-products; AUC, area under the curve; BCRP, breast cancer resistance protein; BSEP, bile salt export pump; C_{max}, peak concentration; CL_{int}, intrinsic clearance; CON, control rats; CYP450s cytochrome P450 enzymes; DM, diabetic rats; FXR, farnesoid X receptor; GLUT9, glucose transporter 9; HFD, high-fat diet; MATEs, multidrug/toxin extrusions; MCTs, monocarboxylate transporters; MRPs, multidrug resistance-associated proteins; NF-κB, nuclear factor kappa-B; NOS, nitric oxide synthase; NPT1/4, sodium-dependent phosphate transport protein 1/4; Nrf2, nuclear factor erythroid 2-related factor 2;

NTCP, sodium taurocholate co-transporting polypeptide; OATPs, Organic anion transporting polypeptides; OATs, organic anion transporters; OCTs, organic cation transporters; PBPK, physiologically-based pharmacokinetic model; P_{eff}, apparent intestinal effective permeability; PepTs, peptide transporters; P-gp, P-glycoprotein; PKCα, protein kinase C alpha; PPAR, peroxisome proliferator activated receptor; PXR, pregnane X receptor; SCFAs, short chain fatty acids; SHP, small heterodimer partner; SGLT2, sodium-glucose cotransporter; SLC, solute carrier; STZ, streptozocin; TSOD, Tsumura, Suzuki, obese, diabetes; UGTs, UDP-glucuronosyltransferases; URAT1, urate transporter 1; ZSF1, Zucker spontaneously hypertensive fatty.

References

1. Lu, C.; Di, L. In vitro and in vivo methods to assess pharmacokinetic drug–drug interactions in drug discovery and development. *Biopharm. Drug Dispos.* **2020**, *41*, 3–31. [CrossRef]
2. Bteich, M.; Poulin, P.; Haddad, S. The potential protein-mediated hepatic uptake: Discussion on the molecular interactions between albumin and the hepatocyte cell surface and their implications for the in vitro-to-in vivo extrapolations of hepatic clearance of drugs. *Expert Opin. Drug Metab. Toxicol.* **2019**, *15*, 633–658. [CrossRef]
3. Liu, X. SLC Family Transporters. *Adv. Exp. Med. Biol.* **2019**, *1141*, 101–202. [CrossRef] [PubMed]
4. Park, J.E.; Kim, K.B.; Bae, S.K.; Moon, B.S.; Liu, K.H.; Shin, J.G. Contribution of cytochrome P450 3A4 and 3A5 to the metabolism of atorvastatin. *Xenobiotica* **2008**, *38*, 1240–1251. [CrossRef] [PubMed]
5. Goosen, T.C.; Bauman, J.N.; Davis, J.A.; Yu, C.; Hurst, S.I.; Williams, J.A.; Loi, C.M. Atorvastatin glucuronidation is minimally and nonselectively inhibited by the fibrates gemfibrozil, fenofibrate, and fenofibric acid. *Drug Metab. Dispos.* **2007**, *35*, 1315–1324. [CrossRef] [PubMed]
6. Li, J.; Volpe, D.A.; Wang, Y.; Zhang, W.; Bode, C.; Owen, A.; Hidalgo, I.J. Use of transporter knockdown Caco-2 cells to investigate the in vitro efflux of statin drugs. *Drug Metab. Dispos.* **2011**, *39*, 1196–1202. [CrossRef] [PubMed]
7. Choi, M.K.; Shin, H.J.; Choi, Y.L.; Deng, J.W.; Shin, J.G.; Song, I.S. Differential effect of genetic variants of Na$^+$-taurocholate co-transporting polypeptide (NTCP) and organic anion-transporting polypeptide 1B1 (OATP1B1) on the uptake of HMG-CoA reductase inhibitors. *Xenobiotica* **2011**, *41*, 24–34. [CrossRef]
8. Keppler, D.; Konig, J. Hepatic secretion of conjugated drugs and endogenous substances. *Semin. Liver Dis.* **2000**, *20*, 265–272. [CrossRef]
9. Shu, N.; Hu, M.; Liu, C.; Zhang, M.; Ling, Z.; Zhang, J.; Xu, P.; Zhong, Z.; Chen, Y.; Liu, L.; et al. Decreased exposure of atorvastatin in diabetic rats partly due to induction of hepatic Cyp3a and Oatp2. *Xenobiotica* **2016**, *46*, 875–881. [CrossRef]
10. Li, F.; Ling, Z.L.; Wang, Z.J.; Zhong, Z.Y.; Shu, N.; Zhang, M.; Liu, C.; Liu, L.; Liu, X.D. Differential effects of pravastatin on the pharmacokinetics of paroxetine in normal and diabetic rats. *Xenobiotica* **2017**, *47*, 20–30. [CrossRef]
11. Wang, Z.; Yang, H.; Xu, J.; Zhao, K.; Chen, Y.; Liang, L.; Li, P.; Chen, N.; Geng, D.; Zhang, X.; et al. Prediction of Atorvastatin Pharmacokinetics in High-Fat Diet and Low-Dose Streptozotocin-Induced Diabetic Rats Using a Semiphysiologically Based Pharmacokinetic Model Involving Both Enzymes and Transporters. *Drug Metab. Dispos.* **2019**, *47*, 1066–1079. [CrossRef] [PubMed]
12. Xu, D.; Li, F.; Zhang, M.; Zhang, J.; Liu, C.; Hu, M.Y.; Zhong, Z.Y.; Jia, L.L.; Wang, D.W.; Wu, J.; et al. Decreased exposure of simvastatin and simvastatin acid in a rat model of type 2 diabetes. *Acta Pharm. Sin.* **2014**, *35*, 1215–1225. [CrossRef] [PubMed]
13. Hasegawa, Y.; Kishimoto, S.; Shibatani, N.; Inotsume, N.; Takeuchi, Y.; Fukushima, S. The disposition of pravastatin in a rat model of streptozotocin-induced diabetes and organic anion transporting polypeptide 2 and multidrug resistance-associated protein 2 expression in the liver. *Biol. Pharm. Bull.* **2010**, *33*, 153–156. [CrossRef] [PubMed]
14. Babalik, A.; Ulus, I.H.; Bakirci, N.; Kuyucu, T.; Arpag, H.; Dagyildizi, L.; Capaner, E. Plasma concentrations of isoniazid and rifampin are decreased in adult pulmonary tuberculosis patients with diabetes mellitus. *Antimicrob. Agents Chemother.* **2013**, *57*, 5740–5742. [CrossRef] [PubMed]
15. Nijland, H.M.; Ruslami, R.; Stalenhoef, J.E.; Nelwan, E.J.; Alisjahbana, B.; Nelwan, R.H.; van der Ven, A.J.; Danusantoso, H.; Aarnoutse, R.E.; van Crevel, R. Exposure to rifampicin is strongly reduced in patients with tuberculosis and type 2 diabetes. *Clin. Infect. Dis.* **2006**, *43*, 848–854. [CrossRef]

16. Kameyama, N.; Arisawa, S.; Ueyama, J.; Kagota, S.; Shinozuka, K.; Hattori, A.; Tatsumi, Y.; Hayashi, H.; Takagi, K.; Wakusawa, S. Increase in P-glycoprotein accompanied by activation of protein kinase Cα and NF- κB p65 in the livers of rats with streptozotocin-induced diabetes. *Biochim. Biophys. Acta* **2008**, *1782*, 355–360. [CrossRef]
17. Lee, J.H.; Lee, A.; Oh, J.H.; Lee, Y.J. Comparative pharmacokinetic study of paclitaxel and docetaxel in streptozotocin-induced diabetic rats. *Biopharm. Drug Dispos.* **2012**, *33*, 474–486. [CrossRef]
18. Zhang, L.L.; Lu, L.; Jin, S.; Jing, X.Y.; Yao, D.; Hu, N.; Liu, L.; Duan, R.; Liu, X.D.; Wang, G.J.; et al. Tissue-specific alterations in expression and function of P-glycoprotein in streptozotocin-induced diabetic rats. *Acta Pharm. Sin.* **2011**, *32*, 956–966. [CrossRef]
19. zhang, L.L.; Jin, S.; Li, J.; Duan, R.; Liu, X.D. Tissue species damage in expression and function of breast cancer resistance protein streptotozocin-induced diabetic rats. *J. China Pharmceut Unversit.* **2011**, *42*, 544–550.
20. He, L.; Yang, Y.; Guo, C.; Yao, D.; Liu, H.H.; Sheng, J.J.; Zhou, W.P.; Ren, J.; Liu, X.D.; Pan, G.Y. Opposite regulation of hepatic breast cancer resistance protein in type 1 and 2 diabetes mellitus. *Eur. J. Pharm.* **2014**, *724*, 185–192. [CrossRef]
21. Aleksunes, L.M.; Xu, J.; Lin, E.; Wen, X.; Goedken, M.J.; Slitt, A.L. Pregnancy represses induction of efflux transporters in livers of type I diabetic mice. *Pharm. Res.* **2013**, *30*, 2209–2220. [CrossRef] [PubMed]
22. van Waarde, W.M.; Verkade, H.J.; Wolters, H.; Havinga, R.; Baller, J.; Bloks, V.; Muller, M.; Sauer, P.J.; Kuipers, F. Differential effects of streptozotocin-induced diabetes on expression of hepatic ABC-transporters in rats. *Gastroenterology* **2002**, *122*, 1842–1852. [CrossRef] [PubMed]
23. Mei, D.; Li, J.; Liu, H.; Liu, L.; Wang, X.; Guo, H.; Liu, C.; Duan, R.; Liu, X. Induction of multidrug resistance-associated protein 2 in liver, intestine and kidney of streptozotocin-induced diabetic rats. *Xenobiotica* **2012**, *42*, 709–718. [CrossRef] [PubMed]
24. Nakashima, E.; Matsushita, R.; Takeda, M.; Nakanishi, T.; Ichimura, F. Comparative pharmacokinetics of cefoperazone and cephradine in untreated streptozotocin diabetic rats. *Drug Metab. Dispos.* **1992**, *20*, 730–735. [PubMed]
25. Watkins, J.B.; Noda, H. Biliary excretion of organic anions in diabetic rats. *J. Pharm. Exp. Ther.* **1986**, *239*, 467–473.
26. Shimojo, N.; Ishizaki, T.; Imaoka, S.; Funae, Y.; Fujii, S.; Okuda, K. Changes in amounts of cytochrome P450 isozymes and levels of catalytic activities in hepatic and renal microsomes of rats with streptozocin-induced diabetes. *Biochem. Pharm.* **1993**, *46*, 621–627. [CrossRef]
27. Hu, N.; Xie, S.; Liu, L.; Wang, X.; Pan, X.; Chen, G.; Zhang, L.; Liu, H.; Liu, X.; Liu, X.; et al. Opposite effect of diabetes mellitus induced by streptozotocin on oral and intravenous pharmacokinetics of verapamil in rats. *Drug Metab. Dispos.* **2011**, *39*, 419–425. [CrossRef]
28. Kim, Y.C.; Lee, A.K.; Lee, J.H.; Lee, I.; Lee, D.C.; Kim, S.H.; Kim, S.G.; Lee, M.G. Pharmacokinetics of theophylline in diabetes mellitus rats: Induction of CYP1A2 and CYP2E1 on 1,3-dimethyluric acid formation. *Eur. J. Pharm. Sci.* **2005**, *26*, 114–123. [CrossRef]
29. Chen, G.M.; Hu, N.; Liu, L.; Xie, S.S.; Wang, P.; Li, J.; Xie, L.; Wang, G.J.; Liu, X.D. Pharmacokinetics of verapamil in diabetic rats induced by combination of high-fat diet and streptozotocin injection. *Xenobiotica* **2011**, *41*, 494–500. [CrossRef]
30. Gawronska-Szklarz, B.; Musial, D.H.; Pawlik, A.; Paprota, B. Effect of experimental diabetes on pharmacokinetic parameters of lidocaine and MEGX in rats. *Pol. J. Pharm.* **2003**, *55*, 619–624.
31. Wang, X.; Wang, F.; Zhang, Y.; Xiong, H.; Zhang, Y.; Zhuang, P.; Zhang, Y. Diabetic cognitive dysfunction is associated with increased bile acids in liver and activation of bile acid signaling in intestine. *Toxicol. Lett.* **2018**, *287*, 10–22. [CrossRef] [PubMed]
32. Drolet, B.; Pilote, S.; Gelinas, C.; Kamaliza, A.D.; Blais-Boilard, A.; Virgili, J.; Patoine, D.; Simard, C. Altered Protein Expression of Cardiac CYP2J and Hepatic CYP2C, CYP4A, and CYP4F in a Mouse Model of Type II Diabetes-A Link in the Onset and Development of Cardiovascular Disease? *Pharmaceutics* **2017**, *9*, 44. [CrossRef] [PubMed]
33. Bae, S.K.; Kim, J.Y.; Yang, S.H.; Kim, J.W.; Kim, T.; Lee, M.G. Pharmacokinetics of oltipraz in rat models of diabetes mellitus induced by alloxan or streptozotocin. *Life Sci.* **2006**, *78*, 2287–2294. [CrossRef] [PubMed]
34. Lee, D.Y.; Lee, M.G.; Shin, H.S.; Lee, I. Changes in omeprazole pharmacokinetics in rats with diabetes induced by alloxan or streptozotocin: Faster clearance of omeprazole due to induction of hepatic CYP1A2 and 3A1. *J. Pharm. Pharm. Sci.* **2007**, *10*, 420–433. [CrossRef]

35. Ueyama, J.; Wang, D.; Kondo, T.; Saito, I.; Takagi, K.; Takagi, K.; Kamijima, M.; Nakajima, T.; Miyamoto, K.; Wakusawa, S.; et al. Toxicity of diazinon and its metabolites increases in diabetic rats. *Toxicol. Lett.* **2007**, *170*, 229–237. [CrossRef]
36. Maksymchuk, O.; Shysh, A.; Rosohatska, I.; Chashchyn, M. Quercetin prevents type 1 diabetic liver damage through inhibition of CYP2E1. *Pharm. Rep.* **2017**, *69*, 1386–1392. [CrossRef]
37. Woodcroft, K.J.; Novak, R.F. Insulin effects on CYP2E1, 2B, 3A, and 4A expression in primary cultured rat hepatocytes. *Chem. Biol. Interact.* **1997**, *107*, 75–91. [CrossRef]
38. Hu, N.; Hu, M.; Duan, R.; Liu, C.; Guo, H.; Zhang, M.; Yu, Y.; Wang, X.; Liu, L.; Liu, X. Increased levels of fatty acids contributed to induction of hepatic CYP3A4 activity induced by diabetes-in vitro evidence from HepG2 cell and Fa2N-4 cell lines. *J. Pharm. Sci.* **2014**, *124*, 433–444. [CrossRef]
39. Elaidy, S.M.; Hussain, M.A.; El-Kherbetawy, M.K. Time-dependent therapeutic roles of nitazoxanide on high-fat diet/streptozotocin-induced diabetes in rats: Effects on hepatic peroxisome proliferator-activated receptor-gamma receptors. *Can. J. Physiol. Pharm.* **2018**, *96*, 485–497. [CrossRef]
40. Zhang, C.; Deng, J.; Liu, D.; Tuo, X.; Xiao, L.; Lai, B.; Yao, Q.; Liu, J.; Yang, H.; Wang, N. Nuciferine ameliorates hepatic steatosis in high-fat diet/streptozotocin-induced diabetic mice through a PPARα/PPARγ coactivator-1α pathway. *Br. J. Pharm.* **2018**, *175*, 4218–4228. [CrossRef]
41. Ahmad, A.; Ali, T.; Kim, M.W.; Khan, A.; Jo, M.H.; Rehman, S.U.; Khan, M.S.; Abid, N.B.; Khan, M.; Ullah, R.; et al. Adiponectin homolog novel osmotin protects obesity/diabetes-induced NAFLD by upregulating AdipoRs/PPARα signaling in ob/ob and db/db transgenic mouse models. *Metabolism* **2019**, *90*, 31–43. [CrossRef] [PubMed]
42. Shi, C.; Min, L.; Yang, J.; Dai, M.; Song, D.; Hua, H.; Xu, G.; Gonzalez, F.J.; Liu, A. Peroxisome Proliferator-Activated Receptor α Activation Suppresses Cytochrome P450 Induction Potential in Mice Treated with Gemfibrozil. *Basic Clin. Pharm. Toxicol.* **2017**, *121*, 169–174. [CrossRef] [PubMed]
43. Liu, Y.; Nakagawa, Y.; Wang, Y.; Sakurai, R.; Tripathi, P.V.; Lutfy, K.; Friedman, T.C. Increased glucocorticoid receptor and 11β-hydroxysteroid dehydrogenase type 1 expression in hepatocytes may contribute to the phenotype of type 2 diabetes in db/db mice. *Diabetes* **2005**, *54*, 32–40. [CrossRef] [PubMed]
44. Liu, Y.; Yan, C.; Wang, Y.; Nakagawa, Y.; Nerio, N.; Anghel, A.; Lutfy, K.; Friedman, T.C. Liver X receptor agonist T0901317 inhibition of glucocorticoid receptor expression in hepatocytes may contribute to the amelioration of diabetic syndrome in db/db mice. *Endocrinology* **2006**, *147*, 5061–5068. [CrossRef] [PubMed]
45. Schuetz, E.G.; Schmid, W.; Schutz, G.; Brimer, C.; Yasuda, K.; Kamataki, T.; Bornheim, L.; Myles, K.; Cole, T.J. The glucocorticoid receptor is essential for induction of cytochrome P-4502B by steroids but not for drug or steroid induction of CYP3A or P-450 reductase in mouse liver. *Drug Metab. Dispos.* **2000**, *28*, 268–278. [PubMed]
46. Gerbal-Chaloin, S.; Daujat, M.; Pascussi, J.M.; Pichard-Garcia, L.; Vilarem, M.J.; Maurel, P. Transcriptional regulation of CYP2C9 gene. Role of glucocorticoid receptor and constitutive androstane receptor. *J. Biol. Chem.* **2002**, *277*, 209–217. [CrossRef]
47. Xu, F.; Zhu, L.; Qian, C.; Zhou, J.; Geng, D.; Li, P.; Xuan, W.; Wu, F.; Zhao, K.; Kong, W.; et al. Impairment of Intestinal Monocarboxylate Transporter 6 Function and Expression in Diabetic Rats Induced by Combination of High-Fat Diet and Low Dose of Streptozocin: Involvement of Butyrate-Peroxisome Proliferator-Activated Receptor-γ Activation. *Drug Metab. Dispos.* **2019**, *47*, 556–566. [CrossRef]
48. Liu, H.; Liu, L.; Li, J.; Mei, D.; Duan, R.; Hu, N.; Guo, H.; Zhong, Z.; Liu, X. Combined contributions of impaired hepatic CYP2C11 and intestinal breast cancer resistance protein activities and expression to increased oral glibenclamide exposure in rats with streptozotocin-induced diabetes mellitus. *Drug Metab. Dispos.* **2012**, *40*, 1104–1112. [CrossRef]
49. Kim, Y.C.; Oh, E.Y.; Kim, S.H.; Lee, M.G. Pharmacokinetics of diclofenac in rat model of diabetes mellitus induced by alloxan or streptozotocin. *Biopharm. Drug Dispos.* **2006**, *27*, 85–92. [CrossRef]
50. Kim, Y.C.; Oh, E.Y.; Kim, S.H.; Lee, M.G. Pharmacokinetics and pharmacodynamics of intravenous torasemide in diabetic rats induced by alloxan or streptozotocin. *Biopharm. Drug Dispos.* **2005**, *26*, 371–378. [CrossRef]
51. Kim, Y.C.; Kang, H.E.; Lee, M.G. Pharmacokinetics of phenytoin and its metabolite, 4'-HPPH, after intravenous and oral administration of phenytoin to diabetic rats induced by alloxan or streptozotocin. *Biopharm. Drug Dispos.* **2008**, *29*, 51–61. [CrossRef] [PubMed]

52. Oh, S.J.; Choi, J.M.; Yun, K.U.; Oh, J.M.; Kwak, H.C.; Oh, J.G.; Lee, K.S.; Kim, B.H.; Heo, T.H.; Kim, S.K. Hepatic expression of cytochrome P450 in type 2 diabetic Goto-Kakizaki rats. *Chem. Biol. Interact.* **2012**, *195*, 173–179. [CrossRef] [PubMed]
53. Shi, R.; Wu, J.; Meng, C.; Ma, B.; Wang, T.; Li, Y.; Ma, Y. Cyp3a11-mediated testosterone-6beta-hydroxylation decreased, while UGT1a9-mediated propofol O-glucuronidation increased, in mice with diabetes mellitus. *Biopharm. Drug Dispos.* **2016**, *37*, 433–443. [CrossRef] [PubMed]
54. Lam, J.L.; Jiang, Y.; Zhang, T.; Zhang, E.Y.; Smith, B.J. Expression and functional analysis of hepatic cytochromes P450, nuclear receptors, and membrane transporters in 10-and 25-week-old db/db mice. *Drug Metab. Dispos.* **2010**, *38*, 2252–2258. [CrossRef]
55. Park, S.Y.; Kim, C.H.; Lee, J.Y.; Jeon, J.S.; Kim, M.J.; Chae, S.H.; Kim, H.C.; Oh, S.J.; Kim, S.K. Hepatic expression of cytochrome P450 in Zucker diabetic fatty rats. *Food Chem. Toxicol.* **2016**, *96*, 244–253. [CrossRef]
56. Patoine, D.; Petit, M.; Pilote, S.; Picard, F.; Drolet, B.; Simard, C. Modulation of CYP3a expression and activity in mice models of type 1 and type 2 diabetes. *Pharm. Res. Perspect.* **2014**, *2*, e00082. [CrossRef]
57. Gravel, S.; Chiasson, J.L.; Turgeon, J.; Grangeon, A.; Michaud, V. Modulation of CYP450 Activities in Patients With Type 2 Diabetes. *Clin. Pharm. Ther.* **2019**, *106*, 1280–1289. [CrossRef]
58. Gade, C.; Dalhoff, K.; Petersen, T.S.; Riis, T.; Schmeltz, C.; Chabanova, E.; Christensen, H.R.; Mikus, G.; Burhenne, J.; Holm, J.C.; et al. Higher chlorzoxazone clearance in obese children compared with nonobese peers. *Br. J. Clin. Pharm.* **2018**, *84*, 1738–1747. [CrossRef]
59. Dostalek, M.; Court, M.H.; Yan, B.; Akhlaghi, F. Significantly reduced cytochrome P450 3A4 expression and activity in liver from humans with diabetes mellitus. *Br. J. Pharm.* **2011**, *163*, 937–947. [CrossRef]
60. Marques, M.P.; Coelho, E.B.; Dos Santos, N.A.; Geleilete, T.J.; Lanchote, V.L. Dynamic and kinetic disposition of nisoldipine enantiomers in hypertensive patients presenting with type-2 diabetes mellitus. *Eur. J. Clin. Pharm.* **2002**, *58*, 607–614. [CrossRef]
61. Moises, E.C.; Duarte Lde, B.; Cavalli Rde, C.; Marques, M.P.; Lanchote, V.L.; Duarte, G.; da Cunha, S.P. Pharmacokinetics of lidocaine and its metabolite in peridural anesthesia administered to pregnant women with gestational diabetes mellitus. *Eur. J. Clin. Pharm.* **2008**, *64*, 1189–1196. [CrossRef] [PubMed]
62. Filgueira, G.C.O.; Filgueira, O.A.S.; Carvalho, D.M.; Marques, M.P.; Moises, E.C.D.; Duarte, G.; Lanchote, V.L.; Cavalli, R.C. Effect of type 2 diabetes mellitus on the pharmacokinetics and transplacental transfer of nifedipine in hypertensive pregnant women. *Br. J. Clin. Pharm.* **2017**, *83*, 1571–1579. [CrossRef] [PubMed]
63. Antunes Nde, J.; Cavalli, R.C.; Marques, M.P.; Moises, E.C.; Lanchote, V.L. Influence of gestational diabetes on the stereoselective pharmacokinetics and placental distribution of metoprolol and its metabolites in parturients. *Br. J. Clin. Pharm.* **2015**, *79*, 605–616. [CrossRef] [PubMed]
64. Adithan, C.; Srinivas, B.; Indhiresan, J.; Shashindran, C.H.; Bapna, J.S.; Thakur, L.C.; Swaminathan, R.P. Influence of type I and type II diabetes mellitus on phenytoin steady-state levels. *Int. J. Clin. Pharm. Ther. Toxicol.* **1991**, *29*, 310–313.
65. Akhlaghi, F.; Dostalek, M.; Falck, P.; Mendonza, A.E.; Amundsen, R.; Gohh, R.Y.; Asberg, A. The concentration of cyclosporine metabolites is significantly lower in kidney transplant recipients with diabetes mellitus. *Ther. Drug Monit.* **2012**, *34*, 38–45. [CrossRef]
66. Mendonza, A.E.; Gohh, R.Y.; Akhlaghi, F. Blood and plasma pharmacokinetics of ciclosporin in diabetic kidney transplant recipients. *Clin. Pharm.* **2008**, *47*, 733–742. [CrossRef]
67. Wadhawan, S.; Jauhari, H.; Singh, S. Cyclosporine trough levels in diabetic and nondiabetic renal transplant patients. *Transplant. Proc.* **2000**, *32*, 1683–1684. [CrossRef]
68. Jamwal, R.; de la Monte, S.M.; Ogasawara, K.; Adusumalli, S.; Barlock, B.B.; Akhlaghi, F. Nonalcoholic Fatty Liver Disease and Diabetes Are Associated with Decreased CYP3A4 Protein Expression and Activity in Human Liver. *Mol. Pharm.* **2018**, *15*, 2621–2632. [CrossRef]
69. Matzke, G.R.; Frye, R.F.; Early, J.J.; Straka, R.J.; Carson, S.W. Evaluation of the influence of diabetes mellitus on antipyrine metabolism and CYP1A2 and CYP2D6 activity. *Pharmacotherapy* **2000**, *20*, 182–190. [CrossRef]
70. Korrapati, M.R.; Vestal, R.E.; Loi, C.M. Theophylline metabolism in healthy nonsmokers and in patients with insulin-dependent diabetes mellitus. *Clin. Pharm. Ther.* **1995**, *57*, 413–418. [CrossRef]
71. Adithan, C.; Danda, D.; Shashindran, C.H.; Bapna, J.S.; Swaminathan, R.P.; Chandrasekar, S. Differential effect of type I and type II diabetes mellitus on antipyrine elimination. *Methods Find. Exp. Clin. Pharm.* **1989**, *11*, 755–758.

72. Zysset, T.; Wietholtz, H. Differential effect of type I and type II diabetes on antipyrine disposition in man. *Eur. J. Clin. Pharm.* **1988**, *34*, 369–375. [CrossRef] [PubMed]
73. Sotaniemi, E.A.; Pelkonen, O.; Arranto, A.J.; Tapanainen, P.; Rautio, A.; Pasanen, M. Diabetes and elimination of antipyrine in man: An analysis of 298 patients classified by type of diabetes, age, sex, duration of disease and liver involvement. *Pharm. Toxicol.* **2002**, *90*, 155–160. [CrossRef] [PubMed]
74. Urry, E.; Jetter, A.; Landolt, H.P. Assessment of CYP1A2 enzyme activity in relation to type-2 diabetes and habitual caffeine intake. *Nutr. Metab. (Lond.)* **2016**, *13*, 66. [CrossRef] [PubMed]
75. Porazka, J.; Szalek, E.; Polom, W.; Czajkowski, M.; Grabowski, T.; Matuszewski, M.; Grzeskowiak, E. Influence of Obesity and Type 2 Diabetes Mellitus on the Pharmacokinetics of Tramadol After Single Oral Dose Administration. *Eur. J. Drug Metab. Pharm.* **2019**, *44*, 579–584. [CrossRef] [PubMed]
76. Shu, N.; Hu, M.; Ling, Z.; Liu, P.; Wang, F.; Xu, P.; Zhong, Z.; Sun, B.; Zhang, M.; Li, F.; et al. The enhanced atorvastatin hepatotoxicity in diabetic rats was partly attributed to the upregulated hepatic Cyp3a and SLCO1B1. *Sci. Rep.* **2016**, *6*, 33072. [CrossRef]
77. Brunner, L.J.; Iyer, L.V.; Vadiei, K.; Weaver, W.V.; Luke, D.R. Cyclosporine pharmacokinetics and effect in the type I diabetic rat model. *Eur. J. Drug Metab. Pharm.* **1989**, *14*, 287–292. [CrossRef]
78. Neuman, M.G.; Cameron, R.G.; Haber, J.A.; Katz, G.G.; Malkiewicz, I.M.; Shear, N.H. Inducers of cytochrome P450 2E1 enhance methotrexate-induced hepatocytotoxicity. *Clin. Biochem.* **1999**, *32*, 519–536. [CrossRef]
79. Malatjalian, D.A.; Ross, J.B.; Williams, C.N.; Colwell, S.J.; Eastwood, B.J. Methotrexate hepatotoxicity in psoriatics: Report of 104 patients from Nova Scotia, with analysis of risks from obesity, diabetes and alcohol consumption during long term follow-up. *Can. J. Gastroenterol. Hepatol.* **1996**, *10*, 369–375. [CrossRef]
80. Liu, X. ABC Family Transporters. *Adv. Exp. Med. Biol.* **2019**, *1141*, 13–100. [CrossRef]
81. Zeng, X.Y.; Dong, S.; He, N.N.; Jiang, C.J.; Dai, Y.; Xia, Y.F. Comparative pharmacokinetics of arctigenin in normal and type 2 diabetic rats after oral and intravenous administration. *Fitoterapia* **2015**, *105*, 119–126. [CrossRef] [PubMed]
82. Yu, S.; Yu, Y.; Liu, L.; Wang, X.; Lu, S.; Liang, Y.; Liu, X.; Xie, L.; Wang, G. Increased plasma exposures of five protoberberine alkaloids from Coptidis Rhizoma in streptozotocin-induced diabetic rats: Is P-GP involved? *Planta Med.* **2010**, *76*, 876–881. [CrossRef] [PubMed]
83. Novak, A.; Godoy, Y.C.; Martinez, S.A.; Ghanem, C.I.; Celuch, S.M. Fructose-induced metabolic syndrome decreases protein expression and activity of intestinal P-glycoprotein. *Nutrition* **2015**, *31*, 871–876. [CrossRef] [PubMed]
84. Watanabe, M.; Kobayashi, M.; Ogura, J.; Takahashi, N.; Yamaguchi, H.; Iseki, K. Alteration of pharmacokinetics of grepafloxacin in type 2 diabetic rats. *J. Pharm. Pharm. Sci.* **2014**, *17*, 25–33. [CrossRef] [PubMed]
85. Nawa, A.; Fujita-Hamabe, W.; Kishioka, S.; Tokuyama, S. Decreased expression of intestinal P-glycoprotein increases the analgesic effects of oral morphine in a streptozotocin-induced diabetic mouse model. *Drug Metab. Pharm.* **2011**, *26*, 584–591. [CrossRef]
86. Joshi, S.D.; Santani, D.D.; Sheth, J.J.; Mehta, H.C.; Dave, K.C.; Goyal, R.K. Investigation into the possible mechanisms involved in altered digoxin levels in diabetic patients. *Indian J. Physiol. Pharm.* **1996**, *40*, 65–69.
87. Gitanjali, B.; Adithan, C.; Raveendran, R.; Shashindran, C.H.; Chandrasekar, S. Pharmacokinetics of single dose oral digoxin in patients with uncomplicated type II diabetes mellitus. *Int. J. Clin. Pharm. Ther. Toxicol.* **1992**, *30*, 113–116.
88. Nawa, A.; Fujita-Hamabe, W.; Tokuyama, S. Involvement of ubiquitination in the decrease of intestinal P-glycoprotein in a streptozotocin-induced diabetic mouse model. *Drug Metab. Pharm.* **2012**, *27*, 548–552. [CrossRef]
89. Nawa, A.; Fujita-Hamabe, W.; Tokuyama, S. Regulatory action of nitric oxide synthase on ileal P-glycoprotein expression under streptozotocin-induced diabetic condition. *Biol. Pharm. Bull.* **2011**, *34*, 436–438. [CrossRef]
90. Nawa, A.; Fujita-Hamabe, W.; Tokuyama, S. Altered intestinal P-glycoprotein expression levels in a monosodium glutamate-induced obese mouse model. *Life Sci.* **2011**, *89*, 834–838. [CrossRef]
91. Nawa, A.; Fujita Hamabe, W.; Tokuyama, S. Inducible nitric oxide synthase-mediated decrease of intestinal P-glycoprotein expression under streptozotocin-induced diabetic conditions. *Life Sci.* **2010**, *86*, 402–409. [CrossRef] [PubMed]
92. Duan, R.; Hu, N.; Liu, H.Y.; Li, J.; Guo, H.F.; Liu, C.; Liu, L.; Liu, X.D. Biphasic regulation of P-glycoprotein function and expression by NO donors in Caco-2 cells. *Acta Pharm. Sin.* **2012**, *33*, 767–774. [CrossRef] [PubMed]

93. Zhang, J.; Xie, Q.; Kong, W.; Wang, Z.; Wang, S.; Zhao, K.; Chen, Y.; Liu, X.; Liu, L. Short-chain fatty acids oppositely altered expressions and functions of intestinal cytochrome P4503A and P-glycoprotein and affected pharmacokinetics of verapamil following oral administration to rats. *J. Pharm. Pharm.* **2020**, *72*, 448–460. [CrossRef] [PubMed]
94. Al-Salami, H.; Butt, G.; Tucker, I.; Skrbic, R.; Golocorbin-Kon, S.; Mikov, M. Probiotic Pre-treatment Reduces Gliclazide Permeation (ex vivo) in Healthy Rats but Increases It in Diabetic Rats to the Level Seen in Untreated Healthy Rats. *Arch. Drug Inf.* **2008**, *1*, 35–41. [CrossRef] [PubMed]
95. Mikov, M.; Al-Salami, H.; Golocorbin-Kon, S.; Skrbic, R.; Raskovic, A.; Fawcett, J.P. The influence of 3alpha,7alpha-dihydroxy-12-keto-5beta-cholanate on gliclazide pharmacokinetics and glucose levels in a rat model of diabetes. *Eur. J. Drug Metab. Pharm.* **2008**, *33*, 137–142. [CrossRef] [PubMed]
96. Xie, Q.S.; Zhang, J.X.; Liu, M.; Liu, P.H.; Wang, Z.J.; Zhu, L.; Liang, L.; Jin, M.M.; Liu, X.N.; Liu, L.; et al. Short-chain fatty acids down-regulate expression and function of p-glycoprotein but up-regulate expression and function of breast cancer resistance protein in intestine of rats. *Acta Pharm. Sin.* **2020**, in press.
97. Hindlet, P.; Bado, A.; Farinotti, R.; Buyse, M. Long-term effect of leptin on H^+-coupled peptide cotransporter 1 activity and expression in vivo: Evidence in leptin-deficient mice. *J. Pharm. Exp. Ther.* **2007**, *323*, 192–201. [CrossRef]
98. Bikhazi, A.B.; Skoury, M.M.; Zwainy, D.S.; Jurjus, A.R.; Kreydiyyeh, S.I.; Smith, D.E.; Audette, K.; Jacques, D. Effect of diabetes mellitus and insulin on the regulation of the PepT 1 symporter in rat jejunum. *Mol. Pharm.* **2004**, *1*, 300–308. [CrossRef]
99. Liang, L.M.; Zhou, J.J.; Xu, F.; Li, X.W.; Liu, P.H.; Qin, L.; Liu, L.; Liu, X.D. Diabetes downregulates peptide transporter 1 in rat jejunum: Possible involvement of cholate-induced FXR activation. *Acta Pharm. Sin.* **2020**, in press.
100. Der-Boghossian, A.H.; Saad, S.R.; Perreault, C.; Provost, C.; Jacques, D.; Kadi, L.N.; Issa, N.G.; Sibai, A.M.; El-Majzoub, N.W.; Bikhazi, A.B. Role of insulin on jejunal PepT1 expression and function regulation in diabetic male and female rats. *Can. J. Physiol. Pharm.* **2010**, *88*, 753–759. [CrossRef]
101. Watanabe, K.; Terada, K.; Jinriki, T.; Sato, J. Effect of insulin on cephalexin uptake and transepithelial transport in the human intestinal cell line Caco-2. *Eur. J. Pharm. Sci.* **2004**, *21*, 87–95. [CrossRef] [PubMed]
102. Thamotharan, M.; Bawani, S.Z.; Zhou, X.; Adibi, S.A. Hormonal regulation of oligopeptide transporter pept-1 in a human intestinal cell line. *Am. J. Physiol.* **1999**, *276*, C821–C826. [CrossRef] [PubMed]
103. Kohyama, N.; Shiokawa, H.; Ohbayashi, M.; Kobayashi, Y.; Yamamoto, T. Characterization of monocarboxylate transporter 6: Expression in human intestine and transport of the antidiabetic drug nateglinide. *Drug Metab. Dispos.* **2013**, *41*, 1883–1887. [CrossRef] [PubMed]
104. Murakami, Y.; Kohyama, N.; Kobayashi, Y.; Ohbayashi, M.; Ohtani, H.; Sawada, Y.; Yamamoto, T. Functional characterization of human monocarboxylate transporter 6 (SLC16A5). *Drug Metab. Dispos.* **2005**, *33*, 1845–1851. [CrossRef] [PubMed]
105. Park, J.H.; Lee, W.I.; Yoon, W.H.; Park, Y.D.; Lee, J.S.; Lee, M.G. Pharmacokinetic and pharmacodynamic changes of furosemide after intravenous and oral administration to rats with alloxan-induced diabetes mellitus. *Biopharm. Drug Dispos.* **1998**, *19*, 357–364. [CrossRef]
106. Park, K.J.; Yoon, W.H.; Shin, W.G.; Lee, M.G. Pharmacokinetics and pharmacodynamics of azosemide after intravenous and oral administration to rats with alloxan-induced diabetes mellitus. *J. Pharm. Pharm.* **1996**, *48*, 1093–1097. [CrossRef] [PubMed]
107. Borbas, T.; Benko, B.; Dalmadi, B.; Szabo, I.; Tihanyi, K. Insulin in flavin-containing monooxygenase regulation. Flavin-containing monooxygenase and cytochrome P450 activities in experimental diabetes. *Eur. J. Pharm. Sci.* **2006**, *28*, 51–58. [CrossRef]
108. Kudo, T.; Toda, T.; Ushiki, T.; Ohi, K.; Ikarashi, N.; Ochiai, W.; Sugiyama, K. Differences in the pharmacokinetics of Cyp3a substrates in TSOD and streptozotocin-induced diabetic mice. *Xenobiotica* **2010**, *40*, 282–290. [CrossRef]
109. Zhang, S.; Pan, X.; Jeong, H. GW4064, an agonist of farnesoid X receptor, represses CYP3A4 expression in human hepatocytes by inducing small heterodimer partner expression. *Drug Metab. Dispos.* **2015**, *43*, 743–748. [CrossRef]
110. Ourlin, J.C.; Lasserre, F.; Pineau, T.; Fabre, J.M.; Sa-Cunha, A.; Maurel, P.; Vilarem, M.J.; Pascussi, J.M. The small heterodimer partner interacts with the pregnane X receptor and represses its transcriptional activity. *Mol. Endocrinol.* **2003**, *17*, 1693–1703. [CrossRef]

111. Ogata, M.; Iizuka, Y.; Murata, R.; Hikichi, N. Effect of streptozotocin-induced diabetes on cyclosporin A disposition in rats. *Biol. Pharm. Bull.* **1996**, *19*, 1586–1590. [CrossRef] [PubMed]
112. Ando, T.; Kusuhara, H.; Merino, G.; Alvarez, A.I.; Schinkel, A.H.; Sugiyama, Y. Involvement of breast cancer resistance protein (ABCG2) in the biliary excretion mechanism of fluoroquinolones. *Drug Metab. Dispos.* **2007**, *35*, 1873–1879. [CrossRef] [PubMed]
113. Jiang, S.; Zhao, W.; Chen, Y.; Zhong, Z.; Zhang, M.; Li, F.; Xu, P.; Zhao, K.; Li, Y.; Liu, L.; et al. Paroxetine decreased plasma exposure of glyburide partly via inhibiting intestinal absorption in rats. *Drug Metab. Pharm.* **2015**, *30*, 240–246. [CrossRef] [PubMed]
114. Liu, X. Overview: Role of Drug Transporters in Drug Disposition and Its Clinical Significance. *Adv. Exp. Med. Biol.* **2019**, *1141*, 1–12. [CrossRef]
115. Phatchawan, A.; Chutima, S.; Varanuj, C.; Anusorn, L. Decreased renal organic anion transporter 3 expression in type 1 diabetic rats. *Am. J. Med. Sci.* **2014**, *347*, 221–227. [CrossRef]
116. Thongnak, L.; Pongchaidecha, A.; Jaikumkao, K.; Chatsudthipong, V.; Chattipakorn, N.; Lungkaphin, A. The additive effects of atorvastatin and insulin on renal function and renal organic anion transporter 3 function in diabetic rats. *Sci. Rep.* **2017**, *7*, 13532. [CrossRef]
117. Babelova, A.; Burckhardt, B.C.; Wegner, W.; Burckhardt, G.; Henjakovic, M. Sex-differences in renal expression of selected transporters and transcription factors in lean and obese Zucker spontaneously hypertensive fatty rats. *J. Diabetes Res.* **2015**, *2015*, 483238. [CrossRef]
118. Sharma, K.; Karl, B.; Mathew, A.V.; Gangoiti, J.A.; Wassel, C.L.; Saito, R.; Pu, M.; Sharma, S.; You, Y.H.; Wang, L.; et al. Metabolomics reveals signature of mitochondrial dysfunction in diabetic kidney disease. *J. Am. Soc. Nephrol.* **2013**, *24*, 1901–1912. [CrossRef]
119. Vallon, V.; Rieg, T.; Ahn, S.Y.; Wu, W.; Eraly, S.A.; Nigam, S.K. Overlapping in vitro and in vivo specificities of the organic anion transporters OAT1 and OAT3 for loop and thiazide diuretics. *Am. J. Physiol. Renal. Physiol.* **2008**, *294*, F867–F873. [CrossRef]
120. Eraly, S.A.; Vallon, V.; Vaughn, D.A.; Gangoiti, J.A.; Richter, K.; Nagle, M.; Monte, J.C.; Rieg, T.; Truong, D.M.; Long, J.M.; et al. Decreased renal organic anion secretion and plasma accumulation of endogenous organic anions in OAT1 knock-out mice. *J. Biol. Chem.* **2006**, *281*, 5072–5083. [CrossRef]
121. Cunha, F.M.; Pereira, J.; Marques, P.; Ribeiro, A.; Bettencourt, P.; Lourenco, P. Diabetic patients need higher furosemide doses: A report on acute and chronic heart failure patients. *J. Cardiovasc. Med. (Hagerstown)* **2020**, *21*, 21–26. [CrossRef] [PubMed]
122. Fu, Y.; Breljak, D.; Onishi, A.; Batz, F.; Patel, R.; Huang, W.; Song, P.; Freeman, B.; Mayoux, E.; Koepsell, H.; et al. Organic anion transporter OAT3 enhances the glucosuric effect of the SGLT2 inhibitor empagliflozin. *Am. J. Physiol. Renal. Physiol.* **2018**, *315*, F386–F394. [CrossRef] [PubMed]
123. Jinnouchi, H.; Nozaki, K.; Watase, H.; Omiya, H.; Sakai, S.; Samukawa, Y. Impact of Reduced Renal Function on the Glucose-Lowering Effects of Luseogliflozin, a Selective SGLT2 Inhibitor, Assessed by Continuous Glucose Monitoring in Japanese Patients with Type 2 Diabetes Mellitus. *Adv. Ther.* **2016**, *33*, 460–479. [CrossRef] [PubMed]
124. Nowicki, M.T.; Aleksunes, L.M.; Sawant, S.P.; Dnyanmote, A.V.; Mehendale, H.M.; Manautou, J.E. Renal and hepatic transporter expression in type 2 diabetic rats. *Drug Metab. Lett.* **2008**, *2*, 11–17. [CrossRef] [PubMed]
125. Grover, B.; Buckley, D.; Buckley, A.R.; Cacini, W. Reduced expression of organic cation transporters rOCT1 and rOCT2 in experimental diabetes. *J. Pharm. Exp. Ther.* **2004**, *308*, 949–956. [CrossRef]
126. Thomas, M.C.; Tikellis, C.; Burns, W.C.; Thallas, V.; Forbes, J.M.; Cao, Z.; Osicka, T.M.; Russo, L.M.; Jerums, G.; Ghabrial, H.; et al. Reduced tubular cation transport in diabetes: Prevented by ACE inhibition. *Kidney Int.* **2003**, *63*, 2152–2161. [CrossRef]
127. Thomas, M.C.; Tikellis, C.; Kantharidis, P.; Burns, W.C.; Cooper, M.E.; Forbes, J.M. The role of advanced glycation in reduced organic cation transport associated with experimental diabetes. *J. Pharm. Exp. Ther.* **2004**, *311*, 456–466. [CrossRef]
128. Lee, M.G.; Choi, Y.H.; Lee, I. Effects of diabetes mellitus induced by alloxan on the pharmacokinetics of metformin in rats: Restoration of pharmacokinetic parameters to the control state by insulin treatment. *J. Pharm. Pharm. Sci.* **2008**, *11*, 88–103. [CrossRef] [PubMed]
129. Tucker, G.T.; Casey, C.; Phillips, P.J.; Connor, H.; Ward, J.D.; Woods, H.F. Metformin kinetics in healthy subjects and in patients with diabetes mellitus. *Br. J. Clin. Pharm.* **1981**, *12*, 235–246. [CrossRef]

130. Bergagnini-Kolev, M.C.; Hebert, M.F.; Easterling, T.R.; Lin, Y.S. Pregnancy Increases the Renal Secretion of N(1)-methylnicotinamide, an Endogenous Probe for Renal Cation Transporters, in Patients Prescribed Metformin. *Drug Metab. Dispos.* **2017**, *45*, 325–329. [CrossRef]
131. Liao, M.Z.; Flood Nichols, S.K.; Ahmed, M.; Clark, S.; Hankins, G.D.; Caritis, S.; Venkataramanan, R.; Haas, D.; Quinney, S.K.; Haneline, L.S.; et al. Effects of Pregnancy on the Pharmacokinetics of Metformin. *Drug Metab. Dispos.* **2020**. [CrossRef] [PubMed]
132. Hughes, R.C.; Gardiner, S.J.; Begg, E.J.; Zhang, M. Effect of pregnancy on the pharmacokinetics of metformin. *Diabet. Med.* **2006**, *23*, 323–326. [CrossRef] [PubMed]
133. Cacini, W.; Singh, Y. Renal metallothionein and platinum levels in diabetic and nondiabetic rats injected with cisplatin. *Proc. Soc. Exp. Biol. Med.* **1991**, *197*, 285–289. [CrossRef] [PubMed]
134. Cacini, W.; Harden, E.A.; Skau, K.A. Reduced renal accumulation and toxicity of cisplatin in experimental galactosemia. *Proc. Soc. Exp. Biol. Med.* **1993**, *203*, 348–353. [CrossRef]
135. Scott, L.A.; Madan, E.; Valentovic, M.A. Attenuation of cisplatin nephrotoxicity by streptozotocin-induced diabetes. *Toxicol. Sci.* **1989**, *12*, 530–539. [CrossRef]
136. da Silva Faria, M.C.; Santos, N.A.; Carvalho Rodrigues, M.A.; Rodrigues, J.L.; Barbosa Junior, F.; Santos, A.C. Effect of diabetes on biodistribution, nephrotoxicity and antitumor activity of cisplatin in mice. *Chem. Biol. Interact.* **2015**, *229*, 119–131. [CrossRef]
137. Valentovic, M.A.; Scott, L.A.; Madan, E.; Yokel, R.A. Renal accumulation and urinary excretion of cisplatin in diabetic rats. *Toxicology* **1991**, *70*, 151–162. [CrossRef]
138. Tramonti, G.; Xie, P.; Wallner, E.I.; Danesh, F.R.; Kanwar, Y.S. Expression and functional characteristics of tubular transporters: P-glycoprotein, PEPT1, and PEPT2 in renal mass reduction and diabetes. *Am. J. Physiol. Renal. Physiol.* **2006**, *291*, F972–F980. [CrossRef]
139. Yeh, S.Y.; Pan, H.J.; Lin, C.C.; Kao, Y.H.; Chen, Y.H.; Lin, C.J. Hyperglycemia induced down-regulation of renal P-glycoprotein expression. *Eur. J. Pharm.* **2012**, *690*, 42–50. [CrossRef]
140. Maximos, S.; Chamoun, M.; Gravel, S.; Turgeon, J.; Michaud, V. Tissue Specific Modulation of cyp2c and cyp3a mRNA Levels and Activities by Diet-Induced Obesity in Mice: The Impact of Type 2 Diabetes on Drug Metabolizing Enzymes in Liver and Extra-Hepatic Tissues. *Pharmaceutics* **2017**, *9*, 40. [CrossRef]
141. Del Villar, E.; Gaule, C.; Vega, P. Kidney drug metabolizing activities in streptozotocin diabetic rats. *Gen. Pharm.* **1995**, *26*, 137–141. [CrossRef]
142. Ding, S.; Huang, J.; Qiu, H.; Chen, R.; Zhang, J.; Huang, B.; Cheng, O.; Jiang, Q. Effects of PPARs/20-HETE on the renal impairment under diabetic conditions. *Exp. Cell Res.* **2019**, *382*, 111455. [CrossRef] [PubMed]
143. Park, J.M.; Moon, C.H.; Lee, M.G. Pharmacokinetic changes of methotrexate after intravenous administration to streptozotocin-induced diabetes mellitus rats. *Res. Commun. Mol. Pathol. Pharm.* **1996**, *93*, 343–352.
144. Kim, S.H.; Kim, W.B.; Lee, M.G. Pharmacokinetics of a new carbapenem, DA-1131, after intravenous administration to rats with alloxan-induced diabetes mellitus. *Biopharm. Drug Dispos.* **1998**, *19*, 303–308. [CrossRef]
145. Valentovic, M.A.; Ball, J.G.; Rogers, B.A. Comparison of cephaloridine renal accumulation and urinary excretion between normoglycemic and diabetic animals. *Toxicology* **1996**, *108*, 93–99. [CrossRef]
146. Kong, W.M.; Sun, B.B.; Wang, Z.J.; Zheng, X.K.; Zhao, K.J.; Chen, Y.; Zhang, J.X.; Liu, P.H.; Zhu, L.; Xu, R.J.; et al. Physiologically based pharmacokinetic-pharmacodynamic modeling for prediction of vonoprazan pharmacokinetics and its inhibition on gastric acid secretion following intravenous/oral administration to rats, dogs and humans. *Acta Pharm. Sin.* **2020**. [CrossRef]
147. Yusuksawad, M.; Chaiyabutr, N. Restoration of renal hemodynamics and functions during black cumin (Nigella sativa) administration in streptozotocin-induced diabetic rats. *J. Exp. Pharm.* **2012**, *4*, 1–7. [CrossRef]
148. Kitani, M.; Ozaki, Y.; Katayama, K.; Kakemi, M.; Koizumi, T. A kinetic study on drug distribution: furosemide in rats. *Chem. Pharm. Bull. (Tokyo)* **1988**, *36*, 1053–1062. [CrossRef]
149. Varma, M.V.; Sarkar, M.; Kapoor, N.; Panchagnula, R. PH-dependent functional activity of P-glycoprotein in limiting intestinal absorption of protic drugs 1. Simultaneous determination of quinidine and permeability markers in rat in situ perfusion samples. *J. Chromatogr. B Analyt. Technol. Biomed. Life Sci.* **2005**, *816*, 243–249. [CrossRef]
150. Choi, D.H.; Chang, K.S.; Hong, S.P.; Choi, J.S.; Han, H.K. Effect of atorvastatin on the intravenous and oral pharmacokinetics of verapamil in rats. *Biopharm. Drug Dispos.* **2008**, *29*, 45–50. [CrossRef]

151. Ruark, C.D.; Hack, C.E.; Robinson, P.J.; Mahle, D.A.; Gearhart, J.M. Predicting passive and active tissue:plasma partition coefficients: Interindividual and interspecies variability. *J. Pharm. Sci.* **2014**, *103*, 2189–2198. [CrossRef] [PubMed]
152. Yang, K.H.; Choi, Y.H.; Lee, U.; Lee, J.H.; Lee, M.G. Effects of cytochrome P450 inducers and inhibitors on the pharmacokinetics of intravenous furosemide in rats: Involvement of CYP2C11, 2E1, 3A1 and 3A2 in furosemide metabolism. *J. Pharm. Pharm.* **2009**, *61*, 47–54. [CrossRef]
153. Li, J.; Guo, H.F.; Liu, C.; Zhong, Z.; Liu, L.; Liu, X.D. Prediction of drug disposition in diabetic patients by means of a physiologically based pharmacokinetic model. *Clin. Pharm.* **2015**, *54*, 179–193. [CrossRef] [PubMed]
154. Sumida, A.; Kinoshita, K.; Fukuda, T.; Matsuda, H.; Yamamoto, I.; Inaba, T.; Azuma, J. Relationship between mRNA levels quantified by reverse transcription-competitive PCR and metabolic activity of CYP3A4 and CYP2E1 in human liver. *Biochem. Biophys. Res. Commun.* **1999**, *262*, 499–503. [CrossRef]

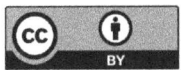

© 2020 by the authors. Licensee MDPI, Basel, Switzerland. This article is an open access article distributed under the terms and conditions of the Creative Commons Attribution (CC BY) license (http://creativecommons.org/licenses/by/4.0/).

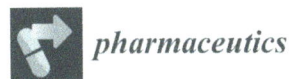

Article

Large Volume Direct Injection Ultra-High Performance Liquid Chromatography–Tandem Mass Spectrometry-Based Comparative Pharmacokinetic Study between Single and Combinatory Uses of *Carthamus tinctorius* Extract and Notoginseng Total Saponins

Jinfeng Chen [1], Xiaoyu Guo [1], Yingyuan Lu [1], Mengling Shi [1], Haidong Mu [1], Yi Qian [1], Jinlong Wang [1], Mengqiu Lu [1], Mingbo Zhao [1], Pengfei Tu [1,2], Yuelin Song [2,*] and Yong Jiang [1,*]

[1] State Key Laboratory of Natural and Biomimetic Drugs, School of Pharmaceutical Sciences, Peking University, Beijing 100191, China; chenjinfeng0513@163.com (J.C.); guoxiaoyu@bjmu.edu.cn (X.G.); luyingyuan2005@126.com (Y.L.); shimenglingbj@126.com (M.S.); a1538933944@163.com (H.M.); yiqian@163.com (Y.Q.); wang-jinlong@pku.edu.cn (J.W.); mengqiulu@163.com (M.L.); zmb_77@163.com (M.Z.); pengfeitu@bjmu.edu.cn (P.T.)
[2] Modern Research Center for Traditional Chinese Medicine, Beijing University of Chinese Medicine, Beijing 100029, China
* Correspondence: syltwc2005@163.com (Y.S.); yongjiang@bjmu.edu.cn (Y.J.); Tel.: + 86-10-82802719 (Y.J.)

Received: 25 December 2019; Accepted: 17 February 2020; Published: 20 February 2020

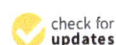

Abstract: The combination of *Carthamus tinctorius* extract (CTE) and notoginseng total saponins (NGTS), namely, CNP, presents a synergistic effect on myocardial ischemia protection. Herein, comparative pharmacokinetic studies between CNP and CTE/NGTS were conducted to clarify their synergistic mechanisms. A large volume direct injection ultra-high performance liquid chromatography–tandem mass spectrometry (LVDI-UHPLC-MS/MS) platform was developed for sensitively assaying the multi-component pharmacokinetic and in vitro cocktail assay of cytochrome p450 (CYP450) before and after compatibility of CTE and NGTS. The pharmacokinetic profiles of six predominantly efficacious components of CNP, including hydroxysafflor yellow A (HSYA); ginsenosides Rg_1 (GRg_1), Re (GRe), Rb_1 (GRb_1), and Rd (GRd); and notoginsenoside R_1 (NGR_1), were obtained, and the results disclosed that CNP could increase the exposure levels of HSYA, GRg_1, GRe, GRb_1, and NGR_1 at varying degrees. The in vitro cocktail assay demonstrated that CNP exhibited more potent inhibition on CYP1A2 than CTE and NGTS, and GRg_1, GRb_1, GRd, quercetin, kaempferol, and 6-hydroxykaempferol were found to be the major inhibitory compounds. The developed pharmacokinetic interaction-based strategy provides a viable orientation for the compatibility investigation of herb medicines.

Keywords: *Carthamus tinctorius* extract; notoginseng total saponins; comparative pharmacokinetic study; large volume direct injection; compatibility mechanism

1. Introduction

Myocardial ischemia-induced infarction is one of the leading causes of human death worldwide. The benefits of either *Carthamus tinctorius* extract (CTE) or notoginseng total saponins (NGTS) towards myocardial ischemia injury on rats have been well defined, and more interestingly, previous studies have demonstrated that better cardio-protective effects were observed when using their combination preparation (CNP) [1–3]. However, the underlying synergetic mechanisms of CTE and NGTS combination, their pharmacokinetic (PK) interactions in particular, still remain unclear.

It is widely accepted that the drug–drug interactions (DDIs) and herb–herb interactions (HHIs) can cause changes of pharmacokinetic profiles, which result in the possible improvement of drug efficacy and in the decrease of side effects, or vice versa [4,5]. However, most of the literature has merely focused on the pharmacokinetic profile variations of these primary components between individual dosing and combined use, but has overlooked the reasons responsible for the changed pharmacokinetic behaviors, which may be caused, at least in part, by cytochrome p450 (CYP450)- and/or transporter-mediated HHIs [6]. Therefore, the objective of this study was to gain insight into the synergistic actions between CTE and NGTS by determination of the pharmacokinetic profiles of six major active components from CTE and NGTS, as well as their CYP450-based synergetic mechanisms. An in vitro cocktail assay, which is an efficient and widely favored approach for CYP450-mediated HHIs, was employed to pursue the factors accounting for the different pharmacokinetic patterns before and after compatibility.

Our previous pharmacological evaluations optimized a relatively low dosage CNP for the anti-myocardial ischemia effect [2]. Furthermore, the cocktail method usually suffers from extensive CYP450 crossover within the probe substrates [7]. Therefore, the emerging demand is to develop a sensitive and efficient method for reliable detection and determination of the trace ingredients for the PK and cocktail studies. Attempts were made herein to propose and apply a large volume direct injection ultra-high performance liquid chromatography–tandem mass spectrometry (LVDI-UHPLC-MS/MS) method for direct and sensitive multiple-component PK and cocktail studies.

2. Materials and Methods

2.1. Plant Materials

Notoginseng total saponins (NGTS), containing ginsenoside Rg_1 (GRg_1, A_1, 26.6%), ginsenoside Rb_1 (GRb_1, A2, 32.5%), ginsenoside Rd (GRd, A3, 6.6%), ginsenoside Re (GRe, A4, 4.1%), and notoginsenoside R_1 (NGR_1, A5, 6.2%), prepared according to the Monograph of NGTS recorded in Chinese Pharmacopoeia [8], was purchased from Yunnan Plant Pharm. Co., Ltd. (Yunnan, China). Besides NGR_1, GRg_1, GRe, GRb_1, and GRd (Han et al., 2010), the remaining amount of around 25% ginsenosides in NGTS were further clarified as previously described [9]. *Carthamus tinctorius* extract, containing hydroxysafflor yellow A (HSYA; A9, 8.0%) and kaempferol-3-O-rutinoside (A11, 0.2%) was prepared following the protocol described in a previous report [1]. The chemical structures of the main components contained in CNP are shown in Figure 1. The chemical profiling based on LC–MS (Figure S1) and the detail chemical composition information were reported in our previous research papers [10]. The detailed information of other chemicals and reagents is shown in the Supplementary Materials section.

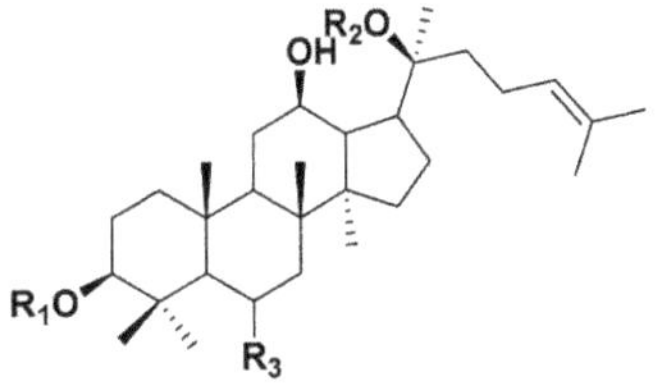

Compound	R_1	R_2	R_3
GRg_1(A1)	H	Glc	OGlc
GRb_1 (A2)	Glc^2-Glc	Glc^6-Glc	H
GRd (A3)	Glc^2-Glc	Glc	H
GRe (A4)	H	Glc	$OGlc^2$-Rha
NGR_1 (A5)	H	Glc	OGlc

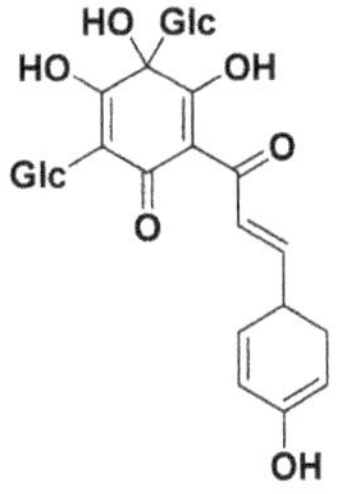

HSYA (A9)

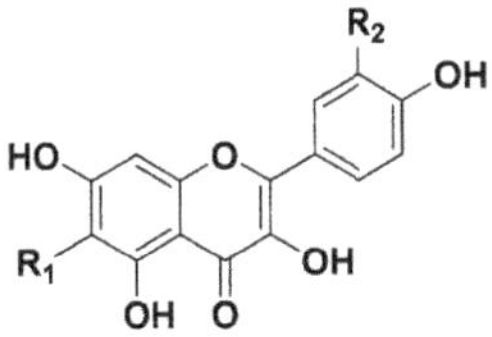

Compound	R_1	R_2
Quercetin (A16)	H	OH
Kaempferol (A17)	H	H
6-Hydoxykaempferol (A18)	OH	H

Figure 1. The chemical structures of the main components contained in the combination of *Carthamus tinctorius* extract and notoginseng total saponins (CNP).

2.2. Animals and Rat Liver Microsomes

Male Sprague-Dawley (SD) rats (12–14 weeks, 200–240 g) were provided by the Experimental Animal Center, Peking University Health Science Center. All animal experimental protocols were approved by the Biomedical Ethical Committee of Peking University Health Science Center (SYXK (Jing) 2016-0041, 23 December 2016). The animal experiments were carried out in accordance with the National Institutes of Health guide for the care and use of laboratory animals (NIH Publications no. 8023, revised 1978).

Pooled SD rat liver microsome (RLM, 20 mg/mL, LM-DS-02M, BDVH) were purchased from the Research Institute for Liver Diseases (Shanghai, China) Co. Ltd.

2.3. Plasma Pharmacokinetic Studies

CTE, NGTS, and CNP powders were dissolved using saline, and were orally dosed at 50 mg·kg^{-1}, 60 mg·kg^{-1}, and 50 mg·kg^{-1} CTE + 60 mg·kg^{-1} NGTS, respectively, whereas saline was administered to the vehicle group. Six rats were used in each group, and all rats fasted overnight but had free access to water prior to treatment. A terminal sampling design was used to collect blood samples at 0 (pre-dose), 0.08, 0.16, 0.25, 0.5, 1, 2, 3, 4, 6, 8, 12, 24, 48, 72, and 96 h. At each time, 0.5 mL of blood was collected in the heparin sodium tubes. Plasma was separated by centrifugation at 4000 rpm for 10 min and stored below −80 °C until bioanalysis. Oasis PRiME HLB SPE cartridges (1 cc/30 mg, Waters, Milford, MA, USA) were used to process the plasma samples (Supplementary Materials).

2.4. Incubation Procedure and CYP450 Activity Assay

The effects of CTE, NGTS, CNP, and 18 representative compounds (A1–A18, Supplementary Materials) on CYP450 activities were investigated using a pool of SD RLM following the procedure in [11]. Incubations were conducted at 37 ± 1 °C in 200 µL of incubation mixtures containing RLM (0.2 mg/mL), phosphate buffer saline (PBS) (pH 7.4, 0.1 mM), $MgCl_2$ (5 mM), nicotinamide adenine dinucleotide phosphate (NADPH) (1 mM), and CYP450 probe substrates (90/1.07/18/0.13/0.02/3.6/90 µM of phenacetin/omeprazole/ tolbutamide/dextromethorphan/midazolam/chlorzoxazone/ bupropion, respectively). CYP450 inhibitors (triethylenethiophosphoramide/sulfaphenazole/ticlopidine/furafylline/

ketoconazole/quinidine/4-methylpyrazole for CYP2B6/2C9/2C19/1A2/3A4/2D6/2E1, respectively) were added as the positive control, and blank solvents (PBS containing methanol and/or dimethyl sulfoxide (DMSO)) were used as the negative control. The incubation mixtures also contained eight concentrations for CTE (2.5–200 µg/mL), NGTS (2.5–200 µg/mL), CNP (2.5–200 µg/mL), A1–A17 (5–200 µM), and A18 (0.25–10 µM). Reactions were initiated by adding the NADPH-generating system and terminated after 15 min by 200 µL of cold methanol containing 105 nM hydroxybupropion-[D_6] (OHBUP-[D_6]) and 5 nM 4'-hydroxydiclofenac-[$^{13}C_6$] (OHDIC-[$^{13}C_6$]) as internal standards (ISs). The mixture was placed in an ice bath for 30 min, and the precipitated protein was removed by centrifugation (12,000 rpm for 10 min at 4 °C) three times. Then an aliquot of 100 µL supernatant was diluted with 100 µL ultrapure water, and centrifuged at 12,000 rpm for 10 min, before being subjected to LVDI-UHPLC-MS/MS analysis.

2.5. LVDI-UHPLC-MS/MS Analysis

The generic layout of instrumentation setup of the LVDI-UHPLC-MS/MS was conducted on a Shimadzu UHPLC system consisting of two LC-20ADXR pumps, a DGU-20A3R degasser, and a CBM-20A controller (Kyoto, Japan) with a SCIEX 4500 QTRAP mass spectrometer mounted with an electron spray ionization (ESI) interface as well as an electronic 6-port/2-channel valve (Foster City, CA, USA). Analyst software package (version 1.6.2, SCIEX) was implemented to control and synchronize the entire system, and also for data acquisition and processing. A single analytical run was fragmented into two phases, namely, loading and elution phases, by switching the electronic valve (Figure 2). At the loading phase, the valve was maintained at A-channel. The specimen aliquot of large volume delivered from the auto-sampler was captured onto a guard column. Meanwhile, the pumps were responsible for delivering the mobile phase at a high flow rate, aiming to dilute the sample solvent, thus facilitating the candidate constituents to concentrate on the pre-guard column. Then, the valve was automatically switched to the B-channel to trigger the elution phase. The trapped components were flushed from the pre-guard column into an analytical column, and underwent multiple reaction monitoring (MRM) analysis on the optimized LC gradients. The detailed information of LVDI-UHPLC-MS/MS analysis for pharmacokinetic and cocktail studies is shown in the Supplementary Materials section.

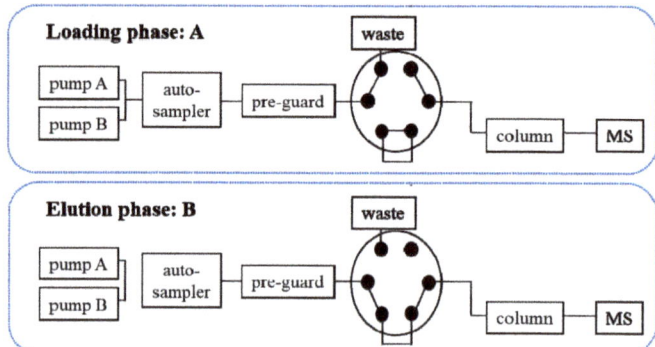

Figure 2. Connectivity sketch of the six-port/two-channel switching valve controlling the large volume direct injection ultra-high performance liquid chromatography–tandem mass spectrometry (LVDI-UHPLC-MS/MS) system. At the loading phase, the valve was maintained at A-channel. The sample delivered from the auto-sampler was captured onto a pre-guard column. Meanwhile, the pumps delivered the mobile phase at a high flow rate. Then, the valve was automatically switched to the B-channel to trigger the elution phase. The trapped components were flushed from the pre-guard column into an analytical column.

2.6. Method Validations

Method validations for the pharmacokinetic and cocktail assays, in terms of specificity, linearity, and sensitivity; precision and accuracy; recovery and matrix effect; and stability, were individually carried out by following the U.S. Food and Drug Administration (FDA) Guidance on Bioanalytical Method Validation and Drug Interaction Studies [12].

2.7. Data Processing

Calibration data were fitted to linear calibration curves using $1/x^2$ weighting. For the PK study, the half-time ($T_{1/2}$), maximum plasma concentration (C_{max}), time to reach the maximum concentration (T_{max}), and area under concentration-time curve (AUC) were determined by non-compartmental method using Drug and Statistics 3.0 (DAS 3.0, Mathematical Pharmacology Professional Committee of China, Shanghai, China). For the cocktail assay, the activity is expressed as the percentage of activity remaining comparing with that of a control sample containing no inhibitor. Substrate inhibition data were analyzed using GraphPad Prism 6 (version 6.01; San Diego, CA, USA) in logistic regression. All the data were described as mean ± standard deviation (SD). Normality assumptions were tested by the Kolmogorov–Smirnov statistic setting $p = 0.10$ as the limit for rejection of the null hypothesis of normality. If the distribution of the data was normal with equal variances, a two-sided test was performed at the 5% level of significance. The Welch's correction was then applied when the underlying variances were not equal. When the assumption of normality must be rejected, the Mann-Whitney test, a non-parametric equivalent of the independent-measures t-test, was used.

3. Results

3.1. Injection Solvent Optimization

It is well known that the sample solvent and volume have large effects on the peak asymmetry and column efficiency [13]. Herein, we established a LVDI-UHPLC-MS/MS method, assisted by injection solvent optimization, for sensitive bioassays of the pharmacokinetic interactions and cocktail analysis of CTE and NGTS. Considering the solubility and the sample pretreatment methods (Supplementary Materials) of the target analytes, the mixed standard solution of the six reference compounds was diluted with methanol (MeOH)/water (H_2O) in a ratio of 20% increment ranging from 100% H_2O to 100% MeOH for the PK study, and all the six standards of the PK study showed the highest responses when using 40% or 60% aqueous MeOH as the injection solvent. The CYP450 probe substrates and their corresponding metabolites for the in vitro cocktail assay were chosen according to the FDA guide [14]. Likewise, the six metabolites for the cocktail assay showed the best chromatograms when the 25% aqueous MeOH was served as the sample solvent, with exception of 1'-hydroxymidazolam, for which 50% aqueous MeOH was selected as the injection solvent (Figure S2).

3.2. Optimization of the Loading Phase for the LVDI-UHPLC-MS/MS-Based Method

The instrument stability of the LVDI-UHPLC-MS/MS setup was first investigated, and the results indicated the LVDI-UHPLC-MS/MS could meet the demands of quantitation (Table S3). An analytical run of the LVDI-UHPLC-MS/MS-based method was fragmented into a loading phase and an elution phase. The gradient condition for the elution phase turned out to be the same as that of the regular UHPLC-MS/MS analysis. Thus, the optimization works were concentrated on the loading phase, including the flow rate, mobile phase, and dilution time. According to the optimized gradient programs of the elution phases, both PK and cocktail studies employed water as the mobile phase for their loading phase after evaluating the solvents ramped from 0% to 20% aqueous acetonitrile. The flow rate of the loading phase for the PK study was finally optimized as 3.0 mL·min^{-1} after assays of 0.4, 1.0, 2.0, and 3.0 mL·min^{-1} flow rates. Because the higher the flow rate, the lower the signal responses of paracetamol and 6-hydroxychlorzoxazone, the cocktail assay finally chose 0.4 mL·min^{-1} as the flow rate of the loading phase. It turned out that the dilution time did not have a profound effect on the total chromatogram by comparing 0.5, 1, and 2 min. Thus, the shortest time, 0.5 min, was chosen to promote the analytical efficiency. The corresponding bioanalytical method validations were carried out by following the FDA guidance [12], and the results demonstrated that the newly developed LVDI-UHPLC-MS/MS-based methods enabled reliable detection and precise determination of the multiple-component in PK and cocktail studies. The lower limits of quantitation (LLOQ) of most analytes (except Rb_1 and Rd) were lower than 60 pg/mL.

3.3. Comparative Multiple-Component PK Studies

Considering the bioavailability improvement of active ingredients is a key point of traditional Chinese medicine compatibility, we executed a multiple-component PK study. HSYA, GRb_1, GRd, GRe, GRg_1, and NGR_1 were the primary circulating compounds and the main cardio-protective components in CNP [15,16], and thus were chosen as the PK markers. Meanwhile, the optimized injection solvent and LVDI-UHPLC-MS/MS method were integrated to achieve a much more sensitive method for reliable quantification of these components in vivo. After validation (Figure 3, Tables S4–S7), the developed method was first applied to characterize the pharmacokinetic characters of HSYA, GRb_1, GRd, GRe, GRg_1, and NGR_1 in rat plasma. Their plasma concentrations versus time profiles are displayed in Figure 4 and Table S8. The combination group showed greater C_{max} and AUC_{0-t} values (Table 1) of HSYA, GRg_1, GRb_1, NGR_1, and GRe over the individual extract groups. Exceptionally, GRd exhibited considerable AUC_{0-t} and C_{max} between NGTS and CNP dosing groups, whereas significantly different $T_{1/2}$ values, which indicated the combination use of CTE and NGTS, may have accelerated the elimination processes of GRd. The reason may have been due to the hydrolysis of GRb_1 to GRd in vivo [17], resulting in a more complicated PK behavior of GRd than other compounds in CNP.

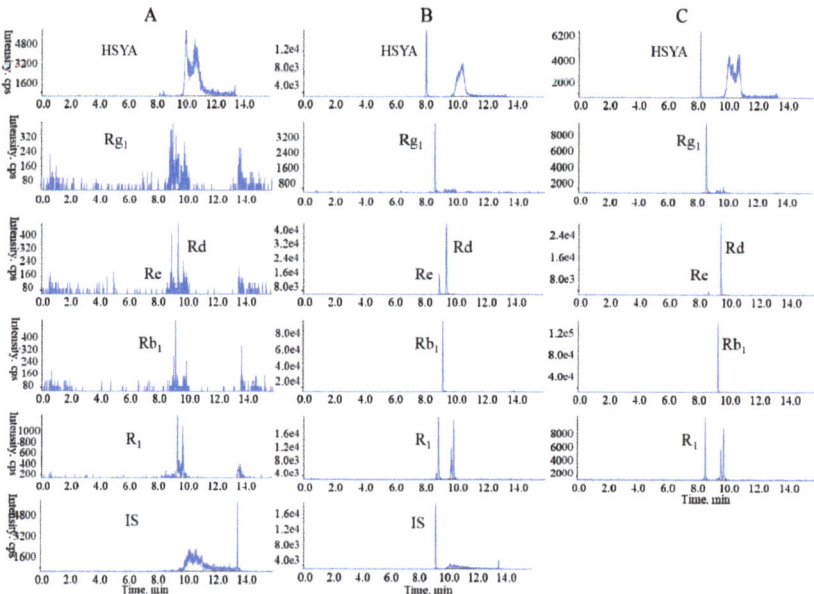

Figure 3. Representative multiple reaction monitoring (MRM) chromatograms of target analytes in rat plasma in a positive mode: (**A**) blank plasma; (**B**) blank plasma spiked with six chemical standards and internal standards (IS); (**C**) plasma sample collected at 2 h following oral administration of extract CNP (*Carthamus tinctorius* extract (CTE) 50 mg/kg + notoginseng total saponins (NGTS) 60 mg/kg) to rats.

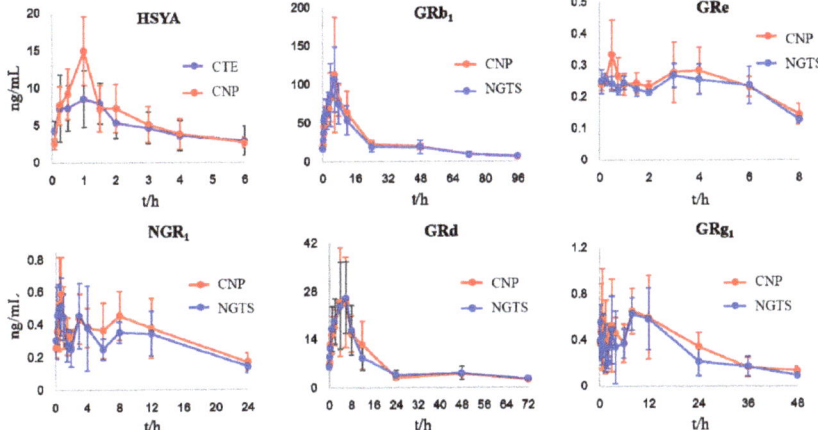

Figure 4. Mean plasma concentration-time profiles of the six analytes in rats after oral administration of CTE, NGTS, and CNP. Each point represents the mean ± SD ($n = 6$).

Table 1. Pharmacokinetic parameters of hydroxysafflor yellow A (HSYA), ginsenoside Re (GRe), ginsenoside Rb1 (GRb$_1$), ginsenoside Rd (GRd), ginsenoside Rg$_1$ (GRg$_1$), and notoginsenoside R$_1$ (NGR$_1$) after oral administration of CTE, NGTS, and CNP to rats. Each point represents the mean ± SD ($n = 6$).

Analyte	Group	$t_{1/2}$ (h)	T_{max} (h)	C_{max} (ng·mL^{-1})	AUC$_{0-t}$ (ng·h·mL^{-1})	AUC$_{0-\infty}$ (ng·h·mL^{-1})
HSYA	CTE	2.01 ± 0.34	0.88 ± 0.54	12.16 ± 3.09	33.05 ± 10.70	33.85 ± 10.78
	CNP	1.68 ± 0.79	1.17 ± 0.41	15.17 ± 4.39	38.33 ± 8.42	38.94 ± 8.60
NGR$_1$	NGTS	10.53 ± 3.06	1.15 ± 1.06	0.64 ± 0.18	6.30 ± 2.41	8.14 ± 3.60
	CNP	12.36 ± 4.48	1.04 ± 0.97	0.79 ± 0.18	8.12 ± 1.53	11.49 ± 3.54
GRb$_1$	NGTS	36.89 ± 9.65	5.50 ± 1.80	113.08 ± 41.78	2317.66 ± 682.70	2808.87 ± 617.99
	CNP	34.47 ± 8.45	6.33 ± 3.45	129.00 ± 65.97	2472.33 ± 394.72	2816.01 ± 563.44
GRd	NGTS	42.75 ± 8.84 *	4.50 ± 1.76	29.43 ± 10.69	460.90 ± 117.22	618.90 ± 157.23
	CNP	27.79 ± 6.94	6.33 ± 3.44	31.07 ± 16.78	459.04 ± 51.04	549.18 ± 58.09
GRg$_1$	NGTS	11.68 ± 2.09 *	4.71 ± 3.71	0.78 ± 0.13	13.99 ± 5.03	16.72 ± 3.93
	CNP	15.11 ± 8.89	5.38 ± 4.66	1.04 ± 0.34	16.69 ± 3.42	20.23 ± 3.35
GRe	NGTS	5.25 ± 2.27	2.60 ± 0.89*	0.29 ± 0.04*	1.82 ± 0.19	2.90 ± 0.60
	CNP	5.99 ± 3.86	0.80 ± 0.41	0.39 ± 0.08	1.93 ± 0.19	3.33 ± 1.13

*: $p < 0.05$, versus the combination group. T_{max}: the time of peak concentration; $t_{1/2}$: half-life; C_{max}: the peak or maximum concentration; AUC: area under concentration-time curve. For abbreviations of analytes A6–A18, please refer to the Supplementary Materials section.

3.4. CYP450-Mediated Herb–Herb Interactions

To investigate the possible HHIs between NGTS and CTE, an in vitro cocktail assay involving seven probe substrates was conducted, with the assistance of LVDI-UHPLC-MS/MS method to avoid CYP450 crossovers (Figure 5, Tables S9–S11). The incubation system was optimized in the aspects of substrate choice, enzyme concentration, incubation time, and substrate concentration (Figures S3–S4, Table S12), following the guidance of the FDA [14]. According to the half inhibiting concentration (IC$_{50}$) values of CTE, NGTS, and CNP (Table 2), CTE showed weak inhibition on CYP1A2, CYP2D6, and CYP2C9 and moderate inhibition on CYP2B6 and CYP2E1, whereas NGTS presented much more potent inhibitions on all these detected CYP450s than CTE (Table 2). After combination, CNP showed more potent inhibition on CYP1A2 than CTE and NGTS, and more potent inhibition on CYP2C9, CYP2C19, CYP3A4, and CYP2D6 than CTE (Table 2).

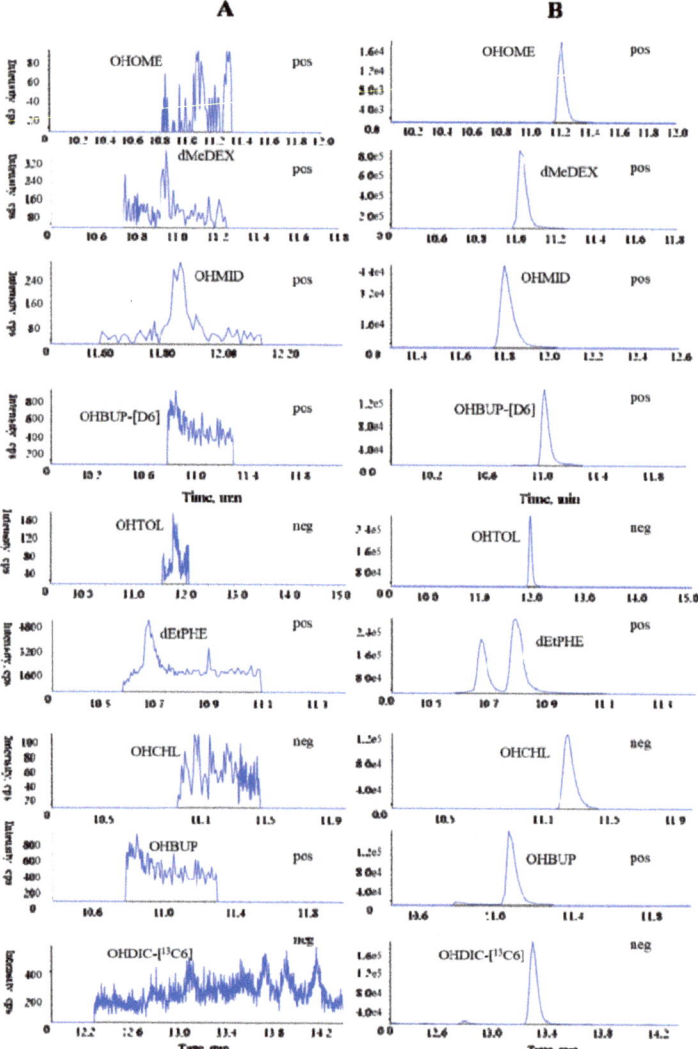

Figure 5. Representative MRM chromatograms of all probe metabolites and two ISs in the incubated rat microsomal sample with no substrate cocktails: (**A**) blank microsomal sample, (**B**) blank microsomal sample spiked with seven chemical standards and two ISs monitored in a polarity switching mode.

Table 2. IC$_{50}$ values of CTE, NGTS, CNP, and the 18 representative compounds for inhibiting cytochrome p450 (CYP450) isozymes.

No.	IC$_{50}$ (µg·mL^{-1}/µM) [#]						
	CYP2C9	CYP2E1	CYP2C19	CYP2D6	CYP2B6	CYP1A2	CYP3A4
CNP	21.66 ± 1.15	31.85 ± 4.15	62.95 ± 1.17	25.27 ± 0.25	52.19 ± 2.24	26.36 ± 6.98	91.77 ± 5.16
CTE	183.30 ± 17.98	35.47 ± 2.98	>200	126.17 ± 17.63	58.09 ± 13.41	138.60 ± 14.36	>200
NGTS	9.32 ± 0.56	16.12 ± 2.59	40.85 ± 6.98	12.23 ± 4.25	43.90 ± 7.91	60.68 ± 2.26	106.27 ± 14.00
GR$_{g1}$ (A1)	36.49 ± 1.32	34.08 ± 4.76	78.12 ± 5.25	55.73 ± 6.08	11.02 ± 0.87	13.09 ± 8.24	39.25 ± 4.57
GR$_{b1}$ (A2)	17.57 ± 2.03	27.96 ± 2.39	16.80 ± 2.52	17.06 ± 1.29	120.83 ± 10.89	5.84 ± 0.14	30.04 ± 2.47
GRd (A3)	73.01 ± 3.71	43.46 ± 0.06	71.36 ± 14.28	64.81 ± 11.68	>200	4.36 ± 2.31	61.43 ± 14.32
GRe (A4)	>200	25.59 ± 9.03	50.53 ± 15.39	>200	39.40 ± 4.81	94.41 ± 4.52	75.11 ± 7.24
NGR$_1$ (A5)	154.47 ± 16.65	121.70 ± 8.96	107.59 ± 29.58	20.42 ± 3.45	>200	112.07 ± 7.72	84.59 ± 1.79
A6	55.84 ± 3.40	40.76 ± 1.65	53.67 ± 0.22	19.46 ± 2.83	114.70 ± 3.04	52.77 ± 1.93	26.45 ± 1.39
A7	80.47 ± 1.05	13.59 ± 0.60	18.50 ± 1.60	31.02 ± 4.17	177.17 ± 4.21	153.27 ± 8.73	126.70 ± 4.24
A8	*1.21 ± 0.51*	*9.06 ± 1.85*	*111.26 ± 21.57*	*10.54 ± 1.11*	*>200*	*>200*	*34.38 ± 9.16*
A9 (HSYA)	*0.17 ± 0.02*	*0.73 ± 0.15*	*49.33 ± 3.28*	*0.14 ± 0.06*	*>200*	*>200*	*9.42 ± 2.26*
A10	39.06 ± 0.09	>200	>200	>200	>200	>200	>200
A11	24.92 ± 4.96	5.45 ± 1.37	>200	64.55 ± 7.71	17.33 ± 0.96	53.17 ± 6.12	16.18 ± 4.30
A12	>200	>200	>200	98.56 ± 12.30	>200	>200	>200
A13	93.00 ± 2.56	10.22 ± 0.65	48.91 ± 4.36	37.12 ± 8.85	21.02 ± 2.31	13.35 ± 2.27	58.52 ± 0.66
A14	>200	>200	>200	>200	>200	>200	>200
A15	>200	>200	>200	>200	>200	127.47 ± 6.55	>200
A16	13.48 ± 2.41	20.29 ± 4.13	46.35 ± 7.05	31.11 ± 3.91	68.48 ± 9.88	41.22 ± 3.18	73.74 ± 13.64
A17	14.92 ± 4.24	32.46 ± 5.79	70.38 ± 1.18	59.17 ± 1.01	>200	21.46 ± 4.50	117.00 ± 6.77
A18	*2.13 ± 0.64*	*4.27 ± 1.30*	*1.79 ± 0.52*	*0.98 ± 0.38*	*4.42 ± 1.31*	*0.12 ± 0.01*	*2.48 ± 0.48*

[#]: Values were obtained from triplicate tests, and presented as mean ± SD. The units of IC$_{50}$ values for CTE, NGTS, and CNP are µg·mL^{-1}, whereas for the 18 single components are µM. Potent inhibitors (IC$_{50}$ < 15 µM for 1A2, 2C9, 2C19, 2D6, 2B6, and 3A4) are presented in italic. For abbreviations of analytes A6–A18, please refer to the Supplementary Materials section.

To identify the major CNP components responsible for the inhibition, 18 representative components from CNP were evaluated by the cocktail assays. The results (Table 2) showed that HSYA and ginsenosides showed high or moderate inhibition activities on the seven CYP450 isozymes. Although flavonoid glycosides showed moderate or weak inhibition activities, or even no inhibition activities (IC_{50} values of >200 μM, Table 2), the flavonoid aglycones quercetin (A16), kaempferol (A17), and 6-hydoxykaempferol (A18), in contrast, exhibited potent inhibitory activities against the seven CYP450 isozymes. In particular, 6-hydroxykaempferol (A18) showed remarkably stronger inhibitory activities on the seven CYP450 isozymes (IC_{50} < 5 μM, Table 2). In conclusion, the ginsenosides GRg_1 (A1), GRb_1 (A2), and GRd (A3), and the flavonoids 6-hydoxykaempferol-3-O-glucoside (A6), kaempferol-3-O-glucoside (A7), anhydroxysafflor yellow B (AHSYB, A8), hydroxysafflor yellow A (HSYA, A9), 6-hydroxykaempferol-3,6-di-O-glucoside (A13), quercetin (A16), kaempferol (A17), and 6-hydroxykaempferol (A18) were presented as being the intensive inhibitors to different CYP450s (IC_{50} ≤ 15 μM). Among them, GRg_1 (A1), GRb_1 (A2), GRd (A3), quercetin (A16), kaempferol (A17), and 6-hydroxykaempferol (A18) were the main active components of CNP for the inhibition of CYP1A2.

3.5. Discussion

Herbal pair, the most fundamental and simplest form of Chinese herbal medicine formula, has been favored for centuries because of its better therapeutic outcomes and fewer side effects [18]. Herein, we primarily aimed to clarify the compatibility mechanisms between NGTS and CTE from PK interactions. Given the low dosage, more efforts were paid onto the detection and quantification of trace CNP-derived components in vivo. We found the injection solvent extensively affected the chromatographic performances. Increasing the injection volume could advance the sensitivity owing to the subjection of larger amounts of analytes [19]. However, the solvent effect might be initiated by directly injecting large volume of solution onto the chromatographic column without any additional treatment. Increasing the flow rate of the mobile phase could guarantee the dilution of the injection solvent and retention of the target analytes, which should be a practical choice to minimize, or even avoid the solvent effect. However, a rapid flow rate gave rise to a higher back pressure. Therefore, the evaporation–reconstitution step often involved loading the sufficient quantity of sample onto the column for LC–MS analysis. Fortunately, the electronic six-port/two-channel valve mounted on the QTRAP system can be applied as a viable solution to split the back pressure. Therefore, LVDI-UHPLC-MS/MS method was proposed. With the LVDI-UHPLC-MS/MS method, the sample can be directly injected into LC-MS analysis without any evaporation–reconstitution step, which is time-consuming and risks crucial chemical degradation during the evaporation procedure. Under the assistance of the injection solvent optimization, the validated LVDI-UHPLC-MS/MS-based method turned out to be extremely sensitive, accurate, and qualified for the bioassay measurement.

The pharmacokinetic results of HSYA, GRg_1, GRe, GRb_1, and NGR_1 indicated that after combination, the absorption of these active components was increased inferred from their higher C_{max} and AUC_{0-t} values over that of the individual extract groups (Table 1). The increment of C_{max} and AUC_{0-t} values suggested that CYP450-mediated HHIs between CTE and NGTS may primarily account for the compatibility mechanisms of CTE and NGTS. An in vitro cocktail assay was then carried out to find the clues being responsible for HHIs between CTE and NGTS. The results showed CNP exhibited more potent inhibition on CYP1A2 (Table 2), the key enzyme involved in the oxidation reactions of most xenobiotics [20], compared with CTE and NGTS. In order to search for the single components contained in CNP responsible for the inhibition of CYP1A2 and other CYP450s, 18 main components from CNP were evaluated for their inhibition on CYP450s.

The results showed that GRg_1 (A1), GRb_1 (A2), GRd (A3), 6-hydoxykaempferol-3-O-glucoside (A6), kaempferol-3-O-glucoside (A7), anhydroxysafflor yellow B (AHSYB, A8), hydroxysafflor yellow A (HSYA, A9), 6-hydroxykaempferol-3,6-di-O-glucoside (A13), quercetin (A16), kaempferol (A17), and 6-hydroxykaempferol (A18) were the main active components for the CYP450 inhibition, and GRg_1

(A1), GRb$_1$ (A2), GRd (A3), quercetin (A16), kaempferol (A17), and 6-hydroxykaempferol (A18) were the main active components for CYP1A2 inhibition.

To further discuss the possibility of in vivo interaction between CTE and NGTS, the inhibitions of GRg$_1$, GRb$_1$, GRd, HSYA, NGR$_1$, and GRe to CYP450s at their C_{max} levels were calculated by their respective "dose–response curve". The results (Table S13) showed GRg$_1$, GRb$_1$, GRd, HSYA, NGR$_1$, and GRe could not significantly inhibit CYP450s at their C_{max} levels, which is in accordance with the results that the combination use of CTE and NGTS can only increase the system exposures of these components to some extent.

4. Conclusions

In conclusion, the findings gained from the comparative pharmacokinetic investigations revealed there were pharmacokinetic interactions between CTE and NGTS, which may explain the integrative mechanisms of CNP and provide the experimental data and theoretical basis for further development and clinical applications of CNP. The developed LVDI-UHPLC-MS/MS method and pharmacokinetic interaction-based strategy provide a viable orientation for the compatibility investigation of herb medicines.

Supplementary Materials: The following are available online at http://www.mdpi.com/1999-4923/12/2/180/s1: Figure S1. The total ion current chromatogram (TIC) of CTE; the corresponding chemical composition information was reported in previous research (Chen, et al., 2014; Analyst 139, 6474–6485). Figure S2. The optimization of sample solvents for the pharmacokinetic analysis (A) and the cocktail assay (B) ($n = 3$). Figure S3. Kinetic profiles for the enzymatic turnover of CYP450-mediated probe reactions. Figure S4. Inhibition curves of the seven positive inhibitors obtained from the substrate cocktail incubation. Table S1. Multiple reaction monitoring transitions and fragmentation parameters of six standards and IS1 for PK analysis. Table S2. Multiple reaction monitoring transitions and fragmentation parameters of seven metabolites and two internal standards (IS2 and IS3) for cocktail assay. Table S3. The instrument stability of the LVDI-UHPLC-MS/MS setup. Table S4. Regression equations, linear ranges, and low limits of quantification (LLOQ) of the six standards in rat plasma for the PK study. Table S5. Intra- and inter-day precisions and determination accuracies of six standards for the pharmacokinetic study. Table S6. Extract recoveries and matrix effects of six target constituents in rat plasma samples for the PK study. Table S7. Stability of the six CNP constituents in rat plasma samples for the PK study. Table S8. Plasma concentration time of the six target constituents after oral administration of CTE, NGTS, and CNP. Table S9. Regression equations, linear ranges, and LLOQs of the seven metabolites for the cocktail analysis. Table S10. Intra- and inter-day precisions and determination accuracies of the seven metabolites for cocktail analysis. Table S11. Extract recoveries and matrix effects of seven target constituents and two ISs for the cocktail analysis. Table S12. Michaelis constant (Km) determined for the enzymatic reaction of the probe substrates and the inhibition IC$_{50}$ values were measured for the positive inhibitors of seven CYP450s. Table S13. Responses (% control) of HSYA, GRb$_1$, GRd, GRe, GRg$_1$, and NGR$_1$ at their C_{max} levels in the rat plasma.

Author Contributions: Conceptualization, P.T. and Y.J.; data curation, J.C.; funding acquisition, X.G. and Y.J.; investigation, J.C., Y.L., M.S., H.M., Y.Q., J.W., and M.L.; methodology, J.C., X.G., Y.L., M.S., and M.Z.; project administration, Y.J.; resources, P.T. and Y.J.; supervision, Y.J.; visualization, J.C.; writing—review and editing, J.C., Y.S., and Y.J. All authors have read and agreed to the published version of the manuscript.

Funding: This work was financially supported by National Natural Science Foundation of China (no. 81573684), Beijing Municipal Science and Technology Project (no. Z181100002218028), and National Key Technology R&D Program "New Drug Innovation" of China (no. 2018ZX09711001-008-003 and 2012ZX09103201-036).

Conflicts of Interest: The authors declare no conflict of interest.

References

1. Han, S.Y.; Li, H.X.; Ma, X.; Zhang, K.; Ma, Z.Z.; Jiang, Y.; Tu, P.F. Evaluation of the anti-myocardial ischemia effect of individual and combined extracts of Panax notoginseng and *Carthamus tinctorius* in rats. *J. Ethnopharmacol.* **2013**, *145*, 722–727. [CrossRef] [PubMed]
2. Meng, Y.; Du, Z.; Li, Y.; Wang, L.; Gao, P.; Gao, X.; Li, C.; Zhao, M.; Jiang, Y.; Tu, P.; et al. Integration of metabolomics with pharmacodynamics to elucidate the anti-myocardial ischemia effects of combination of notoginseng total saponins and safflower total flavonoids. *Front. Pharmacol.* **2018**, *9*, 667. [CrossRef] [PubMed]
3. Han, S.Y.; Li, H.X.; Bai, C.C.; Wang, L.; Tu, P.F. Component analysis and free radical-scavenging potential of Panax notoginseng and *Carthamus tinctorius* extracts. *Chem. Biodivers.* **2010**, *7*, 383–391. [CrossRef] [PubMed]

4. Zhou, D.; Andersson, T.B.; Grimm, S.W. In vitro evaluation of potential drug-drug interactions with ticagrelor: Cytochrome P450 reaction phenotyping, inhibition, induction, and differential kinetics. *Drug Metab. Dispos.* **2011**, *39*, 703–710. [CrossRef] [PubMed]
5. Dong, L.C.; Fan, Y.X.; Yu, Q.; Ma, J.; Dong, X.; Li, P.; Li, H.J. Synergistic effects of rhubarb-gardenia herb pair in cholestatic rats at pharmacodynamic and pharmacokinetic levels. *J. Ethnopharmacol.* **2015**, *175*, 67–74. [CrossRef] [PubMed]
6. Wang, L.; Zhang, D.; Raghavan, N.; Yao, M.; Ma, L.; Frost, C.E.; Maxwell, B.D.; Chen, S.Y.; He, K.; Goosen, T.C.; et al. In vitro assessment of metabolic drug-drug interaction potential of apixaban through cytochrome P450 phenotyping, inhibition, and induction studies. *Drug Metab. Dispos.* **2010**, *38*, 448–458. [CrossRef] [PubMed]
7. Spaggiari, D.; Geiser, L.; Daali, Y.; Rudaz, S. A cocktail approach for assessing the in vitro activity of human cytochrome P450s: An overview of current methodologies. *J. Pharm. Biomed. Anal.* **2014**, *101*, 221–237. [CrossRef] [PubMed]
8. Pharmacopoeia Committee. *Pharmacopoeia of the Peoples's Republic of China*; Part 1; Medical Science and Technology Press: Beijing, China, 2015; pp. 393–394.
9. Chen, J.; Guo, X.; Song, Y.; Zhao, M.; Tu, P.; Jiang, Y. MRM-based strategy for the homolog-focused detection of minor ginsenosides from notoginseng total saponins by ultra-performance liquid chromatography coupled with hybrid triple quadrupole-linear ion trap mass spectrometry. *RSC Adv.* **2016**, *6*, 96376–96388. [CrossRef]
10. Chen, J.; Tu, P.; Jiang, Y. HPLC fingerprint-oriented preparative separation of major flavonoids from safflower extract by preparative pressurized liquid chromatography. *J. Chin. Pharm. Sci.* **2014**, *23*, 6. [CrossRef]
11. Walsky, R.L.; Boldt, S.E. In vitro cytochrome P450 inhibition and induction. *Curr. Drug Metab.* **2008**, *9*, 928–939. [CrossRef] [PubMed]
12. U.S. Food and Drug Administration. Bioanalytical Method Validation Guidance for Industry. 2018. Available online: https://www.fda.gov/regulatory-information/search-fda-guidance-documents/bioanalytical-method-validation-guidance-industry (accessed on 18 February 2020).
13. Tsimidou, M.; Macrae, R. Reversed-phase chromatography of triglycerides-theoretical and practical aspects of the influence of injection solvents. *J. Chromatogr. Sci.* **1985**, *23*, 155–160. [CrossRef] [PubMed]
14. U.S. Food and Drug Administration. Clinical Drug Interaction Studies-Study Design, Data Analysis, and Clinical Implications Guidance for Industry. 2017. Available online: https://www.fda.gov/regulatory-information/search-fda-guidance-documents/clinical-drug-interaction-studies-cytochrome-p450-enzyme-and-transporter-mediated-drug-interactions (accessed on 18 February 2020).
15. Chen, J.F.; Song, Y.L.; Guo, X.Y.; Tu, P.F.; Jiang, Y. Characterization of the herb-derived components in rats following oral administration of *Carthamus tinctorius* extract by extracting diagnostic fragment ions (DFIs) in the MS$^{(n)}$ chromatograms. *Analyst* **2014**, *139*, 6474–6485. [CrossRef] [PubMed]
16. Liu, H.; Yang, J.; Du, F.; Gao, X.; Ma, X.; Huang, Y.; Xu, F.; Niu, W.; Wang, F.; Mao, Y.; et al. Absorption and disposition of ginsenosides after oral administration of *Panax notoginseng* extract to rats. *Drug Metab. Dispos.* **2009**, *37*, 2290–2298. [CrossRef] [PubMed]
17. Hu, Z.; Yang, J.; Cheng, C.; Huang, Y.; Du, F.; Wang, F.; Niu, W.; Xu, F.; Jiang, R.; Gao, X.; et al. Combinatorial metabolism notably affects human systemic exposure to ginsenosides from orally administered extract of *Panax notoginseng* roots (Sanqi). *Drug Metab. Dispos.* **2013**, *41*, 1457–1469. [CrossRef] [PubMed]
18. Ung, C.Y.; Li, H.; Cao, Z.W.; Li, Y.X.; Chen, Y.Z. Are herb-pairs of traditional Chinese medicine distinguishable from others? Pattern analysis and artificial intelligence classification study of traditionally defined herbal properties. *J. Ethnopharmacol.* **2007**, *111*, 371–377. [CrossRef] [PubMed]
19. Song, Y.; Zhang, N.; Jiang, Y.; Li, J.; Zhao, Y.; Shi, S.; Tu, P. Simultaneous determination of aconite alkaloids and ginsenosides using online solid phase extraction hyphenated with polarity switching ultra-high performance liquid chromatography coupled with tandem mass spectrometry. *RSC Adv.* **2015**, *5*, 6419–6428. [CrossRef]
20. Rendic, S.; Guengerich, F.P. Survey of human oxidoreductases and cytochrome p450 enzymes involved in the metabolism of xenobiotic and natural chemicals. *Chem. Res. Toxicol.* **2015**, *28*, 38–42. [CrossRef] [PubMed]

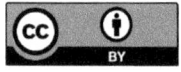

© 2020 by the authors. Licensee MDPI, Basel, Switzerland. This article is an open access article distributed under the terms and conditions of the Creative Commons Attribution (CC BY) license (http://creativecommons.org/licenses/by/4.0/).

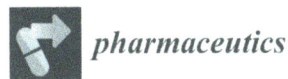

Article

In-Depth Characterization of EpiIntestinal Microtissue as a Model for Intestinal Drug Absorption and Metabolism in Human

Yunhai Cui [1,*], Stephanie Claus [2], David Schnell [1], Frank Runge [1] and Caroline MacLean [2]

1 Department of Drug Discovery Sciences, Boehringer Ingelheim Pharma GmbH & Co KG, 88397 Biberach, Germany
2 Department of Drug Metabolism and Pharmacokinetics, Boehringer Ingelheim Pharma GmbH & Co KG, 88397 Biberach, Germany
* Correspondence: yunhai.cui@boehringer-ingelheim.com; Tel.: +49-7351-54-92193

Received: 6 April 2020; Accepted: 27 April 2020; Published: 28 April 2020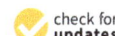

Abstract: The Caco-2 model is a well-accepted in vitro model for the estimation of fraction absorbed in human intestine. Due to the lack of cytochrome P450 3A4 (CYP3A4) activities, Caco-2 model is not suitable for the investigation of intestinal first-pass metabolism. The purpose of this study is to evaluate a new human intestine model, EpiIntestinal microtissues, as a tool for the prediction of oral absorption and metabolism of drugs in human intestine. The activities of relevant drug transporters and drug metabolizing enzymes, including MDR1 P-glycoprotein (P-gp), breast cancer resistance protein (BCRP), CYP3A4, CYP2J2, UDP-glucuronosyltransferases (UGT), carboxylesterases (CES), etc., were detected in functional assays with selective substrates and inhibitors. Compared to Caco-2, EpiIntestinal microtissues proved to be a more holistic model for the investigation of drug absorption and metabolism in human gastrointestinal tract.

Keywords: Caco-2; EpiIntestinal; first-pass; P-gp; BCRP; drug transporter; CYP3A4; UDP-glucuronosyltransferase; carboxylesterase; oral availability

1. Introduction

Despite the recent innovations in drug delivery, oral administration remains the major route of drug administration. Understanding the drug absorption and metabolism in the intestine is thus essential for drug development. To date, several in vitro or ex vivo models are available for the evaluation of drug absorption and metabolism in human intestine. The Caco-2 cell culture model, e.g., is considered the gold standard in vitro model for studies of drug absorption, although there are limitations of this model with regards to drug metabolism [1,2]. Although a number of drug metabolizing enzymes (DME) have been identified in Caco-2 cells, including UDP glucuronosyltransferases (UGT) [3] and carboxylesterases (CES) [4], cytochrome P450 3A4 (CYP3A4), the major drug metabolizing enzyme in human intestine and liver is missing in Caco-2 cells [5]. Alternatively, sections of human intestinal tissue or mucosal biopsy mounted in Ussing chamber can be used to study drug absorption and metabolism in human intestine [6]. The advantage of this method is the combined measurement of permeability/active transport and metabolism. However, throughput, cost and availability of human tissues limit the routine use of this model. In order to integrate CYP3A4 activities into Caco-2 model, Takenaka et al. co-expressed recombinant human CYP3A4 and NADPH-CYP P450 reductase in Caco-2 cells [7]. Although a good correlation between extraction ratios observed in vitro and the gastro-intestinal (GI) extraction ratios in human could be observed for a number of reference compounds, the in vitro model tend to underestimate the GI extraction, indicating a rather low CYP3A4 activity in the model. Since

CYP3A4 activities are readily detected in microsomes prepared from liver or intestine, Gertz et al. used another approach to improve the predictivity of firstpass extraction in human by combining the metabolic clearance of CYP3A4 compounds measured in human intestinal microsomes and the permeability data from Caco-2 or MDCK-MDR1 assay [8]. A clear disadvantage of this approach is that two separate in vitro measurements are needed. In recent years, new in vitro models for human intestine like microfluidic tissue-on-chip [9] or organoids [10] are emerging. These models have been shown as useful models for testing compound toxicity in GI tract or as disease models [9,10]. As an ADME model for human gut, however, a tissue model on a Transwell basis would be more favorable because the equipment for Caco-2 permeability assay could be easily adapted to the new model and would enable the measurement of transcellular permeability and transport in the new model. Two such models have been published recently with basic characterization regarding drug transporters and DMEs: The EpiIntestinal microtissues provided by MatTek [11] and the 3D bioprinted human intestinal tissues provided by Organovo [12]. Due to the earlier availability and easier accessibility we decided to evaluate the EpiIntestinal model as an ADME tool in more detail. The aim of the present study is the in-depth characterization of the EpiIntestinal microtissues as a model for the investigation of activities of drug transporters and DME and for the prediction of GI firstpass availability in human.

2. Materials and Methods

2.1. Material

All marketed drugs used in this manuscript and the metabolites and the deuterated standards thereof are purchased from commercial providers (Sigma, LKT laboratories, Roche, BD Gentest, Toronto Research, Cerilliant or Syncom). Dabigatran etexilate and its metabolites BIBR 951, BIBR 953, BIBR 1087 and internal research compounds of Boehringer Ingelheim are provided by the internal compound management.

2.2. Cell Culture

Caco-2 cells were obtained from Leibniz Institute DSMZ-German Collection of Microorganisms and Cell Cultures (Braunschweig, Germany) and cultured in DMEM containing 10% FCS, 1% NEAA, 2 mM Glutamin, 100 U/mL Penicillin and 100 µg/mL Streptomycin. Caco-2 cells were seeded either onto 24-well Transwell inserts (Corning, #3379) for bidirectional permeability assays or onto 96-well Transwell inserts (Corning #3391) for the screening of DME activities at a density of 160,000 cells/cm^2 and cultured for 3 weeks, with media change on every second day. EpiIntestinal microtissues were obtained from MatTek (Bratislav, Slovakia) and cultured according to the manufacturer's instruction (24-well format for bidirectional permeability assays and GI firstpass availability assays and 96-well format for screening of DME activities).

2.3. Bidirectional Permeability Assay

Bidirectional permeability assays were performed as described previously [13,14]. Briefly, compounds were diluted in transport buffer (128.13 mM NaCl, 5.36 mM KCl, 1 mM MgSO$_4$, 1.8 mM CaCl$_2$, 4.17 mM NaHCO$_3$, 1.19 mM Na$_2$HPO$_4$, 0.41 mM NaH$_2$PO$_4$, 15 mM 2-[4-(2-hydroxyethyl)piperazin-1-yl]ethanesulfonic acid (HEPES), 20 mM glucose, pH 7.4) containing 0.25% bovine serum albumin to a final concentration of 10 µM and added to the apical or basal compartment. In indicated experiments, inhibitors were added to both compartments. Cells were incubated with the compounds for up to 2 h. Samples from the opposite compartment were taken at different timepoints. Compound concentrations in the samples were determined by HPLC-MS/MS (standard equipment: HPLC series 1000 or higher from Agilent, Santa Clara, CA, USA, and mass spectrometers API 4000 or higher from AB Sciex, Toronto, ON, Canada). Prior to bioanalysis samples were spiked with internal standard solution and diluted with acetonitrile (ACN) for protein precipitation. Measurement was operated in multiple reaction monitoring (MRM) mode. Quantification was performed using external calibration. Apparent permeability coefficients in the apical to basal direction ($P_{app,AB}$) and in the basal to apical direction ($P_{app,BA}$) and efflux were calculated as follows

$$P_{app,AB} = \frac{Q_{AB}}{(C_0 \times s \times t)}$$

$$P_{app,BA} = \frac{Q_{BA}}{(C_0 \times s \times t)}$$

$$Efflux = \frac{P_{app,BA}}{P_{app,AB}}$$

where Q is the amount of compound recovered in the receiver compartment after the incubation time t, C_0 the initial compound concentration given to the donor compartment, and s the surface area of the Transwell inserts. Efflux ratio is calculated as the quotient of $P_{app,BA}$ to $P_{app,AB}$. As quality controls, one reference P-gp substrate (apafant) and one low permeable compound (BI internal reference, $P_{app} \approx 3 \times 10^{-7}$ cm/s, no efflux) is included in every assay plate. In addition, Transepithelial electrical resistance (TEER) values are measured for each plate before the permeability assay and total recovery in donor and receiver compartments was determined for each compound. All these parameters (efflux of apafant, P_{app} values of the low permeable compound, TEER values, and total recovery) are used to ensure the quality of the assays.

2.4. Measurement of DME Activities in EpiIntestinal and Caco-2

For measurements of DME activities in EpiIntestinal microtissues and Caco-2 cells, both were cultured in 96-well Transwell inserts. Drugs (Table 1) were dissolved in the respective solvent at 200× concentration and diluted in a pre-warmed transport buffer. Diluted substrate solution was applied to the apical (100 µL) and basal (250 µL) compartment of the Transwell and incubated at 37 °C and 5% CO_2 and 60 rpm continuous shaking. DME activities were determined by monitoring metabolite formation in basal compartment over time (0, 0.5, 1, 2, 3 and 4 h) with LC-MS/MS. For LC-MS/MS, an HTS-xt PAL autosampler (CTC Analytics), LC 1290 infinity G4220A (Agilent Technologies), column oven (Agilent Technologies) and 6500 TripleQuad (AB Sciex) were used. Chromatographic separation of samples was performed on YMC Triart C18 (1.9 µm, 30 × 2 mm; YMC Europe, Dinslaken, Germany) LC analytical column. Quantification of all metabolites listed in Table 1 was achieved by the use of calibration curves for the individual metabolites with appropriate concentration ranges.

Table 1. Drugs applied for drug metabolizing enzymes (DME) activity screen.

Drug	DME/Metabolite	Internal Standard	Drug Concentration (µM)	Solvent
Phenacetin	CYP1A2/Acetaminophen	d4-Acetaminophen	10–100	20% ACN
Bupropion	CYP2B6/2-OH-Bupropion	d8-OH-bupropion	15–300	Aqua bidest.
Amodiaquine	CYP2C8/OH-Desethyl-Amodiaquine	d5-Desethylamodiaquine	20–200	Aqua bidest.
Diclofenac	CYP2C9/4-OH-Diclofenac	(13C6)4'-OH-Diclofenac	20–200	20% ACN
S-Mephenytoin	CYP2C19/4-OH-Mephenytoin	d3-OH-Mephenytoin	20–200	40% ACN
Testosterone	CYP3A4/6β-OH-Testosterone	d3-6β-OH-Testosterone	40–400	ACN/MeOH
Midazolam	CYP3A4/1-OH-Midazolam	d4-1-OH-Midazolam	5–100	Ready-to-use solution
Dextromethorphan	CYP2D6 Dextrorphan	d3-Dextrorphan	10–100	Aqua bidest.
7-OH-Coumarin	UGT/7-OH-Coumarin-Glucuronid	α-Naphtylglucuronid	15–150	40% ACN
7-OH-Coumarin	SULT/7-OH-Coumarin-Sulfat	α-Naphtylglucuronid	15–150	40% ACN
β-Estradiol	UGT1A1/β-Estradiol-3-Glucuronid	α-Naphtylglucuronid	20–200	DMSO
Astemizol	CYP2J2/O-Desmethyl-Astemizol	Dextrorphan tartrate	2–50	30% ACN + 10 mM HCl
BIBF1120	CES/BIBF1202	d8-BIBF1202	10–100	ACN/MeOH

A total of 10 µL of the incubation sample were diluted with 90 µL of water containing 10–20% ACN or methanol, 0.1% formic acid and the respective internal standard. To analyze the intracellular metabolite concentration, cells on Transwell inserts were washed twice with ice-cold PBS and stored at −80 °C for 20 min. Afterwards, 150 µL 50% ACN diluted with transport buffer was added to the cells and incubated at room temperature for 30 min. Cell lysate was transferred to a fresh 96-well plate and centrifuged at 4 °C, 4000 rpm for 10 min. Subsequently, 10 µL of the supernatant were diluted with 90 µl water containing 10–20% ACN or methanol, 0.1% formic acid and the respective internal standard. A total of 2 µL sample was injected into the LC-MS/MS system operated with an electrospray ionization source.

2.5. CES-Mediated Metabolism of Dabigatran Etexilate

CES-mediated metabolism of dabigatran etexilate was measured in cryopreserved human hepatocytes (BioIVT, West Sussex, UK) and cryopreserved human intestinal mucosa (in vitro ADMET laboratories, Columbia, MD, USA) in suspension and in Caco-2 cells and EpiIntestinal microtissues grown on Transwell inserts. Dabigatran etexilate was diluted in culture media for the respective cells or tissues. The final concentrations of dabigatran etexilate were selected in an earlier experiment to ensure reasonable turnover of the compound within the incubation time: 2 µM for hepatocytes and intestinal mucosa, 10 µM for Caco-2 and EpiIntestinal microtissues. In the experiments with Transwell inserts, dabigatran etexilate was given to the apical compartments, metabolites were measured in the basal (receiver) compartments. Concentrations of the metabolites were determined by HPLC-MS/MS (Section 2.3).

2.6. Metabolite Identification

Raloxifene or ezetimibe (10 µM) in culture media was added to the apical compartment of EpiIntestinal microtissues or incubated with cryopreserved human intestinal mucosa (HIM). Samples from basal compartment of EpiIntestinal microtissues or lysates of the incubation mixture with mucosa were prepared for metabolite identification as follows: samples were mixed with the same amount of 0.1% formic acid in ACN and subsequently evaporated and resuspended in water containing 25% methanol and 0.1% formic acid. Analysis was performed on a LC-MS system containing a Vanquish UPLC (ThermoFisher Scientific, San Jose, CA, USA) coupled to an Orbitrap FusionTribrid high resolution mass spectrometer (ThermoFisher Scientific). Structure elucidation was based on exact mass measurements in combination with the interpretation of fragment spectra.

2.7. Measurement of Intestinal First-Pass Availability in EpiIntestinal Microtissues and Caco-2

Compounds were diluted in culture media to a final concentration of 10 µM and added to the apical (donor) compartment (total volume: 100 µL for EpiIntestinal and 200 µL for Caco-2). After the incubation at 37 °C for 2, 4, 6, and 24 h, samples (50 µL) were taken from the basal (receiver) compartment (total volume: 5000 µL for EpiIntestinal and 800 µL for Caco-2). After the last timepoint, samples from the donor compartments and the cell lysates were also collected. Compound concentrations in the samples were determined by HPLC-MS/MS (Section 2.3).

GI first-pass availability of the tested compounds was expressed as fraction (%) of the total amount of a compound added to the donor compartment recovered in the receiver compartment.

2.8. Calculation of $F_a \times F_g$ in Human

The first-pass GI availability ($F_a \times F_g$) of selected drugs was calculated using the equation:

$$F_a \times F_g = F/F_h$$

where F is the total oral availability, F_a the fraction absorbed, F_g the intestinal availability and F_h the hepatic availability. The hepatic availability F_g can be estimated with the equation:

$$F_g = 1 - CL_h/Q_H$$

where CL_h is the hepatic clearance of a drug and Q_H the hepatic blood flow in human (20.7 mL/min/kg). The hepatic clearance CL_h is calculated with the equation:

$$CL_h = CL_b \times (1 - f_e)$$

where CL_b is the blood clearance of a drug and f_e the fraction of renal excretion. Blood CL_b can be converted from plasma clearance CL_p with the blood-to-plasma ratio R_B:

$$CL_b = CL_p / R_B$$

A set of 12 marketed drugs are selected for the evaluation of EpiIntestinal microtissues. The clinical data for the calculation of $F_a \times F_g$ are summarized in Table 2.

Table 2. Clinical pharmacokinetic data of the selected drugs for the calculation of $F_a \times F_g$. Data sources are indicated. Due to a lack of literature data or conflicting data in the literature, R_B values for several compounds are measured in-house (#).

Drug	F	R_B	CL_p (mL/min/kg)	f_e
Atenolol	0.5 [8]	0.95 #	2.5 [15]	1 [16]
Atorvastatin	0.14 [17]	0.85 #	8.93 [8]	0.01 [18]
Buspirone	0.05 [8]	0.81 [8]	28.3 [8]	0.45 [19]
Felodipine	0.15 [8]	0.7 [8]	11 [15]	0 [16]
Indinavir	0.6 [8]	0.84 [8]	18 [20]	0.085 [16]
Irinotecan	0.25 [8]	0.82 [21]	7 [15]	0.32 [16]
Midazolam	0.4 [8]	0.64 #	5.3 [15]	0 [16]
Nifedipine	0.9 [8]	0.67 [8]	7.3 [15]	0 [16]
Oxybutynin	0.06 [8]	0.686 [22]	5.1 [15]	0 *
Quinidine	0.9 [8]	0.87 [8]	4 [15]	0.15 [16]
Rosuvastatin	0.2 [8]	0.75 #	11 [23]	0.3 [23]
Saquinavir	0.04 [8]	0.74 [8]	13 [15]	0.01 *

* Prescription information at fda.gov.

3. Results

3.1. Barrier Function and Transporter Activities

EpiIntestinal microtissues as an intestinal permeability model have been tested in detail by Ayehunie et al. [11]. Our evaluation with in-house compounds and reference drugs (atenolol, fexofenadine, dabigatran, dabigatran etexilate, fenoterol, and otenzepad) showed similar data (not shown). However, the drug rosuvastatin which was used as a P-gp model drug by Ayehunie et al. [11] showed different results in our hands. Both in Caco-2 cells and in EpiIntestinal microtissues, the selective BCRP inhibitor Ko-143 (3 µM) strongly reduced the efflux of rosuvastatin, whereas the selective P-gp inhibitor zosuquidar (5 µM) only showed a minor effect on the efflux of rosuvastatin (Table 3). These data indicate BCRP as the major transporter in both in vitro models.

Table 3. Inhibition of transporter-mediated efflux of rosuvastatin in Caco-2 and EpiIntestinal microtissues. Data are mean values of duplicates (Caco-2) or triplicates (EpiIntestinal microtissues).

Substrate	Inhibitor	Caco-2		EpiIntestinal	
		PappAB (10^{-6} cm/s)	Efflux	PappAB (10^{-6} cm/s)	Efflux
Rosuvastatin	None	0.3	21.0	0.3	100.0
	Ko-143 (3 µM)	0.5	5.5	2.6	3.1
	Zosuqidar (5 µM)	0.3	19.0	0.9	25

3.2. Drug-Metabolising Enzymes (DME) in EpiIntestinal Microtissues

We studied the effect of DME on the GI first-pass availability with two model drugs: Midazolam for CYP3A4 [24] and astemizole for CYP2J2 [25,26]. As shown in Figure 1, midazolam showed a lower availability in EpiIntestinal microtissues than in Caco-2 (recovery in basal/receiver compartment after 24 h: 46.7% vs. 81.0%) when added to the apical compartment of both models. The addition of the covalent CYP3A4 inhibitor CYP3cide [27] increased the availability of midazolam in EpiIntestinal microtissues (46.7% vs. 75.9%), but had almost no effect on the availability in Caco-2 (81.0% vs. 87.9%). Moreover, substantial amount of 1-hydroxymidazolam, the CYP3A4-selective metabolite of midazolam, was detected in EpiIntestinal microtissues and was suppressed by the addition of the selective inhibitor, whereas only a negligible amount of the metabolite was detected in Caco-2, consistent with the low level of CYP3A4 expression in this cell line.

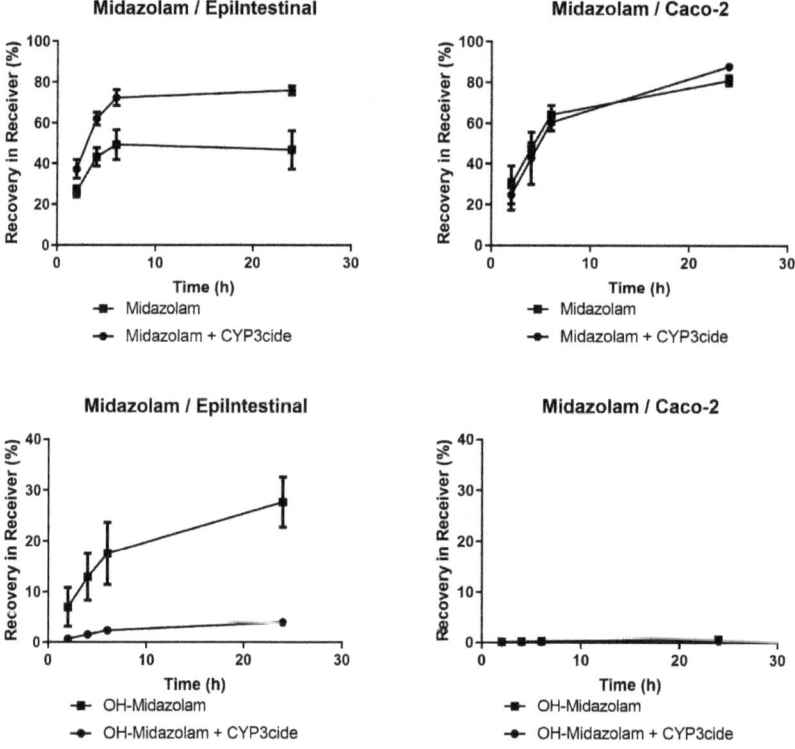

Figure 1. Apical-to-basal transport of midazolam in EpiIntestinal microtissues and Caco-2 cells. Midazolam (10 µM) was added to the apical compartment of EpiIntestinal microtissues (**left panels**) or Caco-2 cells (**right panels**) grown on Transwell inserts and incubated at 37 °C. At the time points as indicated, samples were taken from the basal (receiver) compartment. Midazolam (**upper panels**) and 1-Hydroxymidazolam (**lower panels**) were quantified in the samples via HPLC-MS/MS. The incubation was carried out in the absence or in the presence of the selective covalent CYP3A inhibitor CYP3acide (1 µM). Data are shown as mean values of triplicates. Error bars show standard deviations.

In contrast to CYP3A4, CYP2J2 activities were readily detected both in EpiIntestinal microtissues and in Caco-2 (Figure 2). In both models, co-incubation with the CYP2J2 inhibitor Ebastein (50 µM) [26] increased the availability of astemizole in the receiver compartment.

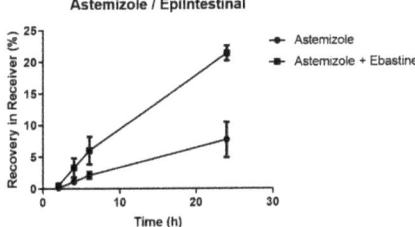
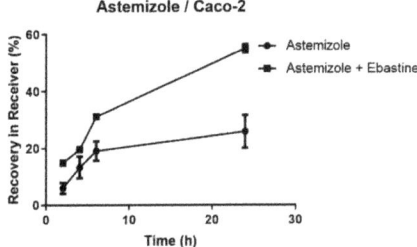

Figure 2. Apical-to-basal transport of astemizole in EpiIntestinal microtissues and Caco-2 cells. Astemizole (10 μM) was added to the apical compartment of EpiIntestinal microtissues (**left**) or Caco-2 cells (**right**) grown on Transwell inserts and incubated at 37 °C. At the indicated timepoints, samples were taken from the basal (receiver) compartment. Astemizole was quantified in the samples via HPLC-MS/MS. The incubation was carried out in the absence or in the presence of the competitive CYP2J2 inhibitor Ebastine (50 μM). Data are shown as mean values of triplicates. Error bars show standard deviations.

Encouraged by the results regarding CYP3A4 and CYP2J2 activities, we screened the activities of DME in EpiIntestinal microtissues more systematically: we quantified the formation of selective metabolite of the respective enzymes at different substrate concentrations (Figure S1). The substrate concentration approaching enzyme saturation (marked dots in Figure S1) was subsequently used to compare the activities in EpiIntestinal microtissues and Caco-2 cells. As shown in Table 4, the most prominent difference in DME activities between both models are the CYP3A4 activities, which could be demonstrated by two different substrates (testosterone and midazolam). In addition, CYP1A2 is the only enzyme with much lower activities in EpiIntestinal than in Caco-2 cells. Furthermore, we measured all metabolites also in the cell lysate. Some of the metabolites showed substantial intracellular accumulation. In order to monitor batch variability with regard to DME activities, experiments shown in Table 4 were repeated with microtissues from a different batch with comparable results (not shown).

Table 4. Determination of activities of DMEs in EpiIntestinal microtissues and Caco-2 cells. Enzyme activities in EpiIntestinal microtissues and Caco-2 cells in 96-well Transwell plates were measured with the respective substrates shown in Figure S1 and at the marked concentration. Data shown as mean and SD from triplicates.

DME/Substrate	Caco-2		EpiIntestinal	
	Enzyme Activities * (pmol/h/cm^2) Mean/SD	>Intracellular Metabolite (% of Total)	Enzyme Activities * (pmol/h/cm^2) Mean/SD	Intracellular Metabolite (% of Total)
CYP1A2/Phenacetin	123.1/4.8	BLQ	17.4/3.0	BLQ
CYP2B6/Bupropion	BLQ	BLQ	2.6/0.9	BLQ
CYP2C8/Amodiaquine	11.2/1.9	36.5	107.9/49.1	37.5
CYP2C9/Diclofenac	20.8/1.6	12.8	28.4/1.6	14.7
CYP2C19/S-Mephenytoin	7.1/0.7	4.5	6.9/0.7	4.3
CYP3A4/Testosterone	26.5/3.6	BLQ	176.4/8.0	0.9
CYP3A4/Midazolam	BLQ	BLQ	1.9/0.5	14.9
CYP2D6/Dextromethorphan	10.9/2.7	BLQ	9.2/1.3	BLQ
UGT/7-OH-Coumarin	10,770.5/721.9	5.5	7583.4/855.2	10.0
SULT/7-OH-Coumarin	508.0/46.1	BLQ	1747.4/140.0	3.4
UGT1A1/β-Estradiol	65.3/6.9	3.2	243.3/6.7	2.8
CYP2J2/Astemizole	4.9/0.3	62.9	17.7/5.2	68.7
CES/BIBF 1120	370.9/31.4	24.7	400.0/12.9	13.3

* Determined as the rate of metabolite formation in supernatant; BLQ: Below limit of quantification.

3.3. Differential Expression of CES1 and CES2 in EpiIntestinal Microtissues and Caco-2 cells

Ishiguro et al. reported that Caco-2 cells, albeit originated from human colorectal carcinoma, resemble rather hepatocytes with regard to expression of the isoforms CES1 and CES2 [4]: Whereas CES2 is predominantly expressed in human intestine, CES1 is the major esterase in human hepatocytes and Caco-2 cells. In order to profile EpiIntestinal microtissues in this regard, we investigated the metabolism of dabigatran etexilate, the same substrate used by Ishiguro et al., in human hepatocytes (huHEP), cryopreserved human intestinal mucosa (HIM), Caco-2 cells and EpiIntestinal microtissues. The metabolic pathway for dabigatran etexilate is depicted in Figure 3a: the formation of the intermediate metabolite BIBR 1087 from the double prodrug dabigatran etexilate and the formation of the active drug from the intermediate metabolite BIBR 951 is catalyzed by CES1. The formation of BIBR 951 from dabigatran etexilate and the formation of the active drug BIBR 953 from BIBR 1087 is catalyzed by CES2. In tissues and cells with predominant expression of CES1 (liver e.g.,), BIBR 1087 should be the major metabolite; in tissues and cells with predominant expression of CES2, BIBR 951 should be the major metabolite (e.g., intestine). As shown in Figure 3b, in human hepatocytes and human intestinal mucosa, the expected metabolite pattern was observed—BIBR 1087 as the main metabolite in hepatocytes, and BIBR 951 as the main metabolite in human intestinal mucosa. Consistent with the data by Ishiguro et al., BIBR 1087 was found to be the main metabolite in Caco-2 cells. Interestingly, the metabolite pattern of dabigatran etexilate in EpiIntestinal microtissues resembles none of the other three models. The active drug BIBR 953 was found as the main metabolite in EpiIntestinal microtissues, suggesting similar CES1 and CES2 enzyme activities in this model.

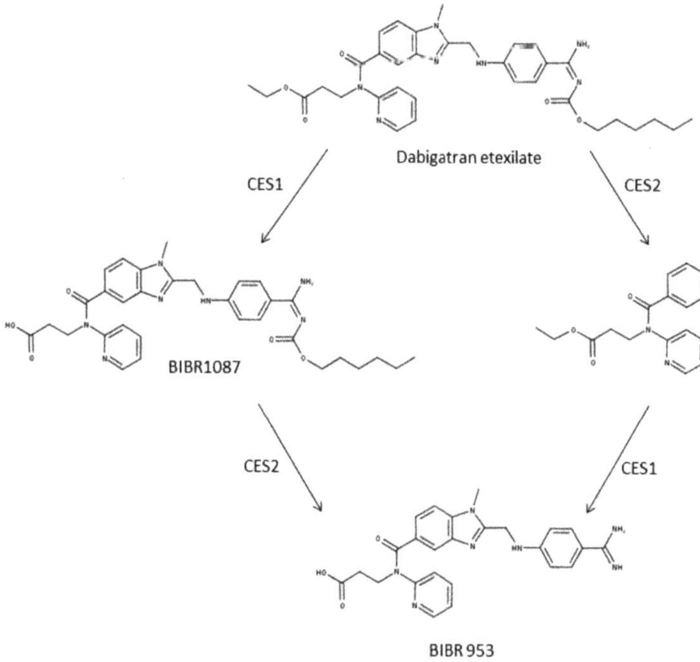

(a)

Figure 3. Cont.

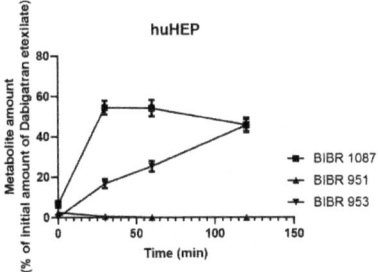
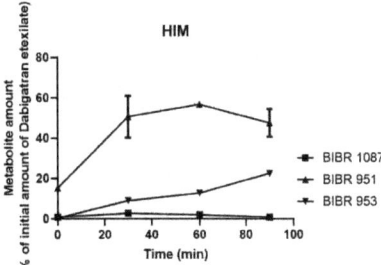
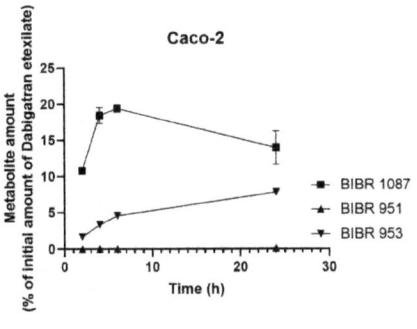
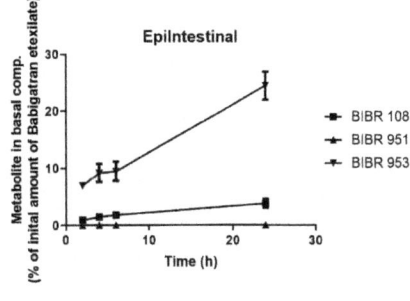

(b)

Figure 3. Metabolic pathways and metabolite pattern of dabigatran etexilate. (**a**) Metabolic pathways of dabigatran involving CES1 and CES2. (**b**) Detection of metabolites of dabigatran etexilate in human hepatocytes (huHEP), human intestinal mucosa (HIM), Caco-2 cells, and EpiIntestinal microtissues. Dabigatran was incubated with hepatocytes and intestinal mucosa in suspension, or given to the apical compartment of Caco-2 cells and EpiIntestinal microtissues and incubated at 37 °C. At the indicated timepoints, samples were taken from the suspension of huHEP and HIM or from the basal compartments of Caco-2 cells and EpiIntestinal microtissues. The metabolites were quantified using LC-MS/MS. Data shown as the mean and SD of triplicates.

3.4. UGT and SULT Activities in EpiIntestinal Microtissues

Extensive glucuronidation in the intestine is one of the major reasons that hamper the oral availability of drugs. Raloxifene and ezetimibe are two examples showing extensive intestinal glucuronidation in human [28–30]. When given to the apical compartment of EpiIntestinal microtissues, two putative glucuronides for both drugs were detected by mass scan (Table 5). We could confirm that these are glucuronides of both drugs by digestion with β-glucuronidase (data not shown). For ezetimibe, glucuronidation was the only metabolism found in EpiIntestinal microtissues. In case of raloxifene, we found an unexpectedly high amount of sulfation products of raloxifene (Table 5). To verify the physiological relevance of this finding, we performed metabolite identification for both drugs also with cryopreserved human intestinal mucosa. As shown in Table 5, the metabolite patterns of both drugs are similar in EpiIntestinal and in HIM: glucuronidation only for ezetimibe; glucuronidation and sulfation for raloxifene.

Table 5. EpiIntestinal microtissues and HIM were incubated with 10 μM ezetimibe or raloxifene. Metabolite scan was performed as described in "Materials and Methods". Amount (Peak areas) of parent drugs and metabolites at the end of the incubation was expressed as percent of peak areas of parent drugs at the beginning of the incubation (T0).

Substrate	EpiIntestinal		Human Intestinal Mucosa (HIM)	
	Ezetimibe	Raloxifene	Ezetimibe	Raloxifene
Parent (% of parent drug at T0)	8.4	2.4	40.3	33.2
Glucuronides (% of parent drug at T0)	39.1	2.2	58.6	18.7
Sulfates (% of parent drug at T0)	n.d.	14.1	n.d.	2.0

n.d.: Not detectable.

3.5. Prediction of $F_a \times F_g$ in Human using EpiIntestinal Microtissues

Since most of the relevant drug transporters and DMEs are present in EpiIntestinal microtissues, we were interested in finding out whether this model could serve as an in vitro model for the prediction of GI firstpass availability of drugs in human ($F_a \times F_g$). For this purpose, we selected a panel of reference drugs with known human data and measured the recovery of these drugs in the basal compartment (equivalent to portal vene) after adding the drugs to the apical compartment (equivalent to GI lumen). The data are summarized in Table 6. We observed a good agreement between the recovery of the drugs in basal compartment of EpiIntestinal microtissues and the $F_a \times F_g$ in human.

Table 6. Comparison of GI firstpass availability measured in EpiIntestinal microtissues and $F_a \times F_g$ in human. GI firstpass availability in EpiIntestinal microtissues was determined as described in 2.7. $F_a \times F_g$ in human for the tested drugs was calculated from the clinical pharmacokinetic data, as described in Section 2.8.

Drug	Recovery in Basal Comp. @ 24h (%)	$F_a \times F_g$ in Human (%)	DMEs/Transporters
Atenolol	86	50	
Atorvastatin	43	61	CYP3A4/BCRP/MRP2
Buspirone	60	70	CYP3A4
Felodipine	47	62	CYP3A4
Indinavir	53	100	CYP3A4
Irinotecan	62	39	Esterases, CYP3A4
Midazolam	47	59	CYP3A4
Nifedipine	110	100	CYP3A4
Oxybutynin	16	9	Esterases, CYP3A4
Quinidine	85	100	CYP3A4, etc.
Rosuvastatin	30	62	CYP2C9/BCRP/MRP2
Saquinavir	18	25	CYP3A4/P-gp

4. Discussion

At present, the Caco-2 cell culture model is the most accepted in vitro model in the pharmaceutical industry for the estimation of drug absorption in human intestine. The lack of the major drug metabolizing enzyme CYP3A4, however, hampers the use of this model for the holistic understanding of drug absorption and metabolism during the first-pass GI transition. Recently, Ayehunie et al. described a new organotypic 3D human intestine model, the EpiIntestinal microtissues, with combined barrier/drug transproter functions and DME activities [11]. In this work, we could confirm the intact barrier function of the EpiIntestinal microtissues with transepithelial electrical resistance (TEER) measurement and with the permeability data of reference drugs and in-house compounds (data not shown). However, our data did not agree with the conclusion by Ayehunie et al. that rosuvastatin is a P-gp substrate. In our opinion, the discordance was mainly due to the different interpretation of the inhibition by Elacridar. Elacridar (GF120918) is a nonselective inhibitor for both BCRP [31] and P-gp [32]. At the concentration of 10 μM used by Ayehunie et al., a strong inhibition of both BCRP and P-gp can be expected. Thus, the inhibition of rosuvastatin efflux by Elacridar cannot be unequivocally attributed to P-gp inhibition. In contrast, the inhibitors we were using in this study are selective [31,33]. Our in-house evaluation showed that, at the concentrations we were using here (5 µM zosuquidar and 3 µM Ko-143), differential inhibition of P-gp and BCRP can be achieved. As shown in Table 3, only Ko-143 reduced in Caco-2 and EpiIntestinal rosuvastatin efflux strongly. Involvement of multiple transporters has been reported in the hepatobiliary transport of rosuvastatin, including OATP1B1, OATP1B3, OATP2B1, MRP2 (ABCC2), MDR1 P-gp (ABCB1), and BCRP (ABCG2) [34]. Except OATP1B1 and OATB1B3, all other transporters are expressed also in human intestine and Caco-2 cells [35–37]. In the clinic, however, only BCRP interaction has been related to increased bioavailability of rosuvastatin [38]. Our results here are in agreement with the clinical observation.

EpiIntestinal microtissues are an improved in vitro model for the intestinal barrier function. A clear advantage of this model over the Caco-2 cellular model is the physiologically relevant activities of CYP3A4 (Figure 1 and Table 4), which accounts for about 80% of total CYP content in human small intestine [39]. We could also detect activities of CYP2B6, CYP2C8, CYP2C9, 2C19, 2D6 and 2J2 in EpiIntestinal microtissues (Table 4), as reported for human intestine [39]. CYP1A2 activity, which is very low in human intestine, were detected in both in vitro models, with Caco-2 showing seven-fold higher activity (Table 4), suggesting that EpiIntestinal microtissues are closer to human intestine. Moreover, enzymes involved in phase 2 biotransformation (UGTs and SULTs) and carboxylesterases are present in EpiIntestinal microtissues at substantial levels (Tables 4 and 5, Figure 3). It is important to note that we measured the respective metabolites of the tested reference drugs both in supernatant and in cell lysate. With the exception of amodiaquine and astemizole, the intracellular accumulation of metabolites was rather low. Since the intracellular accumulation of all measured metabolites is comparable in Caco-2 cells and in EpiIntestinal microtissues, we do not expect a bias in the relative comparison of enzyme activities between Caco-2 and EpiIntesitnal by measuring the metabolite in supernatant only (as shown in Table 4). In the case of carboxylesterase activities, we could demonstrate that EpiIntestinal microtissues are closer to human intestinal mucosa compared to Caco-2 cells, which resemble rather hepatocytes regarding relative CES1/CES2 activities. Because of the rather comprehensive expression of DMEs, EpiIntestinal microtissues can serve as a useful tool for the identification of intestine-specific metabolites, as we demonstrated with raloxifene and ezetimibe (Table 6). One surprising finding was the identification of sulfation of raloxifene not only in EpiIntestinal microtissue, but also in primary human intestinal mucosa. Mono- and diglucuronides were found in human plasma as major metabolites after oral administration; no other metabolites were identified (Prescription information for Evista, Eli Lilly). However, raloxifene was identified as a substrate for various SULTs and the sulfation of raloxifene occurs during incubation with cytosols from human liver and intestine [40,41] and in Caco-2 cells [42]. Moreover, raloxifene is reported to be a potent competitive inhibitor of sulfotransferase 2A1 (SULT2A1) with a K_i value very similar to its K_m value for SULT2A1 [41,43]. The sulfation of raloxifene we observed in EpiIntestinal microtissues was in line with the reported in vitro data in the literature and was obviously not due to a biased expression of SULTs in this model. A possible explanation for the missing raloxifene sulfate in human plasma could be a strong first-pass hepatic extraction and the subsequent excretion of the sulfate into bile.

Although cryopreserved primary human enterocytes and human intestinal mucosa are now available for the investigation of intestinal drug metabolism [44,45], the advantage of EpiIntestinal microtissues is the presence of both intact barrier function and comprehensive DME activities. The combined barrier function and DME activities in EpiIntestinal microtissues make it possible to evaluate intestinal first-pass availability ($F_a \times F_g$) in humans in a single experiment. Indeed, the in vitro intestinal availability of 12 marketed drugs in EpiIntestinal microtissues (% recovery in receiver compartment) is in good agreement with $F_a \times F_g$ calculated from the clinical pharmacokinetic data of these drugs (Table 6). It is important to note that the in vitro availability in our model was obtained after an incubation time of 24 h, while the drug absorption in human intestine is usually completed after a few hours. The longer incubation time in the in vitro model can be mainly attributed to the higher ratio of drug amounts applied to the microtissues (1 nmol) to the surface area of the microtissues (0.6 cm^2). The human small intestine mucosa, in contrast, has a surface area of 30 m^2 [46]. The ratio of drug amounts to surface area is much lower. It would be interesting to compare human intestine tissues mounted in Ussing chambers with the EpiIntestinal microtissues in this regard. One would assume that the primary tissues would perform at least similarly to the EpiIntestinal model, and the low availability of suitable human tissues would limit the broader use of the primary materials in drug screening. There is however one caveat for using the EpiIntestinal model in this regard: the data are only meaningful if the quantities of DMEs and drug transporters in the model are comparable to the human intestine. Investigation into the expression of DMEs and drug transporters in EpiIntestinal microtissues is currently ongoing (transcriptomics) or planned (proteomics).

Although the EpiIntestinal microtissues provide a number of advantages compared to the currently available tools like Caco-2 cells, primary human enterocytes, or human intestinal mucosa, there are some limitations with regard to the use of the model in drug screening. One of the limitations is the unknown donor variability. According to the manufacturer, the microtissues we tested to date were derived from one single donor. For various reasons, we have not been able to get access to microtissues derived from other donors from the manufacturer to date. For drugs involving highly polymorphic metabolizing enzymes, data from a single donor are certainly not representative for the patient population. Therefore, it will be very important to investigate this model further in this regard in the future. Another limitation of this model is the static incubation conditions. Under physiological conditions, both the content in the intestine lumen and the blood at the basal side are under constant flow. The blood flow, for example, can reduce the diffusion of the drugs back into the enterocytes and thus limit the "recycling" of the drugs between blood and intestinal mucosa. Under static conditions, however, the recycling of the drugs might lead to an underestimation of the availability of the drugs, especially for those with extensive metabolic clearance in the intestinal mucosa. Due to the strong dilution effect in the apical-to-basal direction (100 vs. 5000 µL media volume in the apical and the basal compartment, respectively) we consider the effect of recycling, even under the static incubation, to be rather low. We tried to mimic the blood flow by replacing a large part of the media in the basal compartment with fresh media at the indicated sampling time points. The results were comparable to the static incubation (data not shown). Nevertheless, the integration of this model into a microfluidic system might still be interesting because this will make the combination with other organ models (e.g., liver-on-chip) possible.

In summary, our data here demonstrate that the EpiIntestinal microtissues are a useful tool for understanding drug absorption and metabolism in human intestine. The easy access of the model makes it very attractive for drug screening in the drug discovery process. It can also be used for the mechanistic understanding of intestinal drug–drug interaction or for the identification of intestine-specific metabolites.

Supplementary Materials: The following are available online at http://www.mdpi.com/1999-4923/12/5/405/s1, Figure S1: Concentration dependence of activities of drug-metabolising enzymes in EpiIntestinal microtissues.

Author Contributions: Conceptualization, Y.C., S.C., C.M.; methodology, Y.C., S.C., D.S., F.R., C.M.; investigation, Y.C., S.C., D.S., F.R.; writing—original draft preparation, Y.C., S.C.; writing—review and editing, Y.C., S.C., D.S., F.R., C.M.; visualization, Y.C., S.C., D.S.; supervision, Y.C., C.M.; project administration, Y.C. All authors have read and agreed to the published version of the manuscript.

Funding: This research received no external funding.

Acknowledgments: The authors thanks Veronika Diesch, Samira Selman, Sarah Heine, Tilo Goletz, and Jesus Blanco-Santos for technical support and Thomas Ebner, Eva Ludwig-Schwellinger, Jens Borghardt, Achim Sauer, and Klaus Klinder for consulting and fruitful discussion.

Conflicts of Interest: The authors declare no conflict of interest. All authors are employees of Boehringer Ingelheim Pharma GmbH & Co. KG. The company had no role in the design, execution, interpretation, or writing of the study.

References

1. Lennernäs, H.; Palm, K.; Fagerholm, U.; Artursson, P. Comparison between active and passive drug transport in human intestinal epithelial (caco-2) cells in vitro and human jejunum in vivo. *Int. J. Pharm.* **1996**, *127*, 103–107. [CrossRef]
2. Kerns, E.H.; Di, L.; Petusky, S.; Farris, M.; Ley, R.; Jupp, P. Combined Application of Parallel Artificial Membrane Permeability Assay and Caco-2 Permeability Assays in Drug Discovery. *J. Pharm. Sci.* **2004**, *93*, 1440–1453. [CrossRef] [PubMed]
3. Wu, B.; Kulkarni, K.; Basu, S.; Zhang, S.; Hu, M. First-Pass Metabolism via UDP-Glucuronosyltransferase: A Barrier to Oral Bioavailability of Phenolics. *J. Pharm. Sci.* **2011**, *100*, 3655–3681. [CrossRef] [PubMed]
4. Ishiguro, N.; Kishimoto, W.; Volz, A.; Ludwig-Schwellinger, E.; Ebner, T.; Schaefer, O. Impact of Endogenous Esterase Activity on In Vitro P-Glycoprotein Profiling of Dabigatran Etexilate in Caco-2 Monolayers. *Drug Metab. Dispos.* **2013**, *42*, 250–256. [CrossRef]
5. Prueksaritanont, T.; Gorham, L.M.; Hochman, J.H.; O Tran, L.; Vyas, K.P. Comparative studies of drug-metabolizing enzymes in dog, monkey, and human small intestines, and in Caco-2 cells. *Drug Metab. Dispos.* **1996**, *24*, 634–642.
6. Rozehnal, V.; Nakai, D.; Hoepner, U.; Fischer, T.; Kamiyama, E.; Takahashi, M.; Yasuda, S.; Mueller, J. Human small intestinal and colonic tissue mounted in the Ussing chamber as a tool for characterizing the intestinal absorption of drugs. *Eur. J. Pharm. Sci.* **2012**, *46*, 367–373. [CrossRef]
7. Takenaka, T.; Kazuki, K.; Harada, N.; Kuze, J.; Chiba, M.; Iwao, T.; Matsunaga, T.; Abe, S.; Oshimura, M.; Kazuki, Y. Development of Caco-2 cells co-expressing CYP3A4 and NADPH-cytochrome P450 reductase using a human artificial chromosome for the prediction of intestinal extraction ratio of CYP3A4 substrates. *Drug Metab. Pharmacokinet.* **2017**, *32*, 61–68. [CrossRef]
8. Gertz, M.; Harrison, A.; Houston, J.B.; Galetin, A. Prediction of Human Intestinal First-Pass Metabolism of 25 CYP3A Substrates from In Vitro Clearance and Permeability Data. *Drug Metab. Dispos.* **2010**, *38*, 1147–1158. [CrossRef]
9. Bein, A.; Shin, W.; Jalili-Firoozinezhad, S.; Park, M.H.; Sontheimer-Phelps, A.; Tovaglieri, A.; Chalkiadaki, A.; Kim, H.J.; Ingber, D. Microfluidic Organ-on-a-Chip Models of Human Intestine. *Cell. Mol. Gastroenterol. Hepatol.* **2018**, *5*, 659–668. [CrossRef]
10. Rahmani, S.; Breyner, N.; Su, H.-M.; Verdu, E.F.; Didar, T.F. Intestinal organoids: A new paradigm for engineering intestinal epithelium in vitro. *Biomater.* **2019**, *194*, 195–214. [CrossRef]
11. Ayehunie, S.; Landry, T.; Stevens, Z.; Armento, A.; Hayden, P.; Klausner, M. Human Primary Cell-Based Organotypic Microtissues for Modeling Small Intestinal Drug Absorption. *Pharm. Res.* **2018**, *35*, 72. [CrossRef] [PubMed]
12. Madden, L.R.; Nguyen, T.V.; Garcia-Mojica, S.; Shah, V.; Le, A.V.; Peier, A.; Visconti, R.; Parker, E.M.; Presnell, S.C.; Nguyen, D.G.; et al. Bioprinted 3D Primary Human Intestinal Tissues Model Aspects of Native Physiology and ADME/Tox Functions. *iScience* **2018**, *2*, 156–167. [CrossRef] [PubMed]
13. Sieger, P.; Cui, Y.; Scheuerer, S. pH-dependent solubility and permeability profiles: A useful tool for prediction of oral bioavailability. *Eur. J. Pharm. Sci.* **2017**, *105*, 82–90. [CrossRef]
14. Cui, Y.; Lotz, R.; Rapp, H.; Klinder, K.; Himstedt, A.; Sauer, A. Muscle to Brain Partitioning as Measure of Transporter-Mediated Efflux at the Rat Blood–Brain Barrier and Its Implementation into Compound Optimization in Drug Discovery. *Pharmaceutics* **2019**, *11*, 595. [CrossRef]
15. Obach, R.S.; Lombardo, F.; Waters, N. Trend Analysis of a Database of Intravenous Pharmacokinetic Parameters in Humans for 670 Drug Compounds. *Drug Metab. Dispos.* **2008**, *36*, 1385–1405. [CrossRef]
16. Varma, M.V.S.; Feng, B.; Obach, R.S.; Troutman, M.D.; Chupka, J.; Miller, H.R.; El-Kattan, A. Physicochemical Determinants of Human Renal Clearance. *J. Med. Chem.* **2009**, *52*, 4844–4852. [CrossRef]
17. Gibson, D.M.; Stern, R.H.; Abel, R.B.; Whitfield, L.R. Absolute bioavailability of atorvastatin in man. *Pharm. Res.* **1997**, *14*, S253.
18. Stern, R.H.; Yang, B.-B.; Horton, M.; Moore, S.; Abel, R.B.; Olson, S.C. Renal dysfunction does not alter the pharmacokinetics or LDL-cholesterol reduction of atorvastatin. *J. Clin. Pharmacol.* **1997**, *37*, 816–819. [CrossRef]
19. Mahmood, I.; Sahajwalla, C. Clinical Pharmacokinetics and Pharmacodynamics of Buspirone, an Anxiolytic Drug. *Clin. Pharmacokinet.* **1999**, *36*, 277–287. [CrossRef]

20. Yeh, K.C.; Stone, J.A.; Carides, A.D.; Rolan, P.; Woolf, E.; Ju, W.D. Simultaneous investigation of indinavir nonlinear pharmacokinetics and bioavailability in healthy volunteers using stable isotope labeling technique: Study design and model-independent data analysis. *J. Pharm. Sci.* **1999**, *88*, 568–573. [CrossRef]
21. Combes, O.; Barré, J.; Duché, J.-C.; Vernillet, L.; Archimbaud, Y.; Marietta, M.P.; Tillement, J.-P.; Urien, S. In vitro binding and partitioning of irinotecan (CPT-11) and its metabolite, SN-38, in human blood. *Investig. New Drugs* **2000**, *18*, 1–5. [CrossRef] [PubMed]
22. Mizushima, H.; Takanaka, K.; Abe, K.; Fukazawa, I.; Ishizuka, H. Stereoselective pharmacokinetics of oxybutynin and N -desethyloxybutynin in vitro and in vivo. *Xenobiotica* **2007**, *37*, 59–73. [CrossRef] [PubMed]
23. Martin, P. Absolute oral bioavailability of rosuvastatin in healthy white adult male volunteers. *Clin. Ther.* **2003**, *25*, 2553–2563. [CrossRef]
24. Nordt, S.P.; Clark, R.F. Midazolam: A review of therapeutic uses and toxicity. *J. Emerg. Med.* **1997**, *15*, 357–365. [CrossRef]
25. Lee, C.A.; Neul, D.; Clouser-Roche, A.; Dalvie, D.; Wester, M.R.; Jiang, Y.; Jones, J.P.; Freiwald, S.; Zientek, M.; Totah, R.A. Identification of Novel Substrates for Human Cytochrome P450 2J2. *Drug Metab. Dispos.* **2009**, *38*, 347–356. [CrossRef]
26. Matsumoto, S.; Hirama, T.; Matsubara, T.; Nagata, K.; Yamazoe, Y. Involvement of CYP2J2 on the intestinal first-pass metabolism of antihistamine drug, astemizole. *Drug Metab. Dispos.* **2002**, *30*, 1240–1245. [CrossRef]
27. Walsky, R.L.; Obach, R.S.; Hyland, R.; Kang, P.; Zhou, S.; West, M.; Geoghegan, K.F.; Helal, C.J.; Walker, G.; Goosen, T.C.; et al. Selective Mechanism-Based Inactivation of CYP3A4 by CYP3cide (PF-04981517) and Its Utility as an In Vitro Tool for Delineating the Relative Roles of CYP3A4 versus CYP3A5 in the Metabolism of Drugs. *Drug Metab. Dispos.* **2012**, *40*, 1686–1697. [CrossRef]
28. Dalvie, D.; Kang, P.; Zientek, M.; Xiang, C.; Zhou, S.; Obach, R.S. Effect of Intestinal Glucuronidation in Limiting Hepatic Exposure and Bioactivation of Raloxifene in Humans and Rats. *Chem. Res. Toxicol.* **2008**, *21*, 2260–2271. [CrossRef]
29. Kemp, D.C.; Fan, P.W.; Stevens, J.C.; Hill, G.; Cihlar, T.; Oo, C.; Ho, E.S.; Prior, K.; Wiltshire, H.; Barrett, J.; et al. Characterization of Raloxifene Glucuronidation in Vitro: Contribution of Intestinal Metabolism to Presystemic Clearance. *Drug Metab. Dispos.* **2002**, *30*, 694–700. [CrossRef]
30. Van Heek, M.; Farley, C.; Compton, D.S.; Hoos, L.; Alton, K.B.; Sybertz, E.J.; Davis, H.R. Comparison of the activity and disposition of the novel cholesterol absorption inhibitor, SCH58235, and its glucuronide, SCH60663. *Br. J. Pharmacol.* **2000**, *129*, 1748–1754. [CrossRef]
31. Allen, J.D.; Van Loevezijn, A.; Lakhai, J.M.; Van Der Valk, M.; Van Tellingen, O.; Reid, G.; Schellens, J.; Koomen, G.-J.; Schinkel, A.H. Potent and specific inhibition of the breast cancer resistance protein multidrug transporter in vitro and in mouse intestine by a novel analogue of fumitremorgin C. *Mol. Cancer Ther.* **2002**, *1*, 417–425. [PubMed]
32. Luo, F.R.; Paranjpe, P.V.; Guo, A.; Rubin, E.; Sinko, P.J. Intestinal transport of irinotecan in Caco-2 cells and MDCK II cells overexpressing efflux transporters Pgp, cMOAT, and MRP1. *Drug Metab. Dispos.* **2002**, *30*, 763–770. [CrossRef] [PubMed]
33. Shepard, R.L.; Cao, J.; Starling, J.J.; Dantzig, A.H. Modulation of P-glycoprotein but not MRP1- or BCRP-mediated drug resistance by LY335979. *Int. J. Cancer* **2002**, *103*, 121–125. [CrossRef] [PubMed]
34. Kitamura, S.; Maeda, K.; Wang, Y.; Sugiyama, Y. Involvement of Multiple Transporters in the Hepatobiliary Transport of Rosuvastatin. *Drug Metab. Dispos.* **2008**, *36*, 2014–2023. [CrossRef] [PubMed]
35. Brück, S.; Strohmeier, J.; Busch, D.; Droździk, M.; Oswald, S. Caco-2 cells-expression, regulation and function of drug transporters compared with human jejunal tissue. *Biopharm. Drug Dispos.* **2016**, *38*, 115–126. [CrossRef]
36. Nakamura, K.; Hirayama-Kurogi, M.; Ito, S.; Kuno, T.; Yoneyama, T.; Obuchi, W.; Terasaki, T.; Ohtsuki, S. Large-scale multiplex absolute protein quantification of drug-metabolizing enzymes and transporters in human intestine, liver, and kdney microsomes by SWATH-MS: Comparison with MRM/SRM and HR-MRM/PRM. *Proteomics* **2016**, *16*, 2106–2117. [CrossRef]
37. Uchida, Y.; Ohtsuki, S.; Kamiie, J.; Ohmine, K.; Iwase, R.; Terasaki, T. Quantitative targeted absolute proteomics for 28 human transporters in plasma membrane of Caco-2 cell monolayer cultured for 2, 3, and 4 weeks. *Drug Metab. Pharmacokinet.* **2015**, *30*, 205–208. [CrossRef]

38. Elsby, R.; Martin, P.; Surry, D.; Sharma, P.; Fenner, K. Solitary Inhibition of the Breast Cancer Resistance Protein Efflux Transporter Results in a Clinically Significant Drug-Drug Interaction with Rosuvastatin by Causing up to a 2-Fold Increase in Statin Exposure. *Drug Metab. Dispos.* **2015**, *44*, 398–408. [CrossRef]
39. Paine, M.F.; Hart, H.L.; Ludington, S.S.; Haining, R.L.; Rettie, A.E.; Zeldin, D.C. The HUMAN INTESTINAL CYTOCHROME P450 "PIE". *Drug Metab. Dispos.* **2006**, *34*, 880–886. [CrossRef]
40. Hui, Y.; Luo, L.; Zhang, L.; Kurogi, K.; Zhou, C.; Sakakibara, Y.; Suiko, M.; Liu, M.-C. Sulfation of afimoxifene, endoxifen, raloxifene, and fulvestrant by the human cytosolic sulfotransferases (SULTs): A systematic analysis. *J. Pharmacol. Sci.* **2015**, *128*, 144–149. [CrossRef]
41. Falany, C.N.; Pilloff, D.E.; Leyh, T.S.; Falany, C.N. Sulfation of raloxifene and 4-hydroxytamoxifen by human cytosolic sulfotransferases. *Drug Metab. Dispos.* **2005**, *34*, 361–368. [CrossRef] [PubMed]
42. Jeong, E.J.; Lin, H.; Hu, M. Disposition Mechanisms of Raloxifene in the Human Intestinal Caco-2 Model. *J. Pharmacol. Exp. Ther.* **2004**, *310*, 376–385. [CrossRef] [PubMed]
43. Bansal, S.; Lau, A.J. Inhibition of Human Sulfotransferase 2A1-Catalyzed Sulfonation of Lithocholic Acid, Glycolithocholic Acid, and Taurolithocholic Acid by Selective Estrogen Receptor Modulators and Various Analogs and Metabolites. *J. Pharmacol. Exp. Ther.* **2019**, *369*, 389–405. [CrossRef] [PubMed]
44. Li, A.; Alam, N.; Amaral, K.; Ho, M.-C.D.; Loretz, C.; Mitchell, W.; Yang, Q. Cryopreserved Human Intestinal Mucosal Epithelium: A Novel In Vitro Experimental System for the Evaluation of Enteric Drug Metabolism, Cytochrome P450 Induction, and Enterotoxicity. *Drug Metab. Dispos.* **2018**, *46*, 1562–1571. [CrossRef] [PubMed]
45. Wong, S.; Doshi, U.; Vuong, P.; Liu, N.; Tey, S.; Le, H.; Kosaka, M.; Kelly, J.R.; Li, A.; Yan, Z. Utility of Pooled Cryopreserved Human Enterocytes as an In vitro Model for Assessing Intestinal Clearance and Drug-Drug Interactions. *Drug Metab. Lett.* **2018**, *12*, 3–13. [CrossRef]
46. Helander, H.F.; Fändriks, L. Surface area of the digestive tract–revisited. *Scand. J. Gastroenterol.* **2014**, *49*, 681–689. [CrossRef]

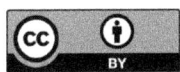

© 2020 by the authors. Licensee MDPI, Basel, Switzerland. This article is an open access article distributed under the terms and conditions of the Creative Commons Attribution (CC BY) license (http://creativecommons.org/licenses/by/4.0/).

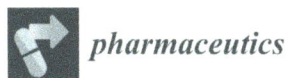

Article

Automated Real-Time Tumor Pharmacokinetic Profiling in 3D Models: A Novel Approach for Personalized Medicine

Jan F. Joseph [1,†], Leonie Gronbach [2,†], Jill García-Miller [2], Leticia M. Cruz [2], Bernhard Wuest [3], Ulrich Keilholz [4], Christian Zoschke [2] and Maria K. Parr [5,*]

1. Core Facility BioSupraMol, Freie Universität Berlin, 14195 Berlin, Germany; jan.joseph@fu-berlin.de
2. Institute of Pharmacy (Pharmacology & Toxicology), Freie Universität Berlin, 14195 Berlin, Germany; leonie.gronbach@fu-berlin.de (L.G.); jillg94@zedat.fu-berlin.de (J.G.-M.); leticia.cruz@fu-berlin.de (L.M.C.); christian.zoschke@fu-berlin.de (C.Z.)
3. Agilent Technologies GmbH, 76337 Waldbronn, Germany; bernhard_wuest@agilent.com
4. Charité–Universitätsmedizin Berlin, corporate member of Freie Universität Berlin, Humboldt-Universität zu Berlin and Berlin Institute of Health, Comprehensive Cancer Center, 10117 Berlin, Germany; Ulrich.Keilholz@charite.de
5. Institute of Pharmacy (Pharmaceutical and Medicinal Chemistry), Freie Universität Berlin, 14195 Berlin, Germany
* Correspondence: maria.parr@fu-berlin.de; Tel.: +49-30-838-51471
† These authors contributed equally to this work.

Received: 31 March 2020; Accepted: 29 April 2020; Published: 30 April 2020

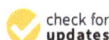

Abstract: Cancer treatment often lacks individual dose adaptation, contributing to insufficient efficacy and severe side effects. Thus, personalized approaches are highly desired. Although various analytical techniques are established to determine drug levels in preclinical models, they are limited in the automated real-time acquisition of pharmacokinetic profiles. Therefore, an online UHPLC-MS/MS system for quantitation of drug concentrations within 3D tumor oral mucosa models was generated. The integration of sampling ports into the 3D tumor models and their culture inside the autosampler allowed for real-time pharmacokinetic profiling without additional sample preparation. Docetaxel quantitation was validated according to EMA guidelines. The tumor models recapitulated the morphology of head-and-neck cancer and the dose-dependent tumor reduction following docetaxel treatment. The administration of four different docetaxel concentrations resulted in comparable courses of concentration versus time curves for 96 h. In conclusion, this proof-of-concept study demonstrated the feasibility of real-time monitoring of drug levels in 3D tumor models without any sample preparation. The inclusion of patient-derived tumor cells into our models may further optimize the pharmacotherapy of cancer patients by efficiently delivering personalized data of the target tissue.

Keywords: automatization; drug absorption; drug dosing; head-and-neck cancer; pharmacokinetics; real-time measurements; taxanes; tissue engineering; UHPLC-MS/MS

1. Introduction

Selecting clinically relevant doses for the evaluation of anticancer drugs remains challenging in preclinical drug development and contributes to the low translatability of effects in vitro to efficacy in patients. While the understanding of cancer biology advances as the complexity of tumor models and analytical techniques increases, the success rate of drug development in oncology remains the lowest among all therapeutic areas.

Historically, anticancer drug doses for clinical trials have been determined by extrapolating the maximum tolerated dose (MTD) in animals to the human patient. Taking the MTD as the starting point, the effective and safe dose for humans was anticipated in the range of −3 to +3, with three concentrations below and three concentrations above. The revision of this concept is urgently needed, since many nonoptimal doses were taken into late stages of drug development. Especially the testing of high-risk drugs requires a more conservative approach, using the minimum anticipated biological effect level (MABEL) in first-in-human trials [1,2].

Up to now, new concepts focused on the improved extrapolation from animal studies to clinical trials, e.g., by introducing drug metabolism and pharmacokinetic studies in early drug development [3]. In particular, model-based, adaptive/Bayesian approaches already helped to better find effective and safe dosage [4]. Nevertheless, animal models are affected by differences in the human pathophysiology and even xenograft models do not fully recapitulate the barriers of drug uptake into human solid tumors [5].

In fact, drug exposure of tumor cells depends on the architecture of solid tumors with cell density, the spatial arrangement of cells and extracellular matrix proteins, interstitial fluid pressure, and vascular supply [6–8]. While 2D monolayer cell culture cannot provide meaningful insights into the pharmacokinetic profiles of solid tumors, sophisticated 3D tumor models such as spheroids or multilayered tumor models could do this, eventually even in a patient-specific manner [9,10].

The introduction of in vitro tumor models into the dose selection for a particular patient requires adapting the protocols to high-content, high-throughput approaches to handle high numbers of tests, e.g., with different drugs and several combinations. However, analytical approaches to quantify drug amounts in tissues comprise imaging- and microdialysis-based methods. While imaging techniques and microdialysis closely map the drug distribution within (tumor) tissues, all methods share the high effort needed in sample preparation [11,12], restricting their use for personalized medicine.

Herein, the development of an in vitro approach for real-time pharmacokinetic investigations in human cell-based models of head-and-neck squamous cell carcinoma is reported. It aims for an automated measurement of docetaxel concentrations within the tumor tissue to quantify the drug absorption. Therefore, an UHPLC-MS/MS method was adapted from clinical practice and optimized for a maximum number of online measurements per time.

2. Materials and Methods

2.1. Materials

Oral fibroblasts and oral fibroblast medium were purchased from ScienCell (Carlsbad, CA, USA). Tongue cancer cells from the SCC-25 cell line (RRID:CVCL_1682) were a generous gift from Howard Green (Dana-Farber Cancer Institute; Boston, MA, USA) [13]. Collagen G was purchased from Biochrom (Berlin, Germany) and consumables for tumor oral mucosa model culture from Greiner bio-one (Leipzig, Germany). Docetaxel was purchased from Selleckchem (Houston, TX, USA). Acetonitrile, formic acid, methanol, and isopropanol, all LC-MS grade, were purchased from Sigma-Aldrich (München, Germany).

2.2. Cell Culture

Oral fibroblasts were precultured in oral fibroblast medium and SCC-25 cells in DMEM/F-12 Ham medium, supplemented with 9% fetal calf serum, 0.9% L-glutamine and 0.9% penicillin/streptomycin at 37 °C and 5% CO_2. The cancer cells were regularly checked by single nucleotide polymorphism authentication (Multiplexion; Heidelberg, Germany). The medium was changed three times a week and the cells were subcultivated after reaching a confluence of 80%. Cell culture was performed according to standard operating procedures and referred to good cell culture practice.

2.3. Sample Port Integration into Tumor Oral Mucosa (TOM) Models

Tumor oral mucosa (TOM) models were prepared as described elsewhere [14] but adopted to a 6-well-plate design to handle the integration of the sample port (Figure 1a). In brief, 0.3×10^6 oral fibroblasts were embedded in collagen G and 1×10^6 SCC-25 cells were seeded on top of these lamina propria equivalents one week after. The model growth medium was changed three times a week and replaced by model differentiation medium one week after seeding the tumor cells [14]. The sampling port was created by placing a 24-well insert (400 nm pore size) into the TOM model before the collagen started to solidify. The tumor cells proliferated and migrated into the collagen matrix around the sampling port for seven days, before docetaxel was applied. The 24-well insert was fixed by a custom-made metal support and filled with 600 µL serum-free growth medium. The top of the 6-well plate was sealed with aluminum foil (VWR, Darmstadt, Germany) instead of using the standard plastic lid. TOM models were incubated at 37 °C inside the autosampler of the UHPLC-MS/MS device (Agilent Technologies GmbH, Waldbronn, Germany) for the 96 h observation period in the final week of TOM model culture.

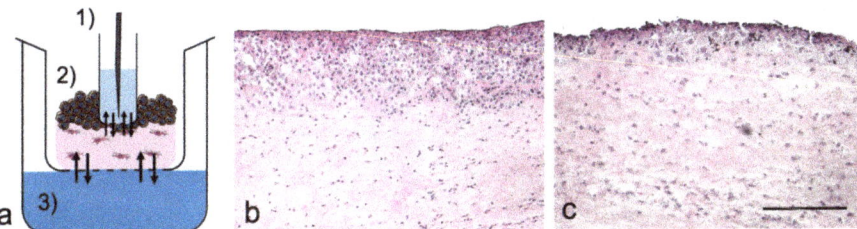

Figure 1. Experimental design and morphology of tumor oral mucosa (TOM) models. (**a**) Schematic cross-section of (1) sampling port with the needle of the autosampler, (2) TOM model with tumor cells (brown) and fibroblasts (magenta) within lamina propria, (3) Reservoir with differentiation medium, supplemented with docetaxel. The arrows indicate drug diffusion equilibria. Hematoxylin and eosin (H&E) staining of TOM models following two applications of (**b**) the vehicle control and (**c**) 7000 ng/mL docetaxel. Images were representative of four batches; scale bar = 250 µm.

2.4. Docetaxel Treatment of TOM Models

Docetaxel was dissolved in DMSO to a 70 mg/mL stock solution and diluted with construct differentiation medium to 7; 70; 700; 7000 ng/mL. DMSO, 0.01% in model differentiation medium, served as vehicle control since this was the maximum DMSO concentration among all samples (0.00001%; 0.0001%; 0.001%; and 0.01% DMSO for 7; 70; 700; 7000 ng/mL docetaxel). Docetaxel solutions were applied two times per construct with an application interval of 48 h.

2.5. Morphological Analysis

TOM models were snap frozen at the end of the 96 h observation period and cut into 7 µm thick slices using a cryotome (Leica CM 1510 S; Leica, Wetzlar, Germany). Cryosections were analyzed by hematoxylin and eosin (H&E) staining and pictures were taken with a microscope (BZ-8000; Keyence, Neu-Isenburg, Germany).

2.6. UHPLC-MS/MS Analyses

Method A: For automated real-time quantitation of docetaxel, an Agilent 1290 UHPLC coupled to an Agilent 6495 triple quadrupole tandem mass spectrometer equipped with a Jet Stream electrospray ionization (ESI) source was used (Agilent Technologies GmbH, Waldbronn, Germany). Separation of docetaxel was achieved on an Agilent Poroshell Phenyl Hexyl column (50 mm × 2.1 mm, 1.9 µm particle size) equipped with a corresponding guard column (5 mm × 2.1 mm, 1.9 µm particle size) using water (solvent A) and acetonitrile (solvent B) each containing 0.1% formic acid (v/v) as mobile phase. At a flow rate of 0.350 mL/min, the following gradient was applied: 5% B for 0.5 min, to 100% B at 4 min, 1 min hold, 5% B at 5.1 min, stop time 6.50 min. The column compartment was kept at 40 °C. The injection volume was 5 µL and the autosampler temperature was set to 37 °C. A needle wash (acetonitrile/methanol/isopropanol/water, 25% each, v/v/v/v) was applied for 20 s while an additional needle seat backflush using an Agilent Flex Cube was used to minimize carry over (15 s at 2 mL/min with needle wash solvent, pure isopropanol, and a mixture of water/acetonitrile (95/5, v/v) containing 0.1% formic acid). The total run time was 9.75 min.

The mass spectrometer was operated in multiple reaction monitoring (MRM) acquisition mode. Positive electrospray ionization mode (ESI+) yielded the sodium adduct of docetaxel [M + Na]$^+$ and was detected at m/z 830.3. Source and MRM parameters were optimized using Mass Hunter Source Optimizer software (version 1.1, Agilent Technologies Inc., Santa Clara, CA, USA). Final source parameters were as follows: drying gas temperature: 230 °C, drying gas flow: 20 L/min (nitrogen), nebulizer pressure: 40 psi (nitrogen), sheath gas temperature: 390 °C, sheath gas flow: 12 L/min (nitrogen), capillary voltage: +4,500 V, nozzle voltage: +300 V, high pressure radio frequency (HPRF): 210 V, low pressure radio frequency (LPRF): 160 V. MRM details are listed in Table 1. MassHunter (Quant) software (version B08, Agilent Technologies Inc., Santa Clara, CA, USA) was used for data acquisition and processing.

Table 1. Multiple reaction monitoring (MRM) transitions of docetaxel sodium adduct, used in method A.

Precursor Ion (m/z)	Product Ion (m/z)	Collision Energy	Cell Accelerator Voltage	Polarity
830.3	549.1	25	4	Positive
830.3	304.1	20	2	Positive

Method B: For identification of degradation products, an Agilent 1290 II HPLC connected to an Agilent 6550 iFunnel QTOF with Agilent Jet Stream source was used (Agilent Technologies Inc., Santa Clara, CA, USA). Separation of docetaxel and its metabolites was achieved on an Agilent Poroshell Phenyl Hexyl column (50 mm × 2.1 mm, 1.9 µm particle size) equipped with a corresponding guard column (5 mm × 2.1 mm, 1.9 µm particle size) using water (solvent A) and acetonitrile (solvent B) each containing 0.1% formic acid (v/v) as mobile phase. At a flow rate of 0.350 mL/min, a longer gradient was applied: 5% B for 0.5 min, to 37% B at 5 min, 50% B at 10 min, to 98% B at 15 min, 2 min hold, back to 5% B at 17.1 min, stop time 19 min. The column compartment was kept at 40 °C. The injection volume was 5 µL. A needle wash (acetonitrile, methanol, isopropanol, water) was applied for 20 s. The mass spectrometric parameters were as follows: drying gas temperature: 230 °C, drying gas flow 14 L/min (nitrogen), nebulizer pressure 40 psi (nitrogen), sheath gas temperature: 375 °C, sheath gas flow: 12 L/min (nitrogen), capillary voltage +4,500 V, nozzle voltage +300 V, high pressure radio frequency 200 V, low pressure radio frequency 100 V, fragmentor 365 V. Data acquisition was performed in auto MS/MS mode using a mass range of m/z 100–1000 at a scan rate of 1 spectrum/s for MS1 and m/z 50–1000 for MS2 experiments at 3 spectra/s. The collision energy was adjusted depending on the target m/z value (offset 4 eV, slope 3 eV/m/z 100).

2.7. Validation

Method A was used for automated real-time quantitation of docetaxel and validated in terms of selectivity, carry-over, lower limit of quantitation (LLOQ), calibration function, accuracy, and precision following the recommendations of the European Medicines Agency's (EMA) guideline on bioanalytical method validation [15]. All calibration (CAL) and quality control (QC) samples were freshly prepared in serum-free model differentiation medium as sample diluents.

Selectivity and carry-over: The guidelines require the analysis of matrix from four different lots. Since the matrix was artificial, no remarkable differences had to be considered. Thus, only one batch was used for assessing selectivity. Blank samples (serum-free model differentiation medium) were analyzed and compared with samples spiked with docetaxel at the LLOQ. Less than 20% detector response of the LLOQ is required for the blank samples. Carry-over was determined by analyzing blank samples after the injection of a high concentration QC (HQC) sample (7,500 ng/mL). Again, less than 20% detector response of the LLOQ is required to comply with the EMA guidelines.

Lower limit of quantitation and calibration: The LLOQ needs to be determined with sufficient accuracy and precision and with at least 5 times higher detector response than a blank sample. For evaluation, matrix-matched samples of 0.1, 0.25, 0.5, 1.0, 5.0 ng/mL were investigated. Additionally, the limit of detection (LOD) was determined based on calculations according to ICH guidelines [16]. Calibration samples in medium ranged from the LLOQ of 0.001 µg/mL to the upper limit of quantitation (ULOQ) of 10 µg/mL. In addition to an analyte free matrix sample, eight levels of calibration samples were prepared in triplicate and analyzed on two consecutive days.

Accuracy and precision: Accuracy and precision were assessed on serum-free medium samples spiked with docetaxel at 4 different QC levels with 5 replicates per level in a concentration range from the LLOQ to the ULOQ covering the calibration range. Samples were analyzed on two different days. Mean concentrations and the coefficient of variation (CV) of QC samples were required to be within ±15% in general, or ±20% at the LLOQ of the nominal concentrations, respectively. Within-run and between-run accuracy and precision were determined.

2.8. Sample Preparation for the Identification of Degradation Products

The degradation products of docetaxel were analyzed in the differentiation medium cultivated with the models (Table 2). To handle these samples, a protein precipitation procedure was performed. Aliquots of 100 µL of the samples were added to 400 µL of cold acetonitrile and centrifuged at 3328× g for 10 min. The serum-free supernatant was then transferred into LC-MS/MS vials for further analysis, according to method B.

Table 2. LC-MS data of docetaxel (highlighted gray) and postulated degradation products, acquired using method B.

Degradation Product	Formula	RT (min)	m/z	Exact Mass	Adduct	Mass Accuracy (ppm)
Carbamate	$C_{38}H_{45}NO_{12}$	4.30	708.3010	708.3015	$[M + H]^+$	0.65
10DABIII	$C_{29}H_{36}O_{10}$	4.55	545.2378	545.2381	$[M + H]^+$	0.60
Epi-carbamate	$C_{38}H_{45}NO_{12}$	4.72	708.3004	708.3015	$[M + H]^+$	1.47
Epi-10DABIII	$C_{29}H_{36}O_{10}$	5.31	567.2196	567.2201	$[M + Na]^+$	0.76
Oxo-10DABIII	$C_{29}H_{34}O_{10}$	5.40	565.2041	565.2044	$[M + Na]^+$	0.56
Epi-oxo-10DABIII	$C_{29}H_{34}O_{10}$	5.84	565.2040	565.2044	$[M + Na]^+$	0.67
1-7 Docetaxel	$C_{43}H_{53}NO_{14}$	7.95	830.3374	830.3358	$[M + Na]^+$	−1.9
Epi-Docetaxel	$C_{43}H_{53}NO_{14}$	9.08	830.3377	830.3358	$[M + Na]^+$	−2.26
Oxo-Docetaxel	$C_{43}H_{51}NO_{14}$	9.94	828.3200	828.3202	$[M + Na]^+$	0.19
Epi-oxo-Docetaxel	$C_{43}H_{51}NO_{14}$	11.07	828.3192	828.3202	$[M + Na]^+$	1.16

2.9. Pharmacokinetic Analysis

Pharmacokinetic analyses were conducted in R [17]. First, a non-compartmental analysis was performed. Assumptions were: (i) dose was calculated by concentration in the reservoir x volume (Figure 1a(3)); (ii) area under the concentration curve (AUC) 0–48 h lasted until 48 h and AUC 48–96 h until the end of the experiment; (iii) for the concentration between 48–96 h the unmeasured concentrations were not considered. Afterwards, interval AUCs were calculated. For 0–48 h, the AUC was calculated from 0.0001 h (start of the experiment) to the end of the 1st cycle; for 48–96 h, the AUC was calculated from the time "end of the 1st cycle" to "end of the 2nd cycle". However, the end

3. Results

3.1. TOM Models with Sampling Port

The TOM models reproducibly showed an unstructured and hyperproliferative epithelial layer with pleomorphic tumor cells, also separating from the epithelial layer into the lamina propria. Neither the sampling port nor the cultivation within the autosampler of the UHPLC-MS/MS device influenced the tumor growth. The effects of docetaxel on the tumor size in TOM models by supplementing the differentiation medium with either two drug doses or the vehicle control were determined. Whereas the vehicle control did not change the tumor morphology (Figure 1b), docetaxel caused a dose-dependent reduction of tumor size with abundant epithelial cell death (Figure 1c). The average tumor size declined from 347 ± 72 µm (untreated) to 100 ± 45 µm (max docetaxel concentration, $n = 4$ each).

3.2. Docetaxel Epimerization and Degradation Products

During electrospray ionization, docetaxel mainly forms a sodium adduct ($[M + Na]^+_{theor}$=830.3358), which is used as precursor ion for all MS/MS experiments. As shown in Figure 2 (top), the product ion spectrum of docetaxel shows three major fragments at m/z 549.2095 (taxane nucleus (10-deacetylbaccatin III, 10DABIII), $[C_{29}H_{34}O_9 + Na]^+$, exact mass m/z 549.2095, mass error $\Delta m/z = 0$ ppm), m/z 304.1159 (phenylpropionic acid side chain, $[C_{14}H_{19}NO+Na]^+$, exact mass m/z 304.1155, $\Delta m/z = -1.17$ ppm), and m/z 248.0537 (side chain with loss of the tert-butyl moiety, $[C_{10}H_{11}NO_5 + Na]^+$, exact mass m/z 248.0529, $\Delta m/z = -3.05$ ppm). The two main fragments m/z 549. 1 and m/z 304.1 were later chosen for MRM transitions in real-time quantitation (method A).

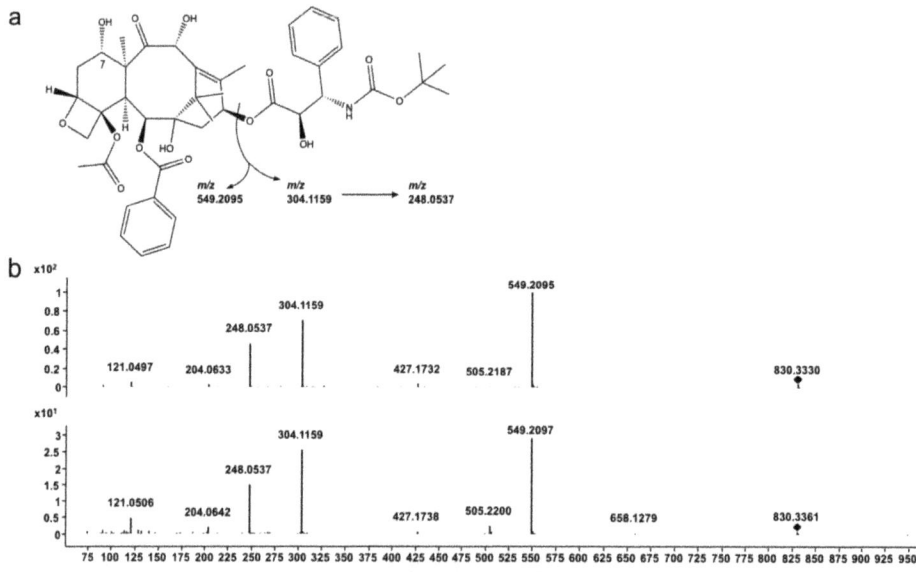

Figure 2. Docetaxel structure fragmentation. (**a**) Chemical structure of docetaxel and main fragmentation products. (**b**) Product ion spectra of docetaxel (top) and its potential 7-epimer (bottom), precursor $[M + Na]^+_{theor} = 830.3358$ indicated with black rhombus.

Analyses of docetaxel reference substance as well as cell culture media without cells, and TOM models, revealed a second peak with almost identical MRM transitions (method A, chromatogram showing transitions in Figure S1) and product ions (method B, Figure 2 (bottom)). It already appeared only minutes after preparing the samples for analysis with serum-free medium as sample diluent. This degradation product is postulated to be the 7-epimer of docetaxel (epi-docetaxel), which is known to occur in basic and acidic conditions [18,19]. Since the epimerization could not be avoided in calibration or quality control samples as well, the combined peak areas of docetaxel and the 7-epimer were considered for all further quantitation experiments of docetaxel.

Based on accurate mass data, we postulated further degradation products beside the main degradant epi-docetaxel. Oxidized species of docetaxel and several hydrolysis products (ester and carbamate hydrolysis), as well as oxidation of the products of ester hydrolysis and their respective epimers (Table 2, Figures S3 and S4) are assigned. Two oxidized species of docetaxel show abundant sodium adducts in MS1 of m/z 828.3200 (oxo-docetaxel, RT: 9.94 min, $[C_{43}H_{51}NO_{14} + Na^+]^+$, exact mass m/z 828.3202, $\Delta m/z$ = 0.19 ppm) and m/z 828.3192 (epi-oxo-docetaxel, RT: 11.07 min, $[C_{43}H_{51}NO_{14} + Na^+]^+$, exact mass m/z 828.3192, $\Delta m/z$ = 1.16 ppm). Their MS/MS spectra show abundant fragments at $m/z_{\text{oxo-docetaxel}}$ 772.2534 and $m/z_{\text{epi-oxo-docetaxel}}$ 772.2584 ($[C_{39}H_{43}NO_{14} + Na]^+$, exact mass m/z 772.2576, $\Delta m/z_{\text{oxo-docetaxel}}$ = −1.07 ppm and $\Delta m/z_{\text{epi-oxo-docetaxel}}$ = 5.41 ppm), which may originate from the loss of the tert-butyl residue. They both show a fragment corresponding to an oxidation at the taxane nucleus at $m/z_{\text{oxo-docetaxel}}$ 547.1927 and $m/z_{\text{epi-oxo-docetaxel}}$ 547.1955 ($[C_{29}H_{32}O_9 + Na]^+$, exact mass m/z 547.1939, $\Delta m/z_{\text{oxo-docetaxel}}$ = 2.11 ppm and $\Delta m/z_{\text{epi-oxo-docetaxel}}$ = −3.01 ppm). Analogously to docetaxel, the fragment m/z 304.1173 originated from the intact phenylpropionic acid side chain ($[C_{14}H_{19}NO_5 + Na]^+$, exact mass m/z 304.1155, $\Delta m/z_{\text{oxo-docetaxel}}$ = −5.77 ppm).

Further degradation products of docetaxel resulted from the ester hydrolysis of the taxane nucleus and the phenylpropionic acid side chain and are postulated here as 10DABIII (m/z 545.2378, RT: 4.55 min, $[C_{29}H_{36}O_{10} + H]^+$, exact mass m/z 545.2381, $\Delta m/z$ = 0.60 ppm) and epi-10DABIII (m/z 567.2196, RT: 5.31 min, $[C_{29}H_{36}O_{10} + Na]^+$, exact mass m/z 567.2201, $\Delta m/z$ = 0.83 ppm). A loss of benzoic acid, acetic acid and two losses of water from 10DABIII resulted in the fragment m/z 327.1587 ($[C_{20}H_{22}O_4 + H]^+$, exact mass m/z 327.1591, $\Delta m/z$ = 1.18 ppm). Epi-10DABIII showed a fragment at m/z 445.1791 ($[C_{22}H_{30}O_8 + Na]^+$, exact mass m/z 445.1833, $\Delta m/z$ = 9.41 ppm) which may correspond to the loss of the benzoic acid moiety and m/z 385.1615 ($[C_{20}H_{26}O_6 + Na]^+$, exact mass m/z 385.1622, $\Delta m/z$ = 1.71 ppm), which indicates a subsequent loss of acetic acid.

These two hydrolyzed esters most likely exist in an oxidized form as well, which are proposed as oxo-10DABIII (m/z 565.2041, RT: 5.40 min, $[C_{29}H_{34}O_{10} + Na]^+$, exact mass m/z 565.2044, $\Delta m/z$ = 0.56 ppm) and epi-oxo-10DABIII (m/z 565.2040, RT: 5.84 min, $[C_{29}H_{34}O_{10} + Na]^+$, exact mass m/z 565.2044, $\Delta m/z$ = 0.74 ppm) based on their accurate mass data. They both show a distinct fragment at $m/z_{\text{oxo-10DABIII}}$ 443.1661 and $m/z_{\text{epi-oxo-10DABIII}}$ 443.1680 ($[C_{22}H_{28}O_8 + Na]^+$, exact mass m/z 443.1676, $\Delta m/z_{\text{oxo-10DABIII}}$ = 3.47 ppm and $\Delta m/z_{\text{epi-oxo-10DABIII}}$ = −0.81 ppm), most likely originating from the loss of the benzoic acid moiety.

Furthermore, the hydrolysis of the carbamate function of docetaxel revealed two more products: 'Carbamate' showed an m/z 708.3010 in MS1 ($[C_{38}H_{45}NO_{12} + H]^+$, exact mass m/z 708.3015, $\Delta m/z$ = 0.64 ppm), and an abundant fragment of m/z 182.0818 in MS/MS which may originate from the cleavage of the remaining phenylpropionic acid side chain and the taxane nucleus ($[C_9H_{11}NO_3 + H]^+$, exact mass m/z 182.0812, $\Delta m/z$ = −3.46 ppm). 'Epi-carbamate' showed a similar product ion spectrum with the same base peak of m/z 182.0820 ($[C_9H_{11}NO_3 + H]^+$, exact mass m/z 182.0812, $\Delta m/z$ = −4.56 ppm) and m/z 708.3004 ($[C_{38}H_{45}NO_{12} + H]^+$, exact mass m/z 708.3015, $\Delta m/z$ = 1.47 ppm) in MS1.

An exemplary chromatogram of the degradation products following two applications of 70 μg/mL docetaxel for 48 h each is shown in Figure S2. We found only trace amounts of docetaxel degradation products in the TOM model media following the two applications of 7 μg/mL docetaxel for 48 h each. Therefore, we did not consider the degradation products in the real-time pharmacokinetic analyses.

3.3. Validation

As method A is used for quantitation in the online hyphenation of the tumor model with UHPLC based analysis, it was validated according to the guideline of the EMA [15].

Selectivity and carry-over: The method fulfilled the criteria for selectivity (<20% response in blank artificial matrix compared to response obtained at LLOQ) with a maximum of 7.45% detector response. Carry-over was a more critical parameter since the concentration range was very broad. Even after the optimization of the injector wash procedures, the detector response of analyte-free matrix samples exceeded the allowed 20% LLOQ detector response with a maximum of 29.42% after injection of HQC samples. Therefore, additional blank sample injections were included after samples of high concentrations resulted in successful prevention of carry-over.

Lower limit of quantitation and calibration: The concentration of 0.001 µg/mL showed acceptable accuracy (92.42–114.17%) and precision (6.58%CV) and was therefore chosen as the lowest point of the calibration. Based on the EMA guideline, the calculated LLOQ was 0.16 ng/mL and LOD 0.05 ng/mL, respectively.

For the calibration function, a quadratic fit after log-log transformation of the data provided the best results in terms of a combination of low residuals and best overall accuracy. All CAL samples met the requirements by EMA.

Accuracy and precision: The method (A) fulfilled the requirements given by EMA. Calculated concentrations of QC and CAL samples were within ±15% of the nominal values (Table 3), only 8.33% (within-day) and 15% (between-day) with only individual values outside.

Table 3. Accuracy and precision. c: docetaxel concentration, CV: coefficient of variation, RE: Relative error as measure of accuracy, LLOQ: lower limit of quantitation, LQC: lower quality control, MQC: middle quality control, HQC: higher quality control.

QC	Within-Day (n = 5)				Between-Day (n = 5)			
	Expected c (ng/mL)	Mean Calculated c (ng/mL)	CV (%)	RE (%)		Mean Calculated c (ng/mL)	CV (%)	RE (%)
LLOQ	1.00	1.06	7.26	5.71		1.01	11.40	1.62
LQC	3.00	2.76	2.27	−7.87		2.67	3.37	−10.94
MQC	3000	3027	7.83	0.89		3254	9.48	8.48
HQC	7500	6982	7.79	−6.91		7676	9.57	2.35

3.4. Docetaxel Pharmacokinetics in TOM Models

The area under the concentration curves (AUC), the maximum concentration (C_{max}), and the time to maximum concentration (t_{max}) as main pharmacokinetic parameters for the concentration versus time profiles of docetaxel within the sampling port are summarized in Table 4.

The course of the concentration versus time curves was comparable between the applied drug doses (Figure 3). Following the administration of docetaxel by supplementing the differentiation medium of TOM models in the reservoir at 0 h, the drug concentration increased until a plateau phase. The time to maximum concentration t_{max}, 39 ± 7.9 h was almost independent of the administered docetaxel dose, while the C_{max} depended on the administered docetaxel dose. Following the exchange of the differentiation medium, again supplemented with the same docetaxel doses, we detected 2.4- to 9.1-fold increased maximum concentrations and 2.4- to 8.8-fold increased AUCs in the sampling port compared to the respective values following the first docetaxel administration. Furthermore, we detected about 4- to 7-fold higher docetaxel concentrations in the sampling port compared to the applied docetaxel concentration (Figure 3b,c). This effect was not observed when applying 7 or 7000 ng/mL docetaxel (Figure 3a,d). Again, the t_{max} values were close to the end of the treatment cycle with values ranging between 82 and 89 h.

Table 4. Main pharmacokinetic parameters following 1st docetaxel application (0–48 h) and 2nd docetaxel application (48–96 h). c: docetaxel concentration, AUC: area under the curve.

c (ng/mL)	AUC (0–48 h) Mean (h × ng/mL)	CV (%)	C_{max} (0–48 h) Mean (ng/mL)	CV (%)	t_{max} (0–48 h) t_{max} (h)	CV (%)
7	66.3	44.6	1.9	194.5	43.9	14.5
70	444.4	12.5	14.4	25.3	39.5	20.7
700	13,324	26.0	461	29.0	41	9.9
7000	85,658	8.3	2492	10.4	32	21.4

c (ng/mL)	AUC (48–96 h) Mean (h × ng/mL)	CV (%)	C_{max} (48–96 h) Mean (ng/mL)	CV (%)	t_{max} (48–96 h) t_{max} (h)	CV (%)
7	151.4	84.4	6.0	65.1	82.8	16.2
70	3915.1	75.0	131.4	78.5	82.7	15.5
700	78,890	75.1	2850	66.3	83	16.6
7000	211,171	12.2	5920	7.3	90	13.7

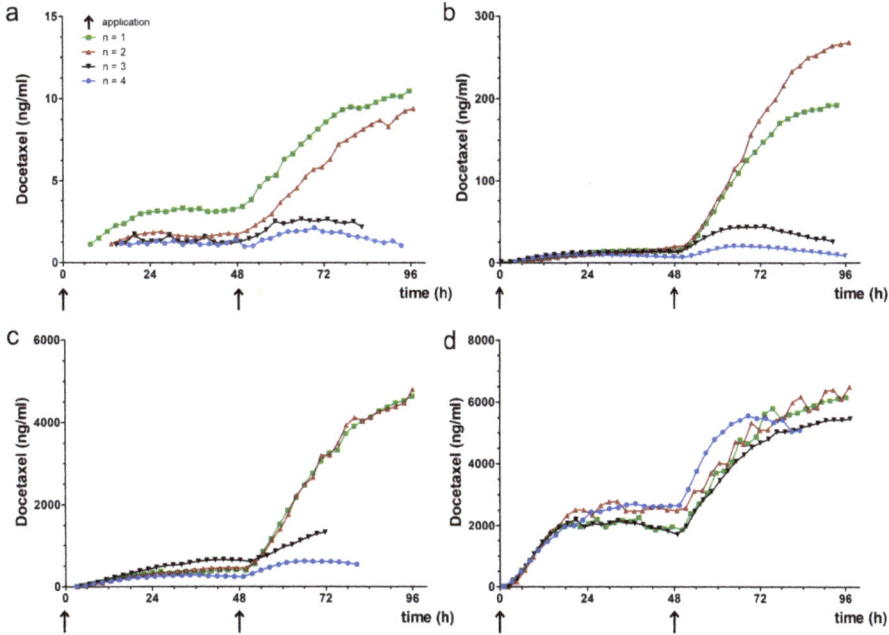

Figure 3. Concentration-time curves of docetaxel. Docetaxel concentrations in the sampling port of TOM models following the application of (**a**) 7, (**b**) 70, (**c**) 700 or (**d**) 7000 ng/mL docetaxel. Docetaxel was supplemented to the differentiation at 0 and 48 h (arrows), $n = 4$ for each concentration.

Moreover, the concentration versus time curves showed a different shape in two experiments (blue and black curve vs. red and green curve in Figure 3a–c). The slope of the blue and black curves markedly differed from the slope of the red and green curves after the second docetaxel administration. The relatively constant docetaxel concentrations within the sampling port could result from evaporation of medium from the reservoir (Figure 1a(3)), causing in loss of contact of the model with the reservoir.

Evaporation also affected the accessibility of the sample fluid for the autosampler needle, since we did not measure docetaxel from certain time points on (e.g., black curve in Figure 3c).

4. Discussion

An automated UHPLC-MS/MS method with online sampling in TOM models is presented here. This proof-of-concept study demonstrated the feasibility of real-time monitoring of drug levels in TOM models without any sample preparation. To achieve this, both the analytical method for docetaxel quantitation in human blood samples [20] and the culture of TOM models [14] needed to be adapted only slightly. Our approach was validated according to EMA guidelines [15] and is easily transferrable to other in vitro disease models.

In vitro studies frequently use drug doses far higher than the maximum tolerated dose in patients [21]. This overdosing causes effects in vitro that are not reproducible in vivo, contributing to the high attrition rate of investigational new drugs in clinical trials. Even if the patients tolerate such high doses, they will be prone to off-target effects. Aside from the bench-to-bedside extrapolation of drug doses, clinical data can be useful to conduct more relevant studies for investigation of personalized adaptations. Considering the maximum plasma concentration at the highest single dose recommended in the drug product of marketed drugs provides an upper limit for in vitro studies [22]. This concept is particularly useful to test potential new indications for approved drugs. We used docetaxel as a model drug to develop our analytical approach since both the efficacy and the pharmacokinetics of docetaxel are well-known [22]. After calculating a steady-state concentration of 74 ng/mL docetaxel in patients following an intravenous application of 75 mg/m^2 (for details, see [14]), we selected 7; 70; 700; and 7000 ng/mL as test concentrations in TOM models. The AUC within the TOM models ranged between 66.32 and 85,658.15 h × ng/mL following the first, and between 151 and 211,171 h×ng/mL following the second docetaxel application. Together with C_{max} values below 2492 and 5920 ng/mL, these in vitro results were in range of the clinical application of 100 mg/m^2, which results in an AUC of 4600 h × ng/mL and C_{max} of 3700 ng/mL [23].

Focusing on the nominal concentration of 70 ng/mL, we detected less docetaxel in the sampling port than has been found in human blood samples. This discrepancy supports the hypothesis of the poor uptake of anticancer drugs into solid tumors [6]. Likewise, paclitaxel penetrates only to the periphery of spheroids [5]. Nevertheless, docetaxel uptake into the TOM models increased following the second drug application. Since apoptosis results in enhanced drug uptake into inner cell layers of solid tumors [8], tumor cells dying after the first application should favor docetaxel uptake into TOM models.

Moreover, our method provides an in-depth insight into the formation of docetaxel degradation products. Since docetaxel epimerization is associated with a loss of potency and tumor resistance development in vivo [24], the considerable epimer formation will affect the efficacy of docetaxel. In contrast, the trace amounts of oxidation products and carbamates should not limit docetaxel effects in TOM models, although they are 10- to 40-fold less active [25]. The degradation products were identified by QTOF-MS and related to degradation products known from the literature [26]. Nevertheless, our approach allows for only limited insights into clinically relevant clearance due to the absence of hepatic metabolism and biliary excretion. If tumor cells metabolize the applied drugs, the quantitation of local metabolites will be feasible as well, but in the case at hand, we observed docetaxel epimerization and formation of degradation products as artifacts also in cell-free medium.

Differences between docetaxel concentrations in human patients and TOM models also arise from differences in protein binding. Whereas plasma protein binding of docetaxel is 97% in the patients [22], protein binding in medium containing fetal bovine serum is saturable. Paclitaxel, close in chemical structure to docetaxel, shows a protein binding between 79% at 500 ng/mL and 20% at 15,000 ng/mL [27]. Thus, we expect higher amounts of free drug available compared to the patients, especially following the application of 7000 ng/mL docetaxel. Nevertheless, we were not able to discriminate free against total docetaxel concentration, since the membrane of the sampling port has a pore size of 400 nm. Most protein sizes range between 1 and 100 nm, making protein diffusion into the sampling port likely. This might also explain higher C_{max} values in the sampling port than the administered concentration in the reservoir, since we quantified all docetaxel within the sampling port. The first docetaxel administration saturated the protein binding and intracellular fluids, the second application directly increased the concentration in the interstitial fluid of TOM models and the sampling port. However, we assume complete equilibration between the interstitial fluid of the TOM model and the sampling fluid within two hours, equal to the time interval we selected between two measurements. Thus, signals of the concentration over time curve earlier between zero and two hours might not recapitulate the concentration within the interstitial fluid of the TOM model, but provide an insight into the lag-time between docetaxel application and first appearance within the sampling port. As to be expected, the lag-time decreases with increasing docetaxel concentrations: 11.1 ± 3 h (7 ng/mL docetaxel application) compared to 1.82 ± 0.6 h (7000 ng/mL docetaxel application).

Since classical microdialysis already allowed insights into tissue-specific drug [28] and cytokine levels [29], the automated determination of pharmacokinetic profiles will enable patient-specific analyses in higher throughput. PK-PD modelling already improved dose selection and characterization of drug effects on tumor growth, overall survival and safety [30], but requires relevant data for the patient and his/her tumor. Nonclinical testing together with pharmacometrics may provide a more detailed insight by testing drugs in patient-specific models and extrapolating drug concentrations in tumors to adapt dose regimen for patients.

UHPLC-MS/MS again proved as the method of choice as it was already useful for a wide range of applications in pharmacology, toxicology, and forensics [31–33]. Despite first dilute and inject attempts to reduce the time-consuming sample preparation [34–39], UHPLC-MS/MS analyses still often utilizes extensive sample preparation to separate the molecule of interest from interfering proteins and potential enzymatic degradation processes [40]. Our method (A) used for quantitation of docetaxel was successfully validated in terms of selectivity, carry-over, lower limit of quantitation (LLOQ), calibration function, accuracy, and precision according to EMA guidelines for bioanalytical method validation. A very broad concentration range of 1–10,000 ng/mL was covered compared to already published methods [20,41], allowing the analysis of docetaxel administered ranging from 7 to 7000 ng/mL. The method proved to be accurate and precise, showed acceptable carry-over after including blank injections between high and low concentration samples, as well as fitness-for purpose in LLOQ. Furthermore, the method was fast, being able to separate docetaxel and 7-epi-docetaxel in less than 3.7 min (total run-time including cleaning of injector 9.75 min).

Future studies will compare differences between the patients' drug responses and drug delivery systems to optimize the dose regimen and application form. For increased efficacy, model size and sampling volume may be further optimized in the direction of high-throughput, and therefore, enhance personalized medicine.

5. Conclusions

We developed and evaluated a real-time approach to automatically measure docetaxel concentrations in TOM models. Partial epimerization and neglectable amounts of degradation products were detected instantaneously upon application of docetaxel to the medium. The courses of concentration versus time curves for 96 h were comparable among four different docetaxel concentrations. The first drug application resulted in an increase of docetaxel concentration, followed by a plateau phase, and exceeded after the second drug application. This proof-of-concept study paves the way for real-time pharmacokinetic and further online investigations in 3D tumor models and beyond, and thus, helps to improve preclinical drug development and personalized medicine.

Supplementary Materials: The following are available online at http://www.mdpi.com/1999-4923/12/5/413/s1, Figure S1: Multiple reaction monitoring (MRM) chromatogram, Figure S2: Overlay of extracted ion chromatograms of docetaxel and degradation products, Figure S3: Product ion spectra of degradation products, Figure S4:

Suggested chemical structure of docetaxel and degradation products, structural differences in comparison to docetaxel are displayed in red color.

Author Contributions: Conceptualization, J.F.J., L.G., B.W., C.Z., and M.K.P.; methodology, J.F.J., L.G., B.W., C.Z., and M.K.P.; validation, J.F.J., L.G., and C.Z.; formal analysis, J.F.J., L.G. and C.Z.; investigation, J.F.J., L.G., J.G., L.M.C..; resources, C.Z., U.K., M.K.P.; data curation, J.F.J., L.G., J.G.-M., L.M.C.; writing—original draft preparation, J.F.J., L.G., C.Z.; writing—review and editing, J.F.J., L.G., U.K., C.Z., M.K.P.; visualization, J.F.J., L.G., J.G., C.Z.; supervision, C.Z., M.K.P.; project administration, U.K., C.Z., M.K.P.; funding acquisition, C.Z., U.K., M.K.P. All authors have read and agreed to the published version of the manuscript.

Funding: This research was funded by the Freie Universität Berlin (Focus Area Disease in Human Aging, "DynAge").

Acknowledgments: The authors thank Kathleen Sauvetre, Université Angers, France, for technical help with the sampling port and Luis Ilia, Freie Universität Berlin, Germany, for help with the pharmacokinetic analyses. The publication of this article was funded by Freie Universität Berlin.

Conflicts of Interest: The authors declare no conflict of interest. The funders had no role in the design of the study; in the collection, analyses, or interpretation of data; in the writing of the manuscript, or in the decision to publish the results.

References

1. Horvath, C.J.; Milton, M.N. The TeGenero incident and the Duff Report conclusions: A series of unfortunate events or an avoidable event? *Toxicol. Pathol.* **2009**, *37*, 372–383. [CrossRef] [PubMed]
2. Zou, P.; Yu, Y.; Zheng, N.; Yang, Y.; Paholak, H.J.; Yu, L.X.; Sun, D. Applications of Human Pharmacokinetic Prediction in First-in-Human Dose Estimation. *AAPS J.* **2012**, *14*, 262–281. [CrossRef] [PubMed]
3. Andrade, E.L.; Bento, A.F.; Cavalli, J.; Oliveira, S.K.; Schwanke, R.C.; Siqueira, J.M.; Freitas, C.S.; Marcon, R.; Calixto, J.B. Non-clinical studies in the process of new drug development—Part II: Good laboratory practice, metabolism, pharmacokinetics, safety and dose translation to clinical studies. *Braz. J. Med. Biol. Res.* **2016**, *49*, e5646. [CrossRef] [PubMed]
4. Nie, L.; Rubin, E.H.; Mehrotra, N.; Pinheiro, J.; Fernandes, L.L.; Roy, A.; Bailey, S.; de Alwis, D.P. Rendering the 3 + 3 Design to Rest: More Efficient Approaches to Oncology Dose-Finding Trials in the Era of Targeted Therapy. *Clin. Cancer Res.* **2016**, *22*, 2623–2629. [CrossRef]
5. Jang, S.H.; Wientjes, M.G.; Lu, D.; Au, J.L. Drug delivery and transport to solid tumors. *Pharm. Res.* **2003**, *20*, 1337–1350. [CrossRef]
6. Dewhirst, M.W.; Secomb, T.W. Transport of drugs from blood vessels to tumour tissue. *Nat. Rev. Cancer* **2017**, *17*, 738–750. [CrossRef]
7. Saleem, A.; Price, P.M. Early tumor drug pharmacokinetics is influenced by tumor perfusion but not plasma drug exposure. *Clin Cancer Res* **2008**, *14*, 8184–8190. [CrossRef]
8. Jang, S.H.; Wientjes, M.G.; Au, J.L. Determinants of paclitaxel uptake, accumulation and retention in solid tumors. *Invest. New Drugs* **2001**, *19*, 113–123. [CrossRef]
9. Fang, Y.; Eglen, R.M. Three-Dimensional Cell Cultures in Drug Discovery and Development. *SLAS Discov* **2017**, *22*, 456–472. [CrossRef]
10. Schütte, M.; Risch, T.; Abdavi-Azar, N.; Boehnke, K.; Schumacher, D.; Keil, M.; Yildiriman, R.; Jandrasits, C.; Borodina, T.; Amstislavskiy, V.; et al. Molecular dissection of colorectal cancer in pre-clinical models identifies biomarkers predicting sensitivity to EGFR inhibitors. *Nat. Commun.* **2017**, *8*, 14262. [CrossRef]
11. Wang, Q.; Zhang, J.; Pi, Z.; Zheng, Z.; Xing, J.; Song, F.; Liu, S.; Liu, Z. Application of online microdialysis coupled with liquid chromatography-tandem mass spectrometry method in assessing neuroprotective effect of Rhizoma coptidis on diabetic rats. *Anal. Methods* **2015**, *7*, 45–52. [CrossRef]
12. Graf, C.; Rühl, E. Imaging Techniques for Probing Nanoparticles in Cells and Skin. In *Biological Responses to Nanoscale Particles*; Springer: Berlin, Germany, 2019; pp. 213–239.
13. Rheinwald, J.G.; Beckett, M.A. Tumorigenic keratinocyte lines requiring anchorage and fibroblast support cultured from human squamous cell carcinomas. *Cancer Res* **1981**, *41*, 1657–1663. [PubMed]
14. Gronbach, L.; Wolff, C.; Klinghammer, K.; Stellmacherc, J.; Jurmeisterd, P.; Alexievc, U.; Schäfer-Kortinga, M.; Tinhofer, I.; Keilholz, U.; Zoschke, C. A multilayered epithelial mucosa model of head neck squamous cell carcinoma for analysis of tumor-microenvironment interactions and drug development. *Clin. Cancer Res..* (in revision).

15. EMA. Guideline on Bioanalytical Method Validation. 2011. Available online: ema.europa.eu/en/documents/scientific-guideline/guideline-bioanalytical-method-validation_en.pdf (accessed on 2 February 2020).
16. EMA. ICH Topic Q 2 (R1) Validation of Analytical Procedures: Text and Methodology. 1995. Available online: ema.europa.eu/en/documents/scientific-guideline/ich-q-2-r1-validation-analytical-procedures-text-methodology-step-5_en.pdf (accessed on 2 February 2020).
17. R Development Core Team. *R: A Language and Environment for Statistical Computing*; R Foundation for Statistical Computing: Vienna, Austria, 2019.
18. Rao, B.M.; Chakraborty, A.; Srinivasu, M.K.; Devi, M.L.; Kumar, P.R.; Chandrasekhar, K.B.; Srinivasan, A.K.; Prasad, A.S.; Ramanatham, J. A stability-indicating HPLC assay method for docetaxel. *J. Pharm. Biomed. Anal.* **2006**, *41*, 676–681. [CrossRef]
19. Kumar, D.; Tomar, R.S.; Deolia, S.K.; Mitra, M.; Mukherjee, R.; Burman, A.C. Isolation and characterization of degradation impurities in docetaxel drug substance and its formulation. *J. Pharm. Biomed.* **2007**, *43*, 1228–1235. [CrossRef]
20. Yamaguchi, H.; Fujikawa, A.; Ito, H.; Tanaka, N.; Furugen, A.; Miyamori, K.; Takahashi, N.; Ogura, J.; Kobayashi, M.; Yamada, T.; et al. A rapid and sensitive LC/ESI–MS/MS method for quantitative analysis of docetaxel in human plasma and its application to a pharmacokinetic study. *J. Chromatogr. B Biomed. Appl.* **2012**, *893-894*, 157–161. [CrossRef]
21. Smith, M.A.; Houghton, P. A proposal regarding reporting of in vitro testing results. *Clin. Cancer Res.* **2013**, *19*, 2828–2833. [CrossRef]
22. Liston, D.R.; Davis, M. Clinically Relevant Concentrations of Anticancer Drugs: A Guide for Nonclinical Studies. *Clin. Cancer Res.* **2017**, *23*, 3489–3498. [CrossRef]
23. EMA. European Public Assessment Report "TAXOTERE", Annex l—Summary of Product. 2019. Available online: ema.europa.eu/documents/product-information/taxotere-epar-product-information_en.pdf (accessed on 2 February 2020).
24. Mohsin, S.; Arellano, I.H.; Choudhury, N.R.; Garg, S. Docetaxel epimerization in silicone films: A case of drug excipient incompatibility. *Drug Test. Anal.* **2014**, *6*, 1076–1084. [CrossRef]
25. Vuilhorgne, M.; Gaillard, C.; Sanderink, G.J.; Royer, I.; Monsarrat, B.; Dubois, J.; Wright, M. Metabolism of Taxoid Drugs. In *Taxane Anticancer Agents*; American Chemical Society: Washington, DC, USA, 1994; Volume 583, pp. 98–110.
26. Tian, J.; Stella, V.J. Degradation of paclitaxel and related compounds in aqueous solutions I: Epimerization. *J. Pharm. Sci.* **2008**, *97*, 1224–1235. [CrossRef]
27. Song, D.; Hsu, L.F.; Au, J.L. Binding of taxol to plastic and glass containers and protein under in vitro conditions. *J. Pharm. Sci.* **1996**, *85*, 29–31. [CrossRef] [PubMed]
28. Schuck, V.J.; Rinas, I.; Derendorf, H. In vitro microdialysis sampling of docetaxel. *J Pharm. Biomed. Anal.* **2004**, *36*, 807–813. [CrossRef] [PubMed]
29. Baumann, K.Y.; Church, M.K.; Clough, G.F.; Quist, S.R.; Schmelz, M.; Skov, P.S.; Anderson, C.D.; Tannert, L.K.; Giménez-Arnau, A.M.; Frischbutter, S.; et al. Skin microdialysis: methods, applications and future opportunities—An EAACI position paper. *Clin. Transl. Allergy* **2019**, *9*, 24. [CrossRef] [PubMed]
30. Pasqua, O.E.D. PKPD and Disease Modeling: Concepts and Applications to Oncology. In *Clinical Trial Simulations: Applications and Trends*; Kimko, H.H.C., Peck, C.C., Eds.; Springer: New York, NY, USA, 2011; pp. 281–306. [CrossRef]
31. Patteet, L.; Maudens, K.E.; Stove, C.P.; Lambert, W.E.; Morrens, M.; Sabbe, B.; Neels, H. The use of dried blood spots for quantification of 15 antipsychotics and 7 metabolites with ultra-high performance liquid chromatography - tandem mass spectrometry. *Drug Test. Anal.* **2015**, *7*, 502–511. [CrossRef]
32. Rodriguez-Aller, M.; Gurny, R.; Veuthey, J.L.; Guillarme, D. Coupling ultra high-pressure liquid chromatography with mass spectrometry: constraints and possible applications. *J. Chromatogr. A* **2013**, *1292*, 2–18. [CrossRef]
33. Novakova, L.; Pavlik, J.; Chrenkova, L.; Martinec, O.; Cerveny, L. Current antiviral drugs and their analysis in biological materials—Part II: Antivirals against hepatitis and HIV viruses. *J Pharm. Biomed. Anal.* **2018**, *147*, 378–399. [CrossRef]

34. Gorgens, C.; Guddat, S.; Schanzer, W.; Thevis, M. Screening and confirmation of myo-inositol trispyrophosphate (ITPP) in human urine by hydrophilic interaction liquid chromatography high resolution / high accuracy mass spectrometry for doping control purposes. *Drug Test. Anal.* **2014**, *6*, 1102–1107. [CrossRef]
35. Ambrosio, G.; Joseph, J.F.; Wuest, B.; Mazzarino, M.; de la Torre, X.; Diel, P.; Botre, F.; Parr, M.K. Detection and quantitation of ecdysterone in human serum by liquid chromatography coupled to tandem mass spectrometry. *Steroids* **2020**, *157*, 108603. [CrossRef]
36. Holder, B.R.; McNaney, C.A.; Luchetti, D.; Schaeffer, E.; Drexler, D.M. Bioanalysis of acetylcarnitine in cerebrospinal fluid by HILIC-mass spectrometry. *Biomed. Chromatogr.* **2015**, *29*, 1375–1379. [CrossRef]
37. Kong, T.Y.; Kim, J.H.; Kim, J.Y.; In, M.K.; Choi, K.H.; Kim, H.S.; Lee, H.S. Rapid analysis of drugs of abuse and their metabolites in human urine using dilute and shoot liquid chromatography-tandem mass spectrometry. *Arch. Pharm. Res.* **2017**, *40*, 180–196. [CrossRef]
38. Bourgogne, E.; Wagner, M. [Sample preparation and bioanalysis in mass spectrometry]. *Ann. Biol. Clin. (Paris)* **2015**, *73*, 11–23. [CrossRef] [PubMed]
39. Parr, M.K.; Ambrosio, G.; Wuest, B.; Mazzarino, M.; de la Torre, X.; Sibilia, F.; Joseph, J.F.; Diel, P.; Botrè, F. Targeting the Administration of Ecdysterone in Doping Control Samples. *bioRxiv* **2019**. [CrossRef]
40. Plock, N.; Kloft, C. Microdialysis–theoretical background and recent implementation in applied life-sciences. *Eur. J. Pharm. Sci.* **2005**, *25*, 1–24. [CrossRef] [PubMed]
41. Hendrikx, J.J.; Hillebrand, M.J.; Thijssen, B.; Rosing, H.; Schinkel, A.H.; Schellens, J.H.; Beijnen, J.H. A sensitive combined assay for the quantification of paclitaxel, docetaxel and ritonavir in human plasma using liquid chromatography coupled with tandem mass spectrometry. *J. Chromatogr. B Analyt. Technol. Biomed. Life Sci.* **2011**, *879*, 2984–2990. [CrossRef]

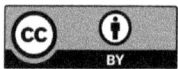

© 2020 by the authors. Licensee MDPI, Basel, Switzerland. This article is an open access article distributed under the terms and conditions of the Creative Commons Attribution (CC BY) license (http://creativecommons.org/licenses/by/4.0/).

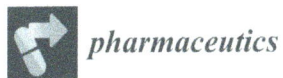

Article

Population Pharmacokinetic Analysis of Tiropramide in Healthy Korean Subjects

Seung-Hyun Jeong [1,†], Ji-Hun Jang [1,†], Hea-Young Cho [2] and Yong-Bok Lee [1,*]

1 College of Pharmacy, Chonnam National University, 77 Yongbong-ro, Buk-Gu, Gwangju 61186, Korea; rhdqn95@naver.com (S.-H.J.); jangji0121@naver.com (J.-H.J.)
2 College of Pharmacy, CHA University, 335 Pangyo-ro, Bundang-gu, Seongnam-si, Gyeonggi-Do 13488, Korea; hycho@cha.ac.kr
* Correspondence: leeyb@chonnam.ac.kr; Tel.: +82-62-530-2931; Fax: +82-62-530-0106
† Both authors contributed equally to this work.

Received: 9 March 2020; Accepted: 17 April 2020; Published: 18 April 2020

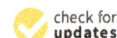

Abstract: The purpose of this study was to perform population pharmacokinetic (PPK) analysis of tiropramide in healthy Korean subjects, as well as to investigate the possible effects of various covariates on pharmacokinetic (PK) parameters of tiropramide. Although tiropramide is commonly used in digestive system-related diseases as an antispasmodic, PPK reporting and factors affecting PKs are not clearly reported. Thus, this study for healthy subjects is very significant because it could find new covariates in patients that had not been reported before or predict PPK for patients in the clinic by establishing PPK in healthy adults. By using Phoenix NLME, PK, demographic, and genetic data (collected to explain PK diversity of tiropramide in population) analyses were performed. As a basic model, a one-compartment with first-order absorption and lag-time was established and extended to include covariates that influenced the inter-subject variability. The total protein significantly influenced the distribution volume and systemic clearance of tiropramide, but genetic factors such as *ABCB1* (1236C>T, 2677G>T/A, and 3435C>T), *CYP2D6* (*1 and *10), *OCT2* (808G>T), and *PEPT1* (1287G>C) genes did not show any significant association with PK parameters of tiropramide. The final PPK model of tiropramide was validated, and suggested that some of the PK diversity in the population could be explained. Herein, we first describe the establishment of the PPK model of tiropramide for healthy Korean subjects, which may be useful as a dosing algorithm for the diseased population.

Keywords: tiropramide; healthy Korean subjects; modeling; population pharmacokinetic

1. Introduction

Tiropramide is a drug that has been used from the past to the present for symptom relief and treatment of diseases of the digestive system such as acute spastic abdominal pain and irritable bowel syndrome. Tiropramide is a structurally equivalent tyrosine derivative and contains amide functional groups in the structure together with tertiary amines. It has been reported that tiropramide is widely metabolized into various metabolites (hydroxytiropramide, *N*-despropyltiropramide, *N*-desethyltiropramide, and *N*-desethyl-*N*-despropyltiropramide) after oral administration to rats and humans [1–3]. The mechanism of action of tiropramide has been reported to directly affect the smooth muscle cells. That is, tiropramide activates intracellular cyclic adenosine monophosphate (cAMP) synthase (adenylcyclase) to increase the amount of cAMP to regulate calcium ions necessary for muscle contraction, thereby controlling the relaxation and contraction of intestinal smooth muscle cells. This mechanism of action is very important for clinical use. Other antispasmodics include anticholinergics or antimuscarinics that relieve abdominal pain by acting on the intestinal nervous system. However, the mechanism of action on the nervous system may cause systemic side effects such as dry mouth, dry eyes, and drowsiness, which may lower the patients' compliance with medication. As a result, tiropramide has been widely used in the clinic for the treatment of diseases related to the digestive system with the reduction of the systemic side effects.

However, reporting of pharmacokinetic (PK) information of tiropramide for humans is still very limited. Above all, tiropramide's population pharmacokinetics (PPK) have not been reported thus far. Tiropramide has been reported to have hypotension and peripheral vasodilation (as side effects) like other anticholinergic or antimuscarinic drugs only when a high dose is administered. Overall, incidences of tiropramide side effects are very low and a very safe profile in humans has been reported [4]. Although the incidence of adverse effects of tiropramide is reported to be low in humans, optimal dosing algorithm may maximize the therapeutic effect of the drug and reduce its adverse effects by using a PPK model. PPK modeling can enable effective dose setting and individualized pharmacotherapy by quantifying the diversity of the drug concentrations among individuals (in the population) with a variety of related physicochemical factors. In addition, identifying the physicochemical factors affecting PKs of tiropramide will be a significant scientific basis for the clinical application (such as usage and dose settings) and formulation of tiropramide in the future.

Tiropramide is usually administered orally to adults at 100 mg (1 tablet) 2-3 times a day in the clinic. In exceptional cases, it is reported that tiropramide may be additionally administered in cases of less symptomatic relief. However, it is difficult to judge whether these levels of capacity and usage are precise when considering the differences among individuals in the population. More scientific evidence and data on the dose setting and safety of tiropramide are needed. Therefore, we thought that a study of the PPK model of tiropramide was necessary. In addition, it begs the question on how the various physicochemical or genetic factors among individuals in the population affect the PKs of tiropramide. Moreover, even if individual physicochemical or genetic factors affect tiropramide's PKs, it is very doubtful as to how large the effect would be. Finding significant covariates of tiropramide is very difficult due to the lack of detailed PK information on the precise metabolic mechanisms, absorption, distribution, and excretion of tiropramide (especially in humans), and no PPK studies have been reported in the past. Therefore, in this study, we set up a variety of candidate covariates early in the study to establish factors that significantly influence the PK of tiropramide. The process was based on the physicochemical or physiological properties of tiropramide that have been reported to date.

Tiropramide has amine groups in its structure and will be basic at pH (about 7.4) in vivo on the basis of its pKa value (of 3.1) [4]. Therefore, the covariate effect was confirmed by genotyping the *OCT* gene, which is known to be related to the absorption, distribution, and excretion of various organic cations [5]. Tiropramide is a substance derived from the amino acid tyrosine [6]. Therefore, the genotyping of the *PEPT* gene, which is known to be involved in the absorption and distribution of the peptide drugs such as peptides and β-lactam antibiotics, was performed to confirm the covariate effect [7]. P-glycoprotein (P-gp) is a transporter with a broad range of substrate specificities of about 170 kDa and is known to be mainly involved in the efflux of neutral or cationic substances. In addition, *ABCB1* has been reported as a gene that encodes the P-gp. In this study, the covariate effect was confirmed by genotyping *ABCB1* [8]. In the past, the metabolism of tiropramide in the liver was examined [1], and the covariate effect was confirmed by genotyping metabolism-related *CYP2D6*. In particular, we focused on single nucleotide polymorphism (SNP) of the *CYP2D6* gene related to phase I metabolism (oxidation, reduction, hydrolysis, etc.) in the liver, and tried to confirm the correlation with PKs [9]. In addition, we collected information on various physicochemical factors (including general functional indicators of the kidney and liver) and sought to find the major covariates affecting PKs.

We report on PPK modeling of tiropramide in this study, together with factors affecting PK diversity in the population, which have not been reported yet. In the tiropramide final PPK model (of this study), we quantitatively reflected on the total protein, physicochemical, or genetic factors with differences between individuals, suggesting that scientific dose setting can be possible. In these aspects, for clinical applications, the tiropramide's PPK model would be a great advantage. As a result, development of a tiropramide's PPK model for use in healthy Korean subjects was the purpose of this study. The developed tiropramide's PPK model is expected to be useful for determining a valuable dosing algorithm for tiropramide in healthy Korean subjects. In addition, the identification of factors affecting PK of tiropramide is expected to be of great help in related future studies.

2. Methods

2.1. Study Design

Samples obtained from a bioequivalence study of tiropramide in 24 healthy Korean males were included in this analysis. The age of these subjects ranged from 19 to 29 years (mean ± standard deviation (SD), 22.96 ± 2.61 years). Their body weights ranged from 55.2 to 82.8 kg (mean ± SD, 67.60 ± 7.28 kg). Their body surface area (BSA) ranged from 1.58 to 1.97 m^2 (mean ± SD, 1.80 ± 0.11 m^2), and their body mass index (BMI) ranged from 17.89 to 29.06 kg/m^2 (mean ± SD, 22.74 ± 2.72 kg/m^2). Each subject had no hypersensitivity to any drugs or previous history of illness and was physically normal. All subjects provided informed written consent to perform bioequivalence and PK studies. All subjects underwent physical examinations, clinical screening, complete blood count, urinalysis, and analysis of blood chemistry prior to the admission of this study to evaluate their physical health status. If subjects were taking any medications, other drugs, and/or alcohol for at least 1 week prior to this study, they were excluded from this study. The Institutional Review Board of the Institute of Bioequivalence and Bridging Study, Chonnam National University, Gwangju, Republic of Korea, reviewed and approved (Bioequivalence Test no. 875; 01.16.2003) this study protocol. Clinical studies were performed in accordance with rules of good clinical practice and the revised Declaration of Helsinki for biomedical research involving human subjects. Bioequivalence studies were performed as randomized, single-dose, open-label, crossover, and two-way studies. The data from reference formulation were only used for the current analysis. The subjects were hospitalized (Chonnam National University Hospital, Gwangju, Korea) at 7:30 p.m. 1 day before the study. The subjects had a heparin-locked catheter installed in the median cubital vein. A single dose (100 mg) of tiropramide was given orally to all subjects (after an overnight fast) in each study group with 240 mL of water. Before administration (0 h) and at 0.33, 0.67, 1, 1.5, 2, 2.5, 3, 4, 6, 8, and 12 h after oral administration, blood samples (8 mL) were collected into Vacutainer tubes. At the time of blood sampling, about 2 mL of blood was drained each time to completely remove the heparinized saline solution remaining in the IV catheter, and about 8 mL of blood was collected. Following centrifugation (for 20 min, at 5000 × g), plasma samples were obtained and transferred to polyethylene tubes. They were then stored at −80 °C until analysis. Another study was repeated in the same manner to complete the crossover design after a washout period of 7 days.

2.2. Determination of Physicochemical Parameters

Plasma samples were used in the determination of physicochemical parameters, including total proteins, aspartate transaminase (AST), albumin, alkaline phosphatase (ALP), alanine transaminase (ALT), and creatinine. The determination of main physicochemical parameters in this study, such as total proteins, albumin, AST, ALT, ALP, and creatinine, was performed in a dry automatic analyzer by microsides VITROS (Ortho Clinical Diagnostics, NJ, USA) operating by reflectance spectrophotometry.

2.3. Determination of Genotypes

The blood samples of 3 mL, obtained from individuals participating in this study, were used for genotyping. The blood samples were centrifuged for 10 min at 1000 × g, and deoxyribonucleic acid (DNA) was extracted from the leukocyte layer using a Wizard Genomic DNA purification kit (Promega Co., Madison, WI, USA). The extracted DNA was dissolved in 100 µL of DNA hydration solution and stored at −70 °C until analysis. In order to amplify a portion of gene containing a SNP by polymerase chain reaction (PCR) from the extracted DNA, each primer was prepared according to the variation of allele. Moreover, the genotypes were determined using appropriate methods that have been reported in the past [5,8,10,11]. We conducted experiments three times to acquire exact genotype data.

2.3.1. Identification of ABCB1 1236C>T (in Exon 12), 2677G>T/A (in Exon 21), and 3435C>T (in Exon 26)

Candidate SNPs (1236C>T, 2677G>T/A, and 3435C>T) in the ABCB1 gene were genotyped by using polymerase chain reaction–restriction fragment length polymorphism (PCR-RFLP). Each primer was prepared according to the variation of allele. Forward primer of 5′-TATCCTGTGTCTGTGAATTGCC-3′ and reverse primer of 5′-CCTGACTCACCACACACCAATG-3′ were used for ABCB1 1236C>T genotypes. Forward primer of 5′-TGCAGGCTATAGGTTCCAGG-3′ and reverse primer of 5′-TTTAG TTTGACTCACCT TCCCG-3′ were used for determination of ABCB1 2677G>T/A genotypes. Forward primer of 5′-TGTTTTCAGCTGCTTGATGG-3′ and reverse primer of 5′-AAGGCATGTAT GTTGGCCTC-3′ were used for ABCB1 3435C>T genotypes. PCR was performed in 20 μL reaction mixture including 1 μL of 10 pmol each primer (forward and reverse), 1 μL extracted DNA, and 17 μL autoclaved distilled water. The PCR program was composed of an initial denaturation at 94 °C for 2 min followed by 35 cycles of denaturation at 94 °C for 30 s, annealing at 59.8 °C for 30 s, and extension at 72 °C for 30 s. The final extension step was performed at 72 °C for 5 min. The DNA fragments amplified by PCR were reacted at 37 °C for 16 h with restriction enzymes HaeIII (for ABCB1 1236C>T), Sau3AI (for ABCB1 3435C>T), and BanI/RsaI (for ABCB1 2677G>T/A), which can recognize and cleave specific sequences. These digested fragments were separated by electrophoresis in 2.5% agarose gel, and were visualized under ultraviolet light after staining the gel with ethidium bromide for 30 min.

2.3.2. Identification of CYP2D6 Alleles

Polymorphisms (*1 and *10) in the CYP2D6 gene of individuals were determined using DNA sequencing analysis. The primers were designed and prepared using the primer3 software. The PCR was performed in 20 μL reaction mixture including 1 μL extracted DNA, 1 μL of 10 pmol of each primer (forward and reverse), and 17 μL autoclaved distilled water. The PCR program was composed of an initial denaturation at 94 °C for 3 min followed by 35 cycles of denaturation at 94 °C for 20 s, annealing for at 62 °C 30 s, and extension at 72 °C for 20 min. A final extension step was conducted at 72 °C for 5 min. The PCR products were then analyzed by direct sequencing using the ABI PRISIM BigDye Terminator Cycle Sequencing Kit and an ABI Prism 3100 Genetic Analyzer (Applied Biosystems, Foster City, CA, USA).

2.3.3. Identification of OCT2 808G>T

Candidate SNP (808G>T) in the OCT2 gene was genotyped using pyrosequencing analysis. Each primer was prepared according to the variation of allele. Forward primer of 5′-CGGAGAACAGT GGGGATTTTTTAC-3′, reverse primer of 5′-CACGTAATTCCTTCCGTCTGAAGA-3′, and sequencing primer of 5′-GGTGGTTGCAGTTCACA-3′ were used for OCT2 808G>T genotype. Forward primer has a 5′ biotin triethylene glycol label necessary for post PCR processing. PCR was performed in 20 μL reaction mixture including 1 μL extracted DNA, 1 μL of 10 pmol each primer (forward and reverse), and 17 μL autoclaved distilled water. The PCR program comprised an initial denaturation at 94 °C for 5 min followed by 45 cycles of denaturation at 94 °C for 20 s, annealing at 52.1 °C for 30 s, and extension at 72 °C for 20 s. A final extension step was performed at 72 °C for 5 min. The biotinylated PCR products were immobilized on streptavidin-coated Sepharose beads (Amersham Biosciences, Uppsala, Sweden). A total of 37 μL of binding buffer (10 mM Tris HCl, 2 M sodium chloride, 1 mM EDTA, 0.1% Tween 20, pH 7.6; Pyrosequencing AB, Uppsala, Sweden), 3 μL of streptavidin-coated Sepharose beads, and 20 μL of water were added to 20 μL PCR product; then, the solution was vigorously shaken for 10 min at room temperature. A 96 pin magnetic tool (Pyrosequencing AB, Uppsala, Sweden) was used to transfer up to 96 samples at a time to solutions as follows. The beads with bound template were first transferred to 70% ethanol solution and 0.2 N sodium hydroxide solution, then to 1X washing buffer (Pyrosequencing AB, Uppsala, Sweden), and finally into a solution of 1X annealing buffer (20 mM Tris acetate, 2 mM magnesium acetate, pH 7.6), including the appropriate sequencing primer of 10 pmol. Lastly, this mixture was heated for 1 min to 95 °C and then cooled to 50 °C and incubated at room temperature for at least 5 min to bind the sequencing primer to the template. After template preparation, a 96-well plate including the samples was loaded into the instrument (PSQ 96MA; Pyrosequencing AB, Uppsala, Sweden) along with the optimal reagents (Pyro Gold; Biotage AB, Uppsala, Sweden). This instrument sequences the templates by dispensing reagents and deoxynucleotide triphosphates in a user-defined order, achieving real-time sequencing by synthesis in an automated fashion. This is achieved by creating and monitoring an enzyme cascade initiated by nucleotide incorporation that produces light emission. Pyrosequencing data were obtained by using Peak Height Determination Software v2.1 (Pyrosequencing AB, Uppsala, Sweden).

2.3.4. Identification of PEPT1 1287G>C (in Exon 16)

Candidate SNP (1287G>C) in the *PEPT1* gene were genotyped by using PCR-RFLP. Each primer was prepared according to the variation of allele. Forward primer of 5'-CCCTTGTCAGGGTTAAGATGA-3' and reverse primer of 5'-GCTTCTCTAAATCCTATTATAACAGGG-3' were used for *PEPT1* 1287G>C genotypes. PCR was performed in 20 µL reaction mixture including 1 µL extracted DNA, 1 µL of 10 pmol each primer (forward and reverse), and 17 µL autoclaved distilled water. The PCR program comprised of an initial denaturation at 95 °C for 5 min followed by 35 cycles of denaturation at 95 °C for 20 s, annealing for at 54.5 °C 30 s, and an extension at 72 °C for 20 s. The final extension step was performed at 72 °C for 5 min. DNA fragments amplified by PCR were reacted at 37 °C for 1 h with restriction enzyme *Sau96I*, which can recognize and cleave specific sequences. The digested fragments were separated by electrophoresis in 2.5% agarose gel, and were visualized under ultraviolet light after staining the gel with ethidium bromide for 30 min.

2.4. Determination of Plasma Tiropramide Concentrations

Plasma concentrations of tiropramide were determined using a validated column-switching semi-micro high-performance liquid chromatography (HPLC) method based on a previous study [12].

2.4.1. Chromatographic Conditions

The analytical system consisted of the Nanospace SI-2 series (Shiseido, Tokyo, Japan) with an ultraviolet-visible (UV–VIS) detector 3002, two 3001 pumps, a 3014 column oven, a high pressure six-way switching valve 3012, a 3010 degasser, and a 3023 autosampler. The system operation and signal processing were operated by Syscon (Shiseido, Tokyo, Japan). The columns used in this on-line extraction system include an analytical column (Capcell Pak C_{18} UG120, 150 × 1.5 mm I.D. Shiseido), a pre-column (Capcell Pak MF Ph-1, 10 × 4 mm I.D. 5 µm Shiseido), and an enrichment column (Capcell Pak C_{18} UG120, 35 × 2 mm I.D. Shiseido). The mobile phase for primary separation of tiropramide in the pre-column and concentration in the enrichment column was phosphate buffer (50 mM, pH 7.0)-acetonitrile (88/12, v/v) with a flow rate of 0.5 mL/min. The mobile phase for analytical column was phosphoric acid–phosphate buffer (50 mM, pH 7.0)-acetonitrile (0.04/59.96/40, v/v/v) with a flow rate of 0.1 mL/min. All the columns were maintained at 25–30 °C. The quantification was performed at 230 nm wavelength. The peak with the retention time of tiropramide was verified using a photodiode array detector (2017 Diode Array, Shiseido, Tokyo, Japan).

2.4.2. Analytical Procedures

The performance of column-switching semi-micro HPLC consists of three steps, as follows: sample loading and primary separation, enrichment of analyte fraction, and chromatographic separation. When the column-switching valve was at the precolumn inlet position, an aliquot of filtered (by 0.22 µm,

Millex-GV syringe filter unit, Millipore, Burlington, MA, USA) plasma sample (80 µL) was loaded to the pre-column, and a primary separation of tiropramide from plasma proteins was conducted by using phosphate buffer (50 mM, pH 7.0)-acetonitrile (88/12, v/v). Subsequently, the valve was switched to the enrichment column inlet position, and the tiropramide fraction was eluted from the pre-column and concentrated in the enrichment column by phosphate buffer (50 mM, pH 7.0)-acetonitrile (88/12, v/v). Afterwards, the valve was switched to analytical column inlet position, and tiropramide was finally isolated and quantified by phosphoric acid–phosphate buffer (50 mM, pH 7.0)-acetonitrile (0.04/59.96/40, v/v/v).

2.5. Pharmacokinetic Analysis

Basic PK parameters of tiropramide were obtained from non-compartmental analysis (NCA) through the Phoenix-WinNonlin (8.1 version, Pharsight, Certara Inc., Princeton, NJ, USA) program. Peak plasma concentration (C_{max}) and the time to reach C_{max} (T_{max}) were individually determined using plasma concentration–time curve. The area under the curve ($AUC_{0-\infty}$) was calculated as the sum of AUC_{0-t} and C_{last}/k, where C_{last} is the final measured concentration and k is the elimination rate constant at terminal phase. AUC_{0-t} was calculated using a linear trapezoidal rule from 0 to t (as 24) h after administration. The half-life ($t_{1/2}$) was calculated as 0.693/k, and the volume of the distribution (V_d/F) was calculated as dose/k·$AUC_{0-\infty}$. The clearance (CL/F) was calculated by dividing the dose of tiropramide by $AUC_{0-\infty}$, where F is the bioavailability of oral administration. All PK parameter values were calculated as mean ± SD, and the statistical differences in the group parameters (according to genotype) were confirmed by the analysis of variance (ANOVA) through the Statistical Package for the Social Sciences (SPSS) program (23 version, IBM). A p-value < 0.05 was established as being statistically significant.

2.6. Model Development

PPK analysis was conducted with a non-linear mixed effects model (NLME) approach through the Phoenix NLME (8.1 version, Pharsight, Certara Inc., Princeton, NJ, USA) program. In addition, PPK model development was performed in the first order conditional estimates method with extended least squares (FOCE-ELS) estimation (with η–ε interaction).

As the first step of PPK modeling, data were fitted to two or one compartment disposition models with first order elimination and absorption kinetics without or with absorption lag-time for determining the structural base model (without covariates). In addition, a multiple transit model with a compartment added to the absorption phase was evaluated to establish the structural base model. The final selection of structural base model was performed by the statistical significance between models using goodness-of-fit (GOF) plots, twice the negative log likelihood (-2LL), and Akaike's information criterion (AIC). The initial values for the parameters used in this process were obtained and referenced using NCA and classic compartment models. As a result, the basic PK parameters were as follows: clearance for the central compartment (CL), absorption lag time (T_{lag}), volume of distribution for the central compartment (V), first oral absorption rate constant (K_{a1}), and second oral absorption rate constant (K_{a2}).

The residual variability was determined to additive error model in log transformed (plasma concentration) data, as shown in the following equation: $C_{obs,ij} = C_{pred,ij} \cdot \exp(\varepsilon_{ij})$, where ε_{ij} is the intra-subject variability (including model misspecification and assay error) with mean 0 and variance σ^2, and $C_{pred,ij}$ and $C_{obs,ij}$ are the jth predicted and observed plasma concentrations in the ith subject, respectively.

The inter-individual variability (IIV) in PK parameters of tiropramide was evaluated by using an exponential error model, as shown in the following equation: $P_i = P_{tv} \cdot \exp(\eta_i)$, where η_i is the random variable for the ith individual, which was normally distributed with mean 0 and variance ω^2; P_i is the parameter value of the ith individual, and P_{tv} is the typical value of the population parameter.

As a second step of PPK modeling, candidate covariates (including demographic and genetic information) screened during this study were considered in reflecting the structural base model to account for PK diversity of tiropramide in the population. Height, body weight, age, BMI, BSA, creatinine, albumin, AST, ALT, ALP, creatinine clearance, and total protein were used as demographic candidate covariates. Here, BMI was determined by using the metric unit system [13]. BSA was determined on the basis of the Mosteller equation [14]. Creatinine clearance was determined on the basis of the Cockcroft–Gault equation [15]. There were also *ABCB1* 1236C>T, *ABCB1* 2677G>T/A, *ABCB1* 3435C>T, *CYP2D6* (*1 and *10), *OCT2* 808G>T, and *PEPT1* 1287G>C as genetic candidate covariates. To confirm the correlation between covariates and PK parameters, these potential covariates were plotted against individual post hoc parameters. In addition, the covariates were divided into categorical and continuous types in order to reflect the identified (correlation with PK parameters) candidate covariates in the PK parameters of the model. Continuous covariates (mainly demographic candidate covariates) were normalized by median values (of observed values). On the other hand, categorical covariates (mainly genetic candidate covariates) were reflected as index variables in the model. The effects of each covariate were confirmed using exponential, power, or additive options. By stepwise backward elimination and forward addition procedure, the covariates were included or eliminated. By change in the objective function value (OFV), the inclusion of covariates was determined. Covariates corresponding to a decrease in the OFV value greater than 3.84 ($p < 0.05$) were included in the base model (in the forward addition procedure). In addition, covariates corresponding to the case where the decrease in OFV value was greater than 6.63 ($p < 0.01$) through the backward elimination process were not removed from the model and were included.

2.7. Model Evaluation

The final established models (in this study) were verified and evaluated both visually and numerically. To evaluate the model, visual predictive check (VPC), bootstrapping, and goodness-of-fit (including distribution of residuals) analyses were used. The goodness-of-fit was confirmed by using diagnostic scatter plots as follows: (a) population-predicted concentrations (PRED) versus observed (DV), (b) individual-predicted concentrations (IPRED) versus DV, (c) PRED versus conditional weighted residuals (CWRES), (d) time (IVAR) versus CWRES, and (e) quantile–quantile plot of the components of CWRES.

By using non-parametric bootstrap analysis, the stability of the final model was confirmed, and the bootstrap option of Phoenix NLME was used. A total of 1000 replicates were generated by the repeated random sampling with replacement from the original dataset. The estimated parameter values, such as the standard errors (SE; including confidence intervals) and medians from the bootstrap procedure, were compared with those estimated from the original dataset.

By using the VPC option of Phoenix NLME, VPCs of the final established models were performed. The time–DV concentration data were graphically superimposed on the median values and the 5th and 95th percentiles of the time-simulated concentration profiles. If the DV concentration data were approximately distributed within the 95th and 5th prediction interval, the model was expected to be precise. Normalized prediction distribution error (NPDE) was used to evaluate the predictive performance of the model on the basis of a Monte Carlo simulation with the R package [16]. NPDE results were summarized graphically using (1) quantile–quantile plot of the NPDE, (2) a histogram of the NPDE, (3) scatterplot of NPDE vs. time, and (4) scatterplot of NPDE vs. PRED. If the predictive performance is satisfied, the NPDE will follow a normal distribution (Shapiro–Wilk test) with a mean value of zero (t-test) and a variance of one (Fisher's test).

3. Results

3.1. Study Design and Demographic Analysis

The bioequivalence data (from reference formulation) collected from 24 healthy Korean males were used in this PK study for tiropramide. For the PK modelling, a total of 288 tiropramide plasma concentrations were available. There was complete information on height, age, and body weight for the 24 participants. Additionally, we successfully collected information on the total proteins, albumin, creatinine, AST, ALT, ALP, and the creatinine clearance levels of each participant, according to the method described above (Section 2.2). The related demographic information about the participants are shown in Table 1.

Table 1. Demographic information of the studied subjects ($n = 24$).

Physicochemical	Median (Range)	Mean ± SD
Age (year)	23 (19–29)	22.96 ± 2.61
Weight (kg)	66.8 (52.5–82.8)	67.60 ± 7.28
Height (cm)	171.45 (164.3–185.4)	172.59 ± 5.85
BSA (m^2) *	1.80 (1.58–1.97)	1.80 ± 0.11
BMI (kg/m^2) **	22.63 (17.89–29.06)	22.74 ± 2.72
Albumin (g/dL)	4.6 (4.2–5.4)	4.64 ± 0.27
Total proteins (g/dL)	7.6 (6.7–8.3)	7.59 ± 0.41
ALT (U/L)	20.5 (8–55)	22.29 ± 11.67
AST (U/L)	20 (10–32)	20.88 ± 5.81
ALP (U/L)	76 (49–126)	81.83 ± 20.66
Creatinine clearance (mL/min) ***	118.49 (91.78–159.77)	122.88 ± 22.25
Creatinine (mg/dL)	0.9 (0.6–1.1)	0.91 ± 0.13

* Body surface area (BSA) was determined on the basis of the Monsteller equation as follows: $\sqrt{\text{height (cm)} \times \text{weight (kg)} / 3600}$; ** body mass index (BMI) was calculated as follows: body weight (kg)/height^2 (m^2); *** creatinine clearance was determined on the basis of the Cockcroft–Gault equation as follows: [(140-age) × body weight (kg)]/[serum creatinine (mg/dL) × 72].

3.2. Genetic Analysis

Genotyping was performed on all 24 individuals who participated in this study. The analyzed genotypes were *ABCB1* (1236C>T, 2677G>T/A, and 3435C>T), *CYP2D6* (*1 and *10), *OCT2* (808G>T), and *PEPT1* (1287G>C) genes. The results are presented in Table 2. The *ABCB1* 1236C>T genotyping revealed that 6 (25.00%) subjects had the mutant type (TT), 13 (54.17%) subjects had the heterozygous type (CT), and 5 (20.83%) subjects had the homozygous wild type (CC). *ABCB1* 2677G>T/A genotyping revealed that eight (33.33%) subjects had the mutant type (TT or AT or TA or AA), nine (37.50%) subjects had the heterozygous type (GT or GA), and seven (29.17%) subjects had the homozygous wild type (GG). *ABCB1* 3435C>T genotyping revealed that 3 (12.50%) subjects had the mutant type (TT), 12 (50.00%) subjects had the heterozygous type (CT), and 9 (37.50%) subjects had the homozygous wild type (CC). *CYP2D6* genotyping revealed that 6 (25.00%) subjects had the homozygous *10 allele (*10/*10), 14 (58.33%) subjects had the heterozygous *10 allele (*1/*10), and 4 (16.67%) subjects had the homozygous *1 allele (*1/*1). *CYP2D6*2, *4, *5, *14A/B, *36, and *47 alleles were not detected in any of the subjects of this study. We classified the *CYP2D6* genotypes into three groups to investigate the impact of *CYP2D6* genotypes on the PKs of tiropramide as follows: extensive metabolizers (EMs) (*1/*1), heterozygous intermediate metabolizers (IMs) (*1/*10), and homozygous IMs (*10/*10), on the basis of the reports of the difference in *CYP2D6* enzyme activity according to *CYP2D6* genotypes [9,17]. *OCT2* 808G>T genotyping revealed that 8 (33.33%) subjects had the heterozygous type (GT) and 16 (66.67%) subjects had the homozygous type (GG). *PEPT1* 1287G>C genotyping revealed that 3 (12.50%) subjects had the mutant type (CC), 2 (8.33%) subjects had the heterozygous type (GC), and 19 (79.17%) subjects had the homozygous wild type (GG).

Table 2. Genetic information of the studied subjects ($n = 24$).

Genotypes		No. (Frequency)
ABCB1		
1236C>T (exon 12)	CC	5 (20.83%)
	CT	13 (54.17%)
	TT	6 (25.00%)
2677G>T/A (exon 21)	GG	7 (29.17%)
	GT, GA	9 (37.50%)
	TT, AT, TA, AA	8 (33.33%)
3435C>T (exon 26)	CC	9 (37.50%)
	CT	12 (50.00%)
	TT	3 (12.50%)
CYP2D6	*1/*1	4 (16.67%)
	*1/*10	14 (58.33%)
	*10/*10	6 (25.00%)
OCT2		
808G>T	GG	16 (66.67%)
	GT	8 (33.33%)
PEPT1		
1287G>C (exon 16)	GG	19 (79.17%)
	GC	2 (8.33%)
	CC	3 (12.50%)

3.3. Determination of Plasma Tiropramide Concentrations

After the oral administration of a 100 mg dose, plasma concentrations of tiropramide were determined by a column-switching semi-micro HPLC method (as mentioned in Section 2.4). This method analyzed tiropramide at a run time of 25 min per sample, enabling PK studies on tiropramide. The linearity of calibration curve for tiropramide was excellent ($r^2 = 0.99$) in human plasma, ranging from 2 to 500 ng/mL. Moreover, the calculation formula of the calibration curve was as follows: $y = 384.51x + 320.45$ ($p < 0.01$), where y is the peak area of tiropramide and x is the concentration (ng/mL) of the tiropramide. In addition, the lower limit of quantitation (LLOQ) for tiropramide was as low as 2 ng/mL, and was sufficient for PK studies after the oral administration of tiropramide tablet to humans. This assay has been validated for specificity, accuracy, precision, and sensitivity in order to be applied to accurate PK studies. There were no significant interferences derived from system or endogenous substances peaks, and we confirmed the identical tiropramide peak spectrum with the diode array detector. Intra-batch ($n = 5$) accuracies for tiropramide ranged from 100.70% to 113.50% with precision (coefficient of variation, CV) of < 13.57%. Inter-batch ($n = 5$) accuracies for tiropramide ranged from 98.00% to 111.42% with precision (CV) of < 9.23%.

3.4. Pharmacokinetic (NCA) Analysis

The observed plasma concentration–time profiles of tiropramide in the 24 subjects after oral administration of the 100 mg dose are presented in Figure 1.

In most individuals, the concentration of tiropramide in blood was measured up to 12 h after dosing. The PK parameters of tiropramide according to the genotypes (*ABCB1* 1236C>T, *ABCB1* 2677G>T/A, *ABCB1* 3435C>T, *CYP2D6*, *OCT2* 808G>T, and *PEPT1* 1287G>C) calculated by NCA are presented in Table 3. According to the NCA results for each genotype, the diversity of PK parameters in each group was not significant ($p > 0.05$). Although the higher mean AUC_{0-t}, $AUC_{0-\infty}$, and C_{max} values but lower mean CL/F values were calculated in the mutant type group (TT) than in the wild homozygous type groups (CC) in the *ABCB1* 1236C>T gene, this was not statistically significant considering the high SD. In the *CYP2D6* gene, higher mean AUC_{0-t}, $AUC_{0-\infty}$, and C_{max} values were calculated for IMs (*1/*10 and *10/*10) than EMs (*1/*1), but this was also not statistically significant considering the high SD. In addition, although the higher mean C_{max}, AUC_{0-t}, and $AUC_{0-\infty}$ values and lower mean CL/F value were calculated in wild homozygous type groups (GG) than in mutant type group (CC) in the *PEPT1* 1287G>C gene, this was not statistically significant considering the high SD. The AUC_{0-t}, $AUC_{0-\infty}$, C_{max}, half-life, and T_{max} values calculated by the NCA analysis of tiropramide were 254.31 ± 197.38 h·ng/mL, 280.34 ± 199.96 h·ng/mL, 69.07 ± 59.74 ng/mL, 3.41 ± 1.99 h, and 1.74 ± 0.63 h, respectively.

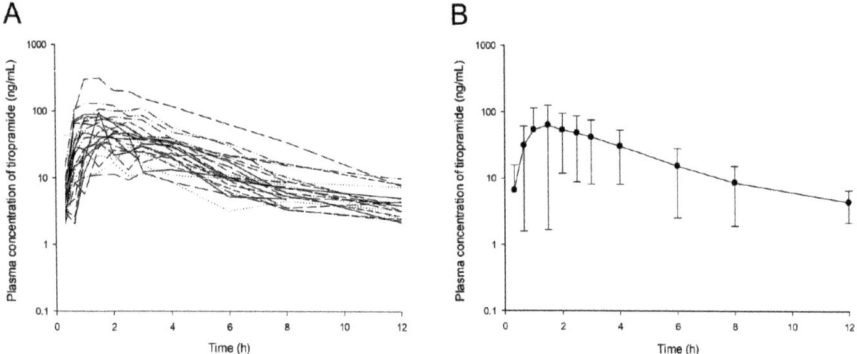

Figure 1. Log-transformed plasma concentration–time profiles of tiropramide in 24 subjects (**A**) and the mean curves (**B**). The vertical bars represent standard deviation of the mean.

Table 3. Pharmacokinetic parameters of tiropramide after a single oral administration of a 100 mg tiropramide tablet according to the genotypes (mean ± SD, $n = 24$).

Genotypes		Half-Life (h⁻¹)	T_{max} (h)	C_{max} (ng/mL)	AUC_{0-t} (h·ng/mL)	$AUC_{0-\infty}$ (h·ng/mL)	CL/F (L/h)
ABCB1 1236C>T							
	CC ($n = 5$)	2.91 ± 1.42	1.90 ± 0.42	104.56 ± 117.25	394.51 ± 376.32	419.54 ± 376.69	380.72 ± 246.10
	CT ($n = 13$)	3.80 ± 2.41	1.67 ± 0.70	49.06 ± 23.81	182.00 ± 60.62	209.85 ± 72.09	551.43 ± 263.69
	TT ($n = 6$)	2.99 ± 1.36	1.75 ± 0.69	82.83 ± 39.09	293.01 ± 149.02	317.08 ± 154.99	419.44 ± 292.77
ABCB1 2677G>T/A							
	GG ($n = 7$)	3.86 ± 3.11	1.38 ± 0.52	52.88 ± 15.94	214.50 ± 69.45	247.94 ± 76.58	439.10 ± 136.89
	GT ($n = 9$)	2.77 ± 0.89	2.06 ± 0.73	88.92 ± 89.16	323.04 ± 294.51	339.44 ± 296.97	481.39 ± 359.30
	TT, AT, TA, AA ($n = 8$)	3.75 ± 1.73	1.69 ± 0.46	60.89 ± 39.69	210.97 ± 122.69	242.22 ± 135.50	522.84 ± 259.46
ABCB1 3435C>T							
	CC ($n = 9$)	2.82 ± 1.11	1.52 ± 0.46	78.29 ± 88.96	294.77 ± 291.67	317.13 ± 293.75	452.72 ± 201.28
	CT ($n = 12$)	3.44 ± 1.45	1.92 ± 0.70	63.79 ± 38.63	235.35 ± 131.42	259.88 ± 136.73	524.94 ± 338.71
	TT ($n = 3$)	5.10 ± 4.82	1.67 ± 0.76	62.51 ± 23.63	206.48 ± 14.18	251.82 ± 44.95	405.08 ± 67.07
CYP2D6							
	*1/*1 ($n = 4$)	4.74 ± 4.00	1.25 ± 0.29	63.24 ± 23.66	240.38 ± 75.18	278.97 ± 67.41	379.92 ± 118.76
	*1/*10 ($n = 14$)	3.14 ± 1.17	1.76 ± 0.59	66.73 ± 72.90	258.15 ± 238.14	280.90 ± 240.02	484.79 ± 223.74
	*10/*10 ($n = 6$)	3.17 ± 1.84	2.00 ± 0.77	78.41 ± 45.97	253.49 ± 168.34	279.97 ± 177.22	547.04 ± 420.10
OCT2 808G>T							
	GG ($n = 16$)	3.62 ± 2.29	1.51 ± 0.53	60.42 ± 29.24	218.24 ± 89.40	247.77 ± 99.03	459.49 ± 166.01
	GT ($n = 8$)	3.00 ± 1.20	2.19 ± 0.59	86.37 ± 96.84	325.60 ± 319.70	345.50 ± 321.06	529.63 ± 414.56
PEPT1 1287G>C							
	GG ($n = 19$)	3.07 ± 1.38	1.82 ± 0.65	62.40 ± 32.14	226.40 ± 109.97	248.21 ± 115.65	506.33 ± 278.61
	GC ($n = 2$)	6.36 ± 6.07	1.25 ± 0.35	181.48 ± 184.26	621.48 ± 609.37	688.85 ± 546.19	211.72 ± 167.87
	CC ($n = 3$)	3.63 ± 0.41	1.50 ± 0.50	36.36 ± 9.98	183.99 ± 65.49	211.54 ± 80.59	515.08 ± 168.25

3.5. Population Pharmacokinetic Model Development

By a one-compartment disposition model with first order elimination and absorption with an absorption lag time, the plasma concentrations of tiropramide were best expressed. Considering the lag time, the numerical values (such as -2LL and AIC) of the model evaluation and graphical data fitting were more improved than otherwise. Although we tried a two-compartment model, it did not show an improved fit when compared with the one-compartment model. In other words, there was a problem (fail to model fit) in fitting the two-compartment model for some individuals, but in the one-compartment model, all individuals were fitted properly. In addition, the -2LL and AIC values significantly decreased in the multiple (two) transit absorption compartment model in which the additional absorption phase was added to the one-compartment model. However, from two or more transit phases of absorption, there was no significant decrease in the -2LL and AIC values (with increasing number of parameters). As a result, the multiple (two) transit absorption phase-one compartment model with an absorption lag time was selected as the base structure model for tiropramide. The model was parameterized in terms of V/F, T_{lag}, CL/F, K_{a1}, and K_{a2}. When the lag-time or model transit time was given to K_{a2} in the parameterization of the model, no significant model improvement was found with the increasing number of parameters. Therefore, significant model improvement was found when parameterization with lag-time was carried out only at K_{a1}, and the rate constant of substance transit in the absorption compartment. Figure 2 shows a schematic of the disposition compartment model presented for tiropramide.

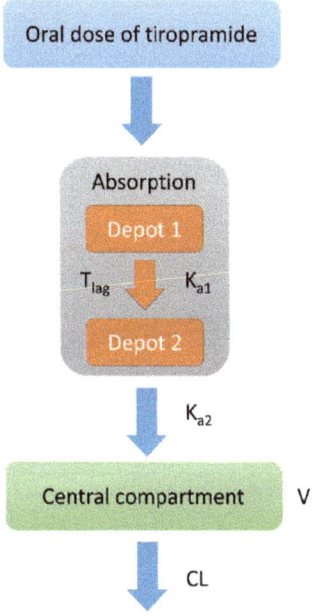

Figure 2. Schematic of tiropramide population pharmacokinetic (PPK) model (two transit absorption phase-one compartment model with an absorption lag time). Depot 1 and 2 represent transit compartments in the absorption phase. K_{a1} refers to the rate constant at which the drug is moved from depot 1 to depot 2. T_{lag} refers to the delay time for the drug to move from depot 1 to depot 2. K_{a2} is the rate constant at which the drug moves from depot 2 to the central compartment. V means the volume of drug distribution in the central compartment, and CL means removal of the drug from the central compartment.

An exponential model was used to describe the IIVs on parameters of T_{lag}, V/F, CL/F, K_{a1}, and K_{a2}. By applying an additive error model on log-transformed data, the residual variability was explained. Table 4 summarizes the steps for developing a basic structural model of tiropramide.

In order to find the covariates affecting the PK parameters of tiropramide, we analyzed the effects of each covariate on the PK parameters. The final potential covariates were selected on the basis of the graphical exploration between candidate covariates and PK parameters. The influence of each selected candidate covariate on the PK parameters of tiropramide was assessed by incorporating the covariates into an established basic structural model. The evaluation was based on OFV, which means model improvement. In this regard, the covariate selection process (according to OFV) to be reflected in the final model of tiropramide is summarized in Table 5.

Table 4. Basic structural model building steps.

Model	Description	n-Parameter	-2LL	AIC	Δ-2LL	ΔAIC	Compared with
	Absorption model						
1	One compartment with first order (no T_{lag})	7	562.27	576.27			
2	One compartment with the first order (add T_{lag})	9	508.80	526.80	−53.48	−49.48	1
3 *	One compartment with the first order (add T_{lag} and additonal absorption transit phase one)	11	420.97	442.97	−87.83	−83.83	2
4	One compartment with the first order (add T_{lag} and additonal absorption transit phase two)	13	419.84	442.11	−1.13	−0.86	3
	Residual error model						
3 *	Log additive	11	420.97	442.97			
5	Additive	11	1964.95	1986.95	1543.98	1543.98	3
6	Proportional	11	1860.33	1882.33	1439.36	1439.36	3
	IIV model						
7	Remove IIV K_{a1}	10	428.64	448.64	7.67	5.67	3
8	Remove IIV K_{a2}	10	428.64	448.64	7.67	5.67	3
9	Remove IIV T_{lag}	10	434.18	454.18	13.21	11.21	3
10	Remove IIV V/F	10	500.86	520.86	79.89	77.89	3
11	Remove IIV CL/F	10	534.10	554.10	113.13	111.13	3

* Selected model.

Table 5. Stepwise search for covariates.

Model	Description	OFV	ΔOFV	n-Parameter	Compared with
1	Base model	420.97		11	
2	Total protein on CL/F	411.72	−9.25	12	1
3 *	Total protein on CL/F and V/F	402.56	−9.16	13	2
4	Total protein on CL/F and V/F, BMI on K_{a1}	400.61	−1.95	14	3
5	Total protein on CL/F and V/F, PEPT1 (1287G>C) on K_{a1}	402.57	0.01	14	3
6	Total protein on CL/F and V/F, ABCB1 (1236C>T) on K_{a1}	401.63	−0.93	14	3
7	Total protein on CL/F and V/F, CYP2D6 (*1 and *10) on K_{a2}	397.15	−5.42	15	3

* Selected final model.

There was a significant correlation between the total protein and tiropramide V/F as well as the total protein and tiropramide CL/F. Figure 3 shows the correlation between the final selected covariates and CL/F of tiropramide.

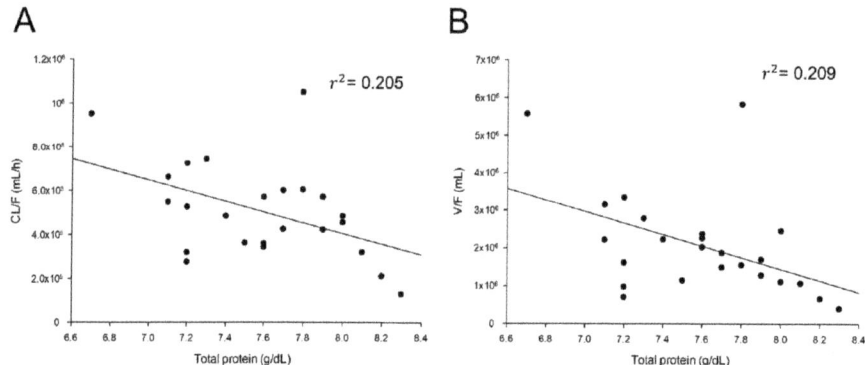

Figure 3. Relationship between subjects' characteristics and individual predicted pharmacokinetic parameters. Clearance (CL/F) of tiropramide according to total protein (**A**). Volume of distribution (V/F) of tiropramide according to total protein (**B**).

When the correlation between the total protein and CL/F was reflected in the PPK model of tiropramide, the ΔOFV was significantly reduced to −9.25 ($p < 0.05$). Furthermore, the addition of total protein and V/F correlation to tiropramide PPK model significantly reduced the ΔOFV to −9.16

($p < 0.05$). However, other covariates including BMI, *PEPT1* 1287G>C, *OCT2* 808G>T, *ABCB1* 1236C>T, *ABCB1* 2677G>T/A, *ABCB1* 3435C>T, and *CYP2D6* (*1 and *10) had no significant effect on model improvement. Even by applying genetic factors (such as *PEPT1* 1287G>C, *OCT2* 808G>T, *ABCB1* 1236C>T, *ABCB1* 2677G>T/A, *ABCB1* 3435C>T, and *CYP2D6* (*1 and *10)) alone to the base model, we examined whether they affected K_{a1}, K_{a2}, CL/F, and V/F, but no significant associations were identified. The final model of tiropramide (reflecting the effects of covariates) is expressed as follows:

$$\begin{aligned}
V/F &= tvV/F \cdot (1 + (Totalproteins - 7.6) \cdot dV/FdTotalproteins) \cdot \exp(\eta_V) \\
CL/F &= tvCL/F \cdot (1 + (Totalproteins - 7.6) \cdot dCL/FdTotalproteins) \cdot \exp(\eta_{CL}) \\
T_{lag} &= tvT_{lag} \cdot \exp(\eta_{Tlag}) \\
K_{a1} &= tvK_{a1} \cdot \exp(\eta_{Ka1}) \\
K_{a2} &= tvK_{a2} \cdot \exp(\eta_{Ka2})
\end{aligned} \quad (1)$$

Population estimates of tiropramide were 466,711 mL/h for CL/F and 1,889,250 mL for V/F. CL/F and V/F values by NCA were 482,567 ± 267,433 mL/h and 2,386,871 ± 1,699,847 mL, respectively. As a result, the CL/F and V/F values estimated in the final model were not significantly different from the NCA values. In the final model, the relative standard error (RSE, %) was 9.53–83.51%. The Eta shrinkage values for the estimated PK parameters were suggested as acceptable at 0.02–0.40%. Compared with the base model, the final model (considering total protein effects) of tiropramide reduced the IIV of V/F from 70.70% to 57.12%, and the IIV of CL/F from 50.55% to 39.95%. Table 6 presents the estimated parameter values in the base model and final PPK model of tiropramide. The AUC_{0-t}, $AUC_{0-\infty}$, C_{max}, half-life, and T_{max} estimated values by the final PPK model of tiropramide were 242.73 ± 175.28 h· ng/mL, 260.92 ± 179.08 h· ng/mL, 54.89 ± 46.18 ng/mL, 2.73 ± 0.88 h, and 1.65 ± 0.53 h, respectively.

Table 6. Population pharmacokinetic parameters for tiropramide in base model and final model.

Parameter	Estimate	SE	RSE (%)	Shrinkage (%)	IIV (%)
Base model					
tvK_{a1} (1/h)	3.160	0.511	16.143		
tvK_{a2} (1/h)	3.171	0.510	16.086		
tvV/F (mL)	1,717,060.491	262,434.751	15.284		
tvCL/F (mL/h)	447,163.154	48,667.242	10.884		
tvT_{lag} (h)	0.196	0.021	10.480		
$\omega^2_{V/F}$	0.500	0.170	33.973	0.044	70.701
$\omega^2_{CL/F}$	0.255	0.103	40.328	0.016	50.546
ω^2_{Tlag}	0.106	0.089	84.320	0.225	32.538
ω^2_{Ka1}	0.608	0.266	43.735	0.399	77.986
ω^2_{Ka2}	0.613	0.261	42.630	0.398	78.269
σ	0.354	0.041	11.673		
Final model					
tvK_{a1} (1/h)	3.187	0.538	16.872		
tvK_{a2} (1/h)	3.183	0.524	16.464		
tvV/F (mL)	1,889,250.002	289,606.633	15.329		
tvCL/F (mL/h)	466,711.101	44,476.962	9.530		
tvT_{lag} (h)	0.196	0.021	10.590		
dCl/FdTotalproteins	−0.804	0.296	36.791		
dV/FdTotalproteins	−1.049	0.232	22.118		
$\omega^2_{V/F}$	0.326	0.158	48.369	0.068	57.118
$\omega^2_{CL/F}$	0.160	0.067	41.977	0.023	39.947
ω^2_{Tlag}	0.107	0.089	83.508	0.225	32.503
ω^2_{Ka1}	0.557	0.276	49.584	0.405	74.627
ω^2_{Ka2}	0.556	0.269	48.406	0.405	74.566
σ	0.357	0.042	11.895		

3.6. Population Pharmacokinetic Model Evaluation

The developed PPK model of the tiropramide was comprehensively evaluated for GOF, bootstrap analysis, and VPC. Figure 4 shows the GOF plots of the base and the final models of tiropramide.

As shown in Figure 4B, the observed and predicted concentrations of tiropramide showed a relatively good agreement in the final model. CWRES was well distributed symmetrically with respect to zero, and CWRES was included in ±4 at all points. In addition, the residuals in the final model were more improved than in the base model. In other words, without any specific bias, the CWRES was randomly well distributed, and the residuals in the final model showed a significant decrease when compared with the base model (larger than ±4).

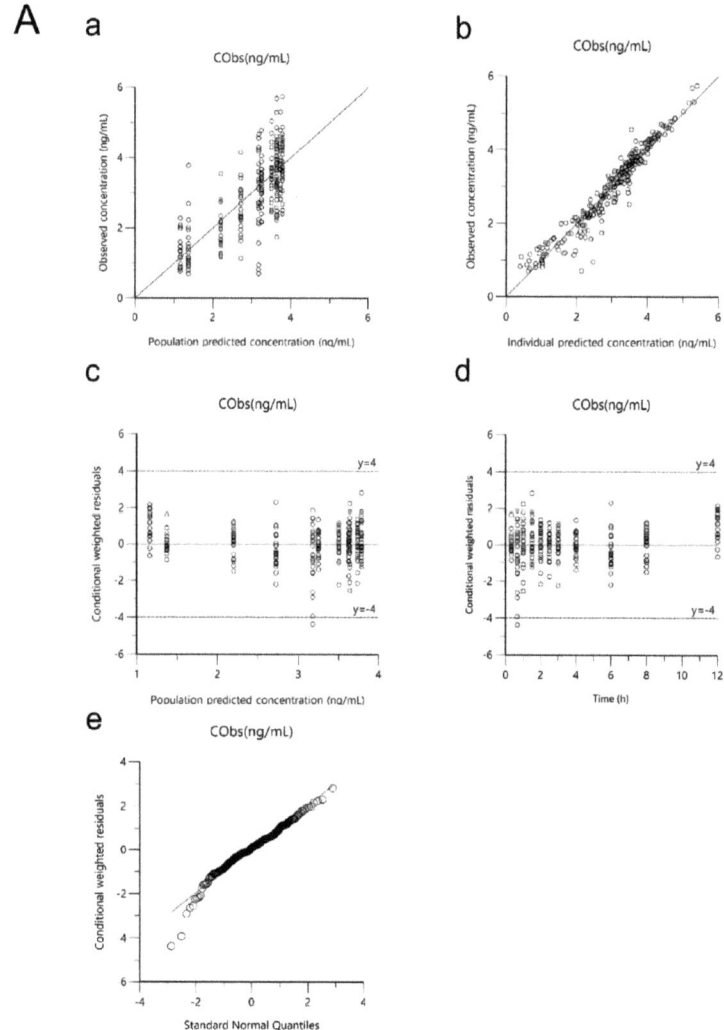

Figure 4. *Cont.*

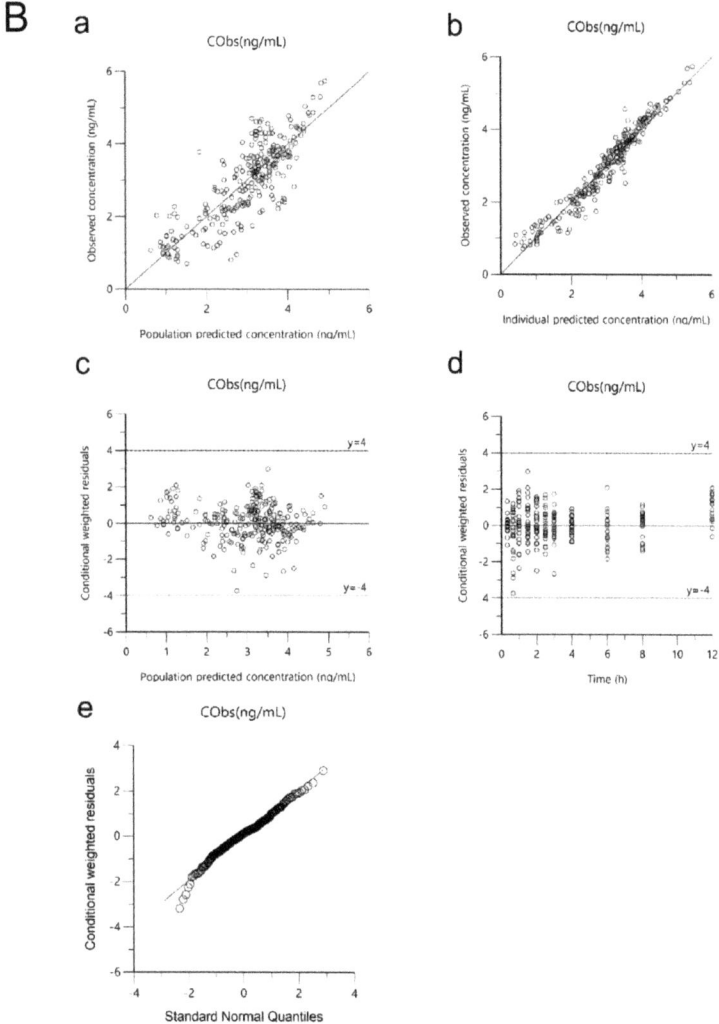

Figure 4. Goodness-of-fit (GOF) plots of base model (**A**) and final model (**B**) for tiropramide. (**a**) Population-predicted concentrations (PRED) against observed plasma concentration (DV), (**b**) individual-predicted concentrations (IPRED) against DV, (**c**) PRED against conditional weighted residuals (CWRES), (**d**) time (IVAR) against CWRES, and (**e**) quantile–quantile plot of components of CWRES.

Bootstrap validation was performed to verify the reproducibility and/or robustness of the final PPK model of tiropramide. Table 7 shows the bootstrapping analysis results. The parameter values estimated in the final model were in the 95% CI range of the bootstrap analysis results, and were similar to the median values of the bootstrap (replicates of 1000).

Table 7. Estimated population pharmacokinetic parameter values of tiropramide and bootstrap validation (*n* = 1000).

Parameter	Final Model		Bootstrapping	
	Estimate	95% CI	Median	95% CI
tvK$_{a1}$ (1/h)	3.187	2.128–4.246	3.187	2.332–4.733
tvK$_{a2}$ (1/h)	3.183	2.151–4.215	3.183	2.273–4.345
tvV/F (mL)	1,889,250.002	1,318,770.124–2,459,730.256	1,889,250.000	1,397,156.042-2,491,555.125
tvCL/F (mL/h)	466,711.101	379,098.212–554,324.163	466,711.000	374,186.003–550,036.012
tvT$_{lag}$ (h)	0.196	0.155–0.237	0.196	0.144–0.234
dCl/FdTotalproteins	−0.804	−1.387–(−0.221)	−0.804	−1.050–0.082
dV/FdTotalproteins	−1.049	−1.506–(−0.592)	−1.049	−1.222–0.246
$\omega^2_{V/F}$	0.326	0.017–0.636	0.296	0.020–0.572
$\omega^2_{Cl/F}$	0.160	0.028–0.291	0.134	0.023–0.245
ω^2_{Tlag}	0.107	0.068–0.282	0.085	0.045–0.215
ω^2_{Ka1}	0.557	0.016–1.098	0.524	0.016–1.063
ω^2_{Ka2}	0.556	0.028–1.084	0.518	0.013–1.049
σ	0.357	0.273–0.441	0.363	0.276–0.428

The VPC simulation results of the final PPK model of tiropramide are presented in Figure 5. Most of the observation values of tiropramide were well distributed within the 90% prediction interval of the prediction values. As a result, this suggests that the final model of the tiropramide is precise and explains the data well.

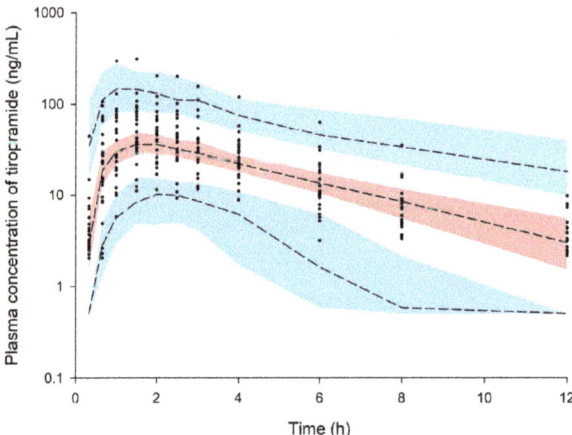

Figure 5. Visual predictive check (VPC) of the final model for tiropramide. Observed concentrations were depicted by the dots. The 95th, 50th, and 5th percentiles of the predicted concentrations are represented by black dashed lines. The 95% confidence intervals (CI) for the predicted 5th and 95th percentiles are represented by the blue shaded regions. The 95% CI for the predicted 50th percentiles are represented by the red shaded regions. The values on the *y*-axis are logarithms.

The NPDE distribution and histogram are presented in Figure S1. The assumption of a normal distribution for the differences between predictions and observations was acceptable. The quantile–quantile plots and histogram also confirmed the normality of the NPDE (Figure S1).

4. Discussion

The mechanism of action of tiropramide, as mentioned in the Introduction section, has been studied relatively well and has been reported in the past. However, studies on the in vivo PK characteristics (including metabolism and excretion) of tiropramide are still insufficient. Therefore, little data was available regarding the dosage and usage of tiropramide in clinical as well as formulation development.

According to Lee et al., despite the frequent use of tiropramide in clinical practice, studies on safety and efficacy are very poor [4]. We conducted a PPK model development study of tiropramide to explore the effective covariates related to PK diversity of tiropramide and to investigate the characteristics of PK in the population. This study was new and was expected to be useful in the evaluation of the safety and efficacy of tiropramide in clinical use. As mentioned in the Abstract section, although tiropramide has a (relatively) broad margin of safety, this study involving healthy subjects was very important because it could find new covariates in healthy subjects that had not been reported before and/or be used to predict PPK for patients in the clinic by establishing PPK in healthy adults. In addition to this, in patients with abdominal pain and irritable bowel syndrome, it is very likely that the absorption process of tiropramide will change. Therefore, if clinical trials are conducted for patients in the future, it is thought that the PK variation of tiropramide between individuals can be explained more specifically through the application of our PPK model.

In this study, the PK of tiropramide was modelled as a two transit absorption phase-one compartment model with an absorption lag time. Various errors (including residual error and IIV) models and covariate effects were evaluated to establish factors that significantly influence the PK parameters of tiropramide and to explain the PK diversity of the tiropramide in the population. As a result of evaluating the model, the final tiropramide PPK model showed relatively good GOF plots, suggesting that the final PPK model had an acceptable predictive power. In addition, all CWRES values over time or predicted concentrations were in the range of -4 and 4, suggesting that the model is relatively stable. In addition, the bootstrap and VPC simulation results suggested that the final tiropramide PPK model was accurate, stable, and precise. We compared the estimated parameter values (of AUC_{0-t}, $AUC_{0-\infty}$, C_{max}, half-life, and T_{max}) by tiropramide's final PPK model with these values by NCA analysis. As a result, there were no significant differences ($p > 0.05$) between the parameter values predicted by the final PPK model of tiropramide and those calculated by NCA analysis. These results suggest that the final PPK model of tiropramide established in this study explains the experimental data relatively well.

The 24 healthy Korean male PK data used to establish the tiropramide PPK model were similar to the previously reported PK results. In other words, the previously reported PK parameter values of tiropramide were similar to our PK results obtained by NCA analysis. After oral administration of 100 mg of tiropramide in humans, the obtained NCA PK parameters (as previously reported values) were 2.34-6.99 h for $t_{1/2}$, 0.66-1.6 h for T_{max}, 77.4-111 ng/mL for C_{max}, and 267.7-812.7 h·ng/mL for AUC [6,12,18–21]. On the other hand, the NCA PK parameters in this study were 3.41 ± 1.99 h for $t_{1/2}$, 1.74 ± 0.63 h for T_{max}, 69.07 ± 59.74 ng/mL for C_{max}, and 280.34 ± 199.96 h·ng/mL for AUC, which were similar to the previously reported values. Table 8 summarizes these results.

As mentioned above, few studies have been done on the metabolic ratio (including pathway) and excretion of tiropramide in humans (especially patient groups), making it difficult to predict candidate covariates. On the basis of previous reports (as drug information provided by the manufacturer) that tiropramide is metabolized in the liver and excreted into urine (about 10–20% of administered dose), the covariate effects were tested in this study by obtaining the physicochemical information of liver function indicators (such as AST, ALT, and ALP) and genotyping the *CYP2D6* gene related to metabolism in the body. The creatinine clearance and the functional indicator of the kidney were collected for each subject, and the covariate effects related to CL/F were tested. In addition, genotyping of genes (such as *ABCB1*, *OCT2*, and *PEPT1*) associated with various transporters known to be widely involved in the distribution, absorption, excretion, and metabolism of drugs in the body has been performed to identify the effects of the covariate associated with the PK parameters. Despite these efforts, only total protein was found to have a significant effect on V/F and CL/F of tiropramide. As shown in Figure 3, the total protein, and the V/F and CL/F showed a significant negative correlation of 45.72% ($r^2 = 0.209$) and 45.28% ($r^2 = 0.205$), respectively. The correlation values of the total protein to CL/F and V/F were the largest of all the covariates we collected in this study.

Table 8. Previously reported pharmacokinetic (PK) parameter values of tiropramide obtained by non-compartmental analysis (NCA) analysis.

References	Subjects	PK Parameters				
		Half-life (h)	Tmax (h)	Cmax (ng/mL)	$AUC_{0-\infty}$ (h·ng/mL)	CL/F (L/h)
Kwon et al. (2003) [21]	Human ($n = 2$, 100 mg dose)	-	0.66–2	87.3–191.3	267.7–812.7	-
Kwon et al. (2003) [20]	Human ($n = 16$, 100 mg dose)	2.34–2.61	-	96.4 ± 51.6	380.8 ± 239.0	-
Lee et al. (2003) [6]	Human ($n = 4$, 100 mg dose)	2.7 ± 0.5	1.6 ± 0.6	77.4 ± 33.0	319 ± 147	-
Baek et al. (2003) [12]	Human ($n = 14$, 100 mg dose)	6.3 ± 2.0	1.6 ± 0.6	111 ± 62	377 ± 220	-
Jhee et al. (2006) [19]	Human ($n = 18$, 100 mg dose)	6.99 ± 0.83	1.33 ± 0.34	98.77 ± 30.23	434.39 ± 102.35	-
Imran et al. (2007) [18]	Human ($n = 12$, 100 mg dose)	3.3 ± 1.0	1.5 ± 0.2	105.35 ± 15.7	375.4 ± 76.7	-
In this study	Human ($n = 24$, 100 mg dose)	3.41 ± 1.99	1.74 ± 0.63	69.07 ± 59.74	280.34 ± 199.96	482.87 ± 267.25

Although the plasma protein binding ratio of tiropramide in humans has not been reported accurately, it has been reported that the plasma protein binding ratio of tiropramide in rats is about 48–51% [22]. This suggests that the amount of plasma protein may affect the in vivo PK properties of tiropramide by binding to the plasma proteins in the blood. According to our tiropramide PPK model, higher total protein levels in the blood mean a smaller distribution of tiropramide in the body and a lower excretion. This can be explained by the fact that tiropramide binds to proteins in the blood and affects the distribution and excretion of substances from the body. Tiropramide combined with proteins in the blood will make it difficult to filter the glomerulus of the kidney and distribute from blood to many organs. The reflection of the total protein covariates in tiropramide PPK model reduced V/F IIV and CL/F IIV by 13.58% and 10.60%, respectively. These results suggested that the variabilities of tiropramide plasma concentrations could be partly explained by individual variances of total protein level related with V/F and CL/F of tiropramide. On the other hand, other candidate covariates (such as AST, ALT, ALP, and creatinine clearance) had no significant effect on the PK parameter values and IIV improvement of tiropramide. Although tiropramide is metabolized in the liver and excreted in the kidney, our results suggest that tiropramide is a drug that does not require dose control depending on the liver and renal function. However, because our PPK model was based on the data from healthy men, further studies (for patient groups) will be needed for further clarification. That is, if PK data significantly different from the normal group (like our study) was obtained from the patient groups, and if the PPK analysis was conducted in the same manner as in this study with our model (from patient groups), other significant covariates may be identified. Therefore, PK studies or PPK analysis of tiropramide in patient groups will need to be performed in the future. Nevertheless, this study was important because it is a PPK model study of tiropramide that has not been previously conducted, and other related studies (such as clinical dose setting, formulation development, and PK comparison with certain other groups) on tiropramide may be possible in the future, on the basis of our findings. In addition, another limitation of our study was that PK analysis and PPK model studies were conducted for limited ages (between 19 and 29 years old). In the future, PK analysis and/or PPK model studies of tiropramide for more diverse age groups will need to be conducted in this regard.

As shown in Table 6, unexplained variability (as IIV) still exists in K_a (74.63% for K_{a1} and 74.57% for K_{a2}) and T_{lag} (32.50%). These results meant that multi-complex gastrointestinal (GI) tract absorption processes of tiropramide including the variabilities of each individual gastric emptying time, GI tract transit time, and other transporters, among others, could considerably affect the variabilities of tiropramide plasma concentrations. This study could not find any significant covariates that could explain K_a IIV and T_{lag} IIV. Perhaps, despite collecting various genetic and demographic information, there was still not enough information to explain the K_a and T_{lag} IIVs of tiropramide. Therefore, further studies are needed to explore significant covariates related to the absorption of tiropramide in the body.

5. Conclusions

A PPK model for tiropramide was developed on the basis of PK data for healthy Korean men in this study. The plasma concentration profiles for tiropramide were described well by a two transit absorption phase-one compartment model with an absorption lag time. The total protein was identified by significant covariates of CL/F and V/F for tiropramide, and their correlation was finally reflected in the PPK model of tiropramide. On the other hand, no significant correlation was found between genetic information such as *ABCB1*, *CYP2D6*, *OCT2*, *PEPT1*, and the PK parameters of tiropramide. To the best of our knowledge, this is the first time a PPK model has been studied for tiropramide, and it is expected to be a valuable resource for future studies (such as in clinical use, as well as dose control and formulation development).

Supplementary Materials: The following are available online at http://www.mdpi.com/1999-4923/12/4/374/s1, Figure S1: Normalized prediction distribution error (NPDE) for the final model.

Author Contributions: Research idea planning, S.-H.J., J.-H.J., and Y.-B.L.; method planning, S.-H.J. and J.-H.J.; method and data validation, S.-H.J. and H.-Y.C.; literature search, S.-H.J.; investigation, S.-H.J. and J.-H.J.; data analysis and modeling, S.-H.J. and J.-H.J.; original manuscript writing, S.-H.J. and J.-H.J.; review and editing of manuscript, S.-H.J., J.-H.J., H.-Y.C., and Y.-B.L.; supervision, Y.-B.L. All authors have read and agreed to the published version of the manuscript.

Funding: This research did not receive any specific grant from funding agencies in the public, commercial, or not-for-profit sectors.

Conflicts of Interest: The authors declare that they have no conflicts of interest relevant to this study.

References

1. Setnikar, I.; Makovec, F.; Chiste, R.; Giachetti, C.; Zanolo, G. Tiropramide and metabolites in blood and plasma after intravenous or peroral administration of 14C-tiropramide to the rat. *Arzneim. Forsch.* **1988**, *38*, 1815–1819.
2. Arigoni, R.; Chiste, R.; Drovanti, A.; Makovec, F.; Senin, P.; Setnikar, I. Pharmacokinetics of tiropramide after single doses in man. *Arzneim. Forsch.* **1986**, *36*, 738–744.
3. Arigoni, R.; Chiste, R.; Makovec, F.; Setnikar, I.; Benfenati, E.; Fanelli, R. Identification of metabolites of tiropramide in human urine. *Biomed. Environ. Mass Spectrom.* **1988**, *15*, 205–209. [CrossRef] [PubMed]
4. Lee, K.N.; Lee, O.Y.; Choi, M.-G.; Sohn, C.I.; Huh, K.C.; Park, K.S.; Kwon, J.G.; Kim, N.; Rhee, P.-L.; Myung, S.-J.; et al. Efficacy and safety of tiropramide in the treatment of patients with irritable bowel syndrome: A multicenter, randomized, double-blind, non-inferiority trial, compared with octylonium. *J. Neurogastroenterol. Motil.* **2014**, *20*, 113–121. [CrossRef] [PubMed]
5. Kim, S.-M.; Lee, S.-N.; Yoon, H.; Kang, H.-A.; Cho, H.-Y.; Lee, I.-K.; Lee, Y.-B. Haplotype analysis and single nucleotide polymorphism frequency of organic cation transporter gene (OCT1 and 2) in Korean subjects. *J. Pharm. Investig.* **2009**, *39*, 345–351. [CrossRef]
6. Lee, H.W.; Ji, H.Y.; Kim, H.H.; Cho, H.-Y.; Lee, Y.-B.; Lee, H.S. Determination of tiropramide in human plasma by liquid chromatography–tandem mass spectrometry. *J. Chromatogr. B* **2003**, *796*, 395–400. [CrossRef]
7. Kim, S.-M.; Lee, S.-N.; Kang, H.-A.; Cho, H.-Y.; Lee, I.-K.; Lee, Y.-B. Haplotype analysis and single nucleotide polymorphism frequency of PEPT1 gene (Exon 5 and 16) in Korean. *J. Pharm. Investig.* **2009**, *39*, 411–416. [CrossRef]

8. Kim, S.-M.; Park, S.-A.; Cho, H.-Y.; Lee, Y.-B. Haplotype analysis of MDRI gene (Exon 12, 21 and 26) in Korean. *J. Pharm. Investig.* **2008**, *38*, 365–372.
9. Gaedigk, A.; Simon, S.; Pearce, R.; Bradford, L.; Kennedy, M.; Leeder, J. The CYP2D6 activity score: Translating genotype information into a qualitative measure of phenotype. *Clin. Pharmacol. Ther.* **2008**, *83*, 234–242. [CrossRef]
10. Lee, S.-Y.; Sohn, K.M.; Ryu, J.Y.; Yoon, Y.R.; Shin, J.G.; Kim, J.-W. Sequence-based CYP2D6 genotyping in the Korean population. *Ther. Drug Monit.* **2006**, *28*, 382–387. [CrossRef]
11. Byeon, J.-Y.; Kim, Y.-H.; Lee, C.-M.; Kim, S.-H.; Chae, W.-K.; Jung, E.-H.; Choi, C.-I.; Jang, C.-G.; Lee, S.-Y.; Bae, J.-W. CYP2D6 allele frequencies in Korean population, comparison with East Asian, Caucasian and African populations, and the comparison of metabolic activity of CYP2D6 genotypes. *Arch. Pharm. Res.* **2018**, *41*, 921–930. [CrossRef] [PubMed]
12. Baek, S.K.; Lee, S.S.; Park, E.J.; Sohn, D.H.; Lee, H.S. Semi-micro high-performance liquid chromatographic analysis of tiropramide in human plasma using column-switching. *J. Pharm. Biomed. Anal.* **2003**, *31*, 185–189. [CrossRef]
13. Deurenberg, P.; Weststrate, J.A.; Seidell, J.C. Body mass index as a measure of body fatness: Age-and sex-specific prediction formulas. *Br. J. Nutr.* **1991**, *65*, 105–114. [CrossRef] [PubMed]
14. Mosteller, R. Simplified calculation of body surface area. *N. Engl. J. Med.* **1987**, *317*, 1098.
15. Cockcroft, D.W.; Gault, M.H. Prediction of creatinine clearance from serum creatinine. *Nephron* **1976**, *16*, 31–41. [CrossRef]
16. Comets, E.; Brendel, K.; Mentré, F. Computing normalised prediction distribution errors to evaluate nonlinear mixed-effect models: The npde add-on package for R. *Comput. Methods Programs Biomed.* **2008**, *90*, 154–166. [CrossRef]
17. Deardorff, O.G.; Jenne, V.; Leonard, L.; Ellingrod, V.L. Making sense of CYP2D6 and CYP1A2 genotype vs. phenotype. *Curr. Psychiatry* **2018**, *17*, 41–45.
18. Imran, K.; Punnamchand, L.; Natvarlal, S.M. A simple sample preparation with HPLC–UV method for estimation of tiropramide from plasma: Application to bioequivalence study. *J. Pharm. Biomed. Anal.* **2007**, *43*, 1135–1140. [CrossRef]
19. Jhee, O.H.; Jeon, Y.C.; Choi, H.S.; Lee, M.H.; Om, A.S.; Lee, J.-W.; Hong, J.W.; Kim, Y.S.; Kang, J.C.; Lee, Y.S. Quantitative analysis of tiropramide in human plasma by gas chromatography coupled to mass spectrometry for application to a bioequivalence test. *Clin. Chim. Acta* **2006**, *366*, 179–184. [CrossRef]
20. Kwon, O.-S.; Park, Y.-J.; Chung, Y.-B. Pharmacokinetics and bioequivalence of tiropramide in healthy volunteers. *Arzneim. Forsch.* **2003**, *53*, 578–583. [CrossRef]
21. Kwon, O.-S.; Park, Y.-J.; Ryu, J.-C.; Chung, Y.B. Quantitative analysis of tiropramide in human blood by gas chromatography with nitrogen-phosphorus detector. *Arch. Pharm. Res.* **2003**, *26*, 416–420. [CrossRef] [PubMed]
22. Abe, H.; Inokawa, Y.; Yasuda, E.; Nishioka, Y.; Esumi, Y.; Nemoto, H.; Inaba, A.; Jin, Y.; Ninomiya, S. Pharmacokinetic studies of tiropramide in rats (I). Absorption, distribution, metabolism and excretion after single administration. *Yakuri Chiryo* **1992**, *20*, 113–129.

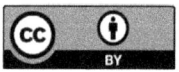

© 2020 by the authors. Licensee MDPI, Basel, Switzerland. This article is an open access article distributed under the terms and conditions of the Creative Commons Attribution (CC BY) license (http://creativecommons.org/licenses/by/4.0/).

MDPI
St. Alban-Anlage 66
4052 Basel
Switzerland
Tel. +41 61 683 77 34
Fax +41 61 302 89 18
www.mdpi.com

Pharmaceutics Editorial Office
E-mail: pharmaceutics@mdpi.com
www.mdpi.com/journal/pharmaceutics

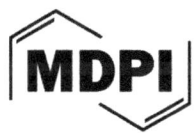

www.ingramcontent.com/pod-product-compliance
Lightning Source LLC
LaVergne TN
LVHW070442100526
838202LV00014B/1650